p.202 - philosophical
uthor prefers
losophical

c

p.213 - autonomy +
unpredictability
└ different cultural stances
on autonomy

The Philosophy of Medicine Reborn

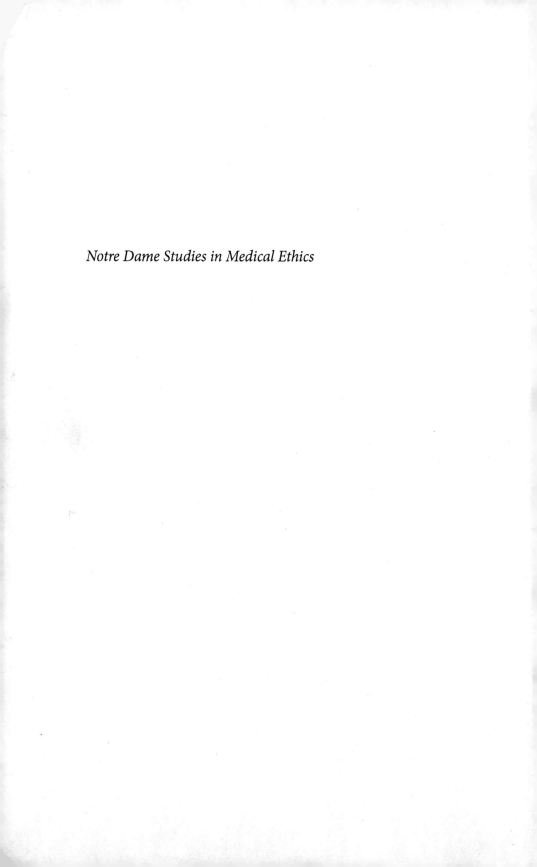

Notre Dame Studies in Medical Ethics

The Philosophy of Medicine Reborn

A Pellegrino Reader

EDMUND D. PELLEGRINO

Edited by H. Tristram Engelhardt, Jr., and Fabrice Jotterand

University of Notre Dame Press
Notre Dame, Indiana

Apologia and Introduction © 2008 by University of Notre Dame
Notre Dame, Indiana 46556
www.undpress.nd.edu
All Rights Reserved

Reprinted in 2011

Designed by Wendy McMillen
Set in 10.3/14 Minion by EM Studio

Library of Congress Cataloging-in-Publication Data

Pellegrino, Edmund D., 1920–
The philosophy of medicine reborn : a Pellegrino reader / Edmund D. Pellegrino ;
edited by H. Tristram Engelhardt, Jr., and Fabrice Jotterand.
     p. ; cm. — (Notre Dame studies in medical ethics)
Includes bibliographical references and index.
ISBN-13: 978-0-268-03834-2 (pbk. : alk. paper)
ISBN-10: 0-268-03834-1 (pbk. : alk. paper)
1. Medicine—Philosophy. 2. Medical ethics. I. Engelhardt, H. Tristram
(Hugo Tristram), 1941– II. Jotterand, Fabrice, 1967– III. Title. IV. Series.
[DNLM: 1. Philosophy, Medical—Collected Works. 2. Ethics, Medica—
Collected Works. W 61 P386P 2008]
R723.P3815   2008
174.2—dc22

                                                        2008000419

∞ *This book printed on acid-free paper.*

To Edmund D. Pellegrino,

Friend, Teacher, and Colleague

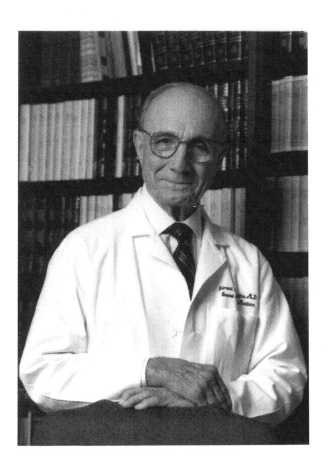

CONTENTS

Hippocratic Tradition

ACKNOWLEDGMENTS

With gratitude it is acknowledged that the following has been reprinted with permission:

What the Philosophy *of* Medicine *Is. Theoretical Medicine and Bioethics* 19 (1998): 315–336. © Kluwer Academic Publishers, with kind permission of Springer Science and Business Media.

Philosophy of Medicine: Should It Be Teleologically or Socially Construed? *Kennedy Institute of Ethics Journal* 11 (2001): 169–180. © The Johns Hopkins University Press.

The Internal Morality of Clinical Medicine: A Paradigm for the Ethics of the Helping and Healing Professions. *Journal of Medicine and Philosophy* 26 (2001): 559–579. © Swets & Zeitlinger.

Humanistic Basis of Professional Ethics. In *Humanism and the Physician*, 117–129. Knoxville: University of Tennessee Press, 1979. © Edmund D. Pellegrino.

The Commodification of Medical and Health Care: The Moral Consequences of a Paradigm Shift from a Professional to a Market Ethic. *Journal of Medicine and Philosophy* 24 (1999): 243–266. © Swets & Zeitlinger.

Medicine Today: Its Identity, Its Role, and the Role of Physicians. *Itinerarium* 10 (2002): 57–79. © Istituto Teologico "S. Tommaso."

From Medical Ethics to a Moral Philosophy of the Professions. In *The Story of Bioethics: From Seminal Works to Contemporary Explorations*, ed. J. K. Walter and E. P. Klein, 3–15. Washington, DC: Georgetown University Press, 2003. © Georgetown University Press.

Moral Choice, the Good of the Patient, and the Patient's Good. In *Ethics and Critical Care Medicine*, ed. J. C. Moskop and L. Kopelman, 117–138. Dordrecht: D. Reidel, 1985. © D. Reidel Publishing Company, with kind permission of Springer Science and Business Media.

The Four Principles and the Doctor-Patient Relationship: The Need for a Better Linkage. In *Principles of Health Care Ethics,* ed. R. Gillon, 353–367. New York: John Wiley, 1994. © John Wiley & Sons Ltd.

Patient and Physician Autonomy: Conflicting Rights and Obligations in the Physician-Patient Relationship. *Journal of Contemporary Health Law and Policy* 10 (1994): 47–68. © Catholic University of America Press.

Character, Virtue, and Self-Interest in the Ethics of the Professions. *Journal of Contemporary Health Law and Policy* 5 (1989): 53–73. © Catholic University of America Press.

Toward a Virtue-Based Normative Ethics for the Health Professions. *Kennedy Institute of Ethics Journal* 5 (1995): 253–277. © The Johns Hopkins University Press.

The Physician's Conscience, Conscience Clauses, and Religious Belief: A Catholic Perspective. *Fordham Urban Law Journal* 30 (2002): 221–244. © Fordham University School of Law.

The Most Humane of the Sciences, the Most Scientific of the Humanities. In *Humanism and the Physician,* 16–37. Knoxville: University of Tennessee Press, 1979. © University of Tennessee Press.

The Humanities in Medical Education: Entering the Post-Evangelical Era. *Theoretical Medicine* 5 (1984): 253–266. © D. Reidel Publishing Company, with kind permission of Springer Science and Business Media.

Agape and Ethics: Some Reflections on Medical Morals from a Catholic Christian Perspective. In *Catholic Perspectives on Medical Morals,* ed. Edmund D. Pellegrino et al., 277–300. Dordrecht: Kluwer Academic Publishers, 1989. © Kluwer Academic Publishers, with kind permission of Springer Science and Business Media.

Bioethics at Century's Turn: Can Normative Ethics Be Retrieved? *Journal of Medicine and Philosophy* 25 (2000): 655–675. © Swets & Zeitlinger.

Toward an Expanded Medical Ethics: The Hippocratic Ethic Revisited. In *In Search of the Modern Hippocrates,* ed. Roger J. Bulger, 45–64. Iowa City: University of Iowa Press, 1987. © University of Iowa Press.

Medical Ethics: Entering the Post-Hippocratic Era. *Journal of the American Board of Family Practice* 1 (1988): 230–237. © American Board of Family Practice.

APOLOGIA FOR A MEDICAL TRUANT

Edmund D. Pellegrino

The more our time seems to force us into an inherently confused relationship of doctor and patient, the more firmly must we recall what a true physician is like.

—Karl Jaspers, *Philosophy and the World*

I am grateful to the editors of this collection for their generous invitation to write a brief introduction to these readings. This gives me the opportunity to thank them for sifting assiduously through my writings for what might be significant. It is no small honor to be taken seriously by two bona fide philosophers—especially when one of them, Tristram Engelhardt, is a colleague whom I have admired for many years for his erudition and the vigor and rigor of his thought.

I would be remiss if I did not also express my gratitude to David Thomasma, my collaborator for 25 years. The marks of his philosophical scholarship are everywhere embedded in these readings (Pellegrino 2005). Finally, I thank, also, my colleagues at the Kennedy Institute of Ethics and the Department of Philosophy at Georgetown for their intellectual courtesy which permitted me to explore some of my thinking with them in collegial discourse.

These associations have special meaning for a philosophizing nonphilosopher. There is no small disdain these days for physicians who transgress the perimeters of their clinical expertise. Like them, I have been a trespasser in the olive groves of Academia. This was not always the case. Physicians and philosophers were not easily distinguishable in ancient Greece. Hippocrates grossly overstated the case with his grandiose dictum: "Iatros philosophus Iso Theos" (The physician who is a philosopher is like a god). He was trying to say that good medical care needs more than its scientific orientation.

Grandiosity aside, it is worth remembering that medicine was one of the original nine liberal arts, until the fifth century AD, when it was banished by Martianus Capella. But even after its exile, university-trained physicians were well educated in the liberal arts from the Middle Ages through the Renaissance and up to the latter half of the twentieth century. They often wrote and spoke as members of a "learned profession" in fields beyond medicine.

This was still the case well into the twentieth century, when the enormous power and productivity of the physical and biological sciences made a scientific education more relevant for many. As medical specialization expanded, it became ever more difficult for physicians to wander beyond the perimeters of their own expertise. But these trends did not quench the intellectual wanderlust of physicians for the humanities and the arts.

This is probably because medicine is in fact the most humanistic of the sciences (Pellegrino 1979, pp. 11–39). Any physician who goes beyond technique to contemplate the human object of his ministrations must turn to the humanities for those meanings which medical science alone cannot give. It is this compulsion that has made some physicians "medical truants," trespassers beyond the bounds of medicine.

Lord Moynahan, one of Britain's most distinguished surgeons, used this term to describe physicians who, in his words, "deserted" medicine (Moynahan 1936). A. M. Cook (1986) and John Bowers (2004) also described this phenomenon. They had in mind such worthies as Borodin and Berlioz in music, Chekhov in drama, Thomas Linacre and William Osler in the classics, John Keats and William Carlos Williams in poetry, Walker Percy, Somerset Maugham, William Osler, Richard Selzer, and Lewis Thomas in literature and belles lettres. In philosophy, a short list would include John Locke, La Mettrie, Maurice Blondel, William James, Karl Jaspers, Erwin Straus, and, of course, H. Tristram Engelhardt, Jr., himself.

Some of these "truants" abandoned medicine, some continued to practice it, and some developed such expertise in their truancy as to triumph within it. Medicine in one way or another either stimulated, enriched, or provoked their incursions into other fields. I was once asked whether a physician can ever forget he is a physician. I am not sure. But the odds are high that the special existential phenomena of having a medical education and caring for other humans in distress leaves an indelible mark on any but the most insensate of physicians.

Without suggesting any achievements even remotely comparable to those of the medical truants I have mentioned, I feel a kinship with them in my efforts to reflect philosophically on the realities of healing, helping, curing, comforting, counseling and educating. These are ineradicable elements that are part of the lived world of the good clinician. I have been a medical truant, but one who remains primarily a physician. Without being a professional philosopher, I have shared Jaspers's convictions that we must have two commitments—to a scientific attitude and to philosophical reflection on the meaning of that science (Jaspers 1963, p. 234).

These convictions have shaped these readings and encouraged me to search for a moral philosophy of medicine based in the nature of medicine. Without this, medical ethics becomes what social convention, politics, economics, or sheer pragmatics makes it to be. Given its enormous power for good and evil, medical ethics cannot serve the personal and common good without clarity about its ends and purposes.

My inquiry into the ends and nature of medicine has inevitably taken me into the terrain of philosophy. I am not a professional philosopher, of course, but a philosophically inquisitive physician. I will not dilate here on the methodologies I have employed. The convergence of classical and medieval philosophy, enriched by some elements of a realist phenomenology, has seemed most appropriate for my project.

So far as bioethics is concerned, I appreciate its interdisciplinary nature. But if ethics is to be normative, it must be justified by ethical argumentation, not by descriptive disciplines only. In the relationships among the disciplines of bioethics, moral philosophy remains the guiding discipline. Without it, as is increasingly the case today, "ethics" in bioethics is so severely attenuated as to be on the verge of disappearance.

I have left the selection of readings entirely to Engelhardt and Jotterand. Authors in any case make poor critics of their own work. Moreover, as a medical truant, I can learn more from how they make their selections than by selecting my own.

Being a medical truant is an ambiguous but rewarding undertaking. There is the pleasure of the occasional compliment on a good idea or line of argument. Another reward is the colleague, student, or resident who is stimulated to read philosophy or contemporary bioethics on his own. Finally, there is the pleasure of seeing the ordinary phenomena of medicine in new and more profound ways.

These pleasures are not bought cheaply. The truant may bring more enthusiasm than light to his argument. He may misuse common terms, be ignorant of or misquote the literature. Or, less fairly, the truant may be ruled out of the debate on grounds of lack of expertise. The medical truant is often discredited on grounds that physicians are technicians not intellectuals. The truant himself may easily weaken his own thinking by arguing that only a physician can understand his point of view on the philosophy of medicine.

Acknowledging the perils of self-deception and the sometimes ludicrous errors, the role of medical truant has value, not just to the truant himself, but to medicine and health care. In the last decade, bioethics has more or less swallowed traditional medical ethics whole. There will always be a need for physicians who will engage in critical reflection, as physicians, and enter into dialogue with representatives of the humanistic disciplines. Few though they may be, medical truants have a leavening effect on both the philosophers who see nothing special in medicine as a human activity, and the physicians who see medicine as so special that it is closed to non-clinicians.

I hope these readings will stimulate critical thought on the part of physicians and more informed philosophizing on the part of ethicists and moral philosophers. Given the ephemeral nature of most writing, I hope this is not too much to ask.

balance of insider vs. outsider perspectives

References

Bowers, John Z. 2004. "Truants from Medicine." *Maryland Medical Alumni Bulletin.*

Cooke, A. M. 1986. "Doctors in Other Walks of Life." In J. N. Walton, et al. (Eds.), *The Oxford Companion to Medicine*, Vol. 1. New York: Oxford University Press.

Jaspers, K. 1963. *Philosophy and the World: Selected Essays and Lectures.* (E. B. Ashton, trans.) Chicago: Regnery.

Moynahan, Berkeley. 1936. *Truants: The Story of Some Who Deserted Medicine Yet Triumphed.* New York: Cambridge University Press.

Pellegrino, E. D. 2005. "Homage to David Thomasma: Introduction." Special issue of *Theoretical Medicine and Bioethics* 26: 437–439.

Pellegrino, E. D. 1979. "The Most Humane Science: Some Notes on Liberal Education in Medicine and the University." The Sixth Sanger Lecture. *Bulletin of the Medical College of Virginia* 67(4):11–39.

philosophy of medicine

medical humanities

bioethics

An Introduction

Edmund D. Pellegrino's Project

H. Tristram Engelhardt, Jr., and Fabrice Jotterand

Framing a Collage of Fields

Bioethics and the medical humanities, especially their emergence in the latter part of the twentieth century, cannot be understood apart from Edmund D. Pellegrino. He shaped the character of these fields. He placed bioethics and health care policy within an innovative vision of the philosophy of medicine. He recognized that one cannot rightly appreciate the medical humanities, bioethics, the philosophy of medical law, and medical-moral theology unless one also understands the core of the philosophy of medicine: the internal morality and the *telos* of medicine. Pellegrino's work compasses important explorations of the healing relationship, medicine as a profession, the patient's good, the role of autonomy, the place of money, and the importance of a virtue-based normative ethics for health care. This volume offers a comprehensive vision of Pellegrino's work. His work is important in its own right and because of the influence it has had and continues to have on the philosophy of medicine and bioethics.

This volume is composed of a critical selection from Pellegrino's corpus. It is aimed at providing the student, the scholar, the physician, and

1

the educated inquirer with a rich presentation of fundamental issues in the reflective consideration of medicine. To date, these essays have been unavailable in one work. This collection integrates essays scattered among various journals spanning a period of over a quarter of a century. This Pellegrino Reader provides insight into the emergence of a field, as well as analyses of issues, including the definition of the philosophy of medicine, the role of humanism in medicine, and the place of a virtue ethics in medicine.

The essays explore the philosophy of medicine, the medical humanities, and bioethics. The order of the fields is important. Pellegrino's work has been dedicated to showing that bioethics cannot be understood outside of the context of the medical humanities, and that the medical humanities cannot be understood outside of the context of the philosophy of medicine. Pellegrino correctly appreciates that bioethics should not be narrowly restricted to the usual fare of topics, ranging from abortion, third-party-assisted reproduction, physician-assisted suicide, and euthanasia, to genetic engineering, cloning, organ sales, and the allocation of medical resources. He appreciates that all of these issues are shaped by foundational views regarding the nature of the physician-patient relationship and the goals of medicine, all of which are the proper focus of the philosophy of medicine.

Autonomy, beneficence, non-maleficence, justice, solidarity, property rights, and vulnerability are set within a conceptual and value scaffolding that has structured medicine for millennia: medicine's dedication to the good of the patient. Pellegrino takes seriously medicine as a practice that carries with it its own teleological commitments, internal morality, presuppositions regarding the nature and significance of the physician/patient relationship, views concerning the nature of the virtuous physician, and the prerequisites for human flourishing. Because of the implicit role played by understandings of human flourishing, of what it is as a human to live properly and fully, the medical humanities are essential to locating and giving content to bioethics. That is, a particular bioethics presupposes a particular understanding of that which is truly human, the core notion of the humanities. One's view of what is normatively human, of what constitutes the *humanum,* lies at the roots of culture and morality. Concerns with the humanities bring together an interest in that which is most truly human (i.e., *humanissimus*) and in what it is to act in the fullness of one's humanity (i.e., *humaniter*), as well as in those engagements in study (e.g., art, history, and literature) that aid one to appreciate that which is truly human.[1] Because this area of scholarship discloses the hidden content and implicit presuppositions of bioethics, a bioethics is not understandable apart from the medical humanities. The humanities disclose the implicit assumptions regarding human flourishing that supply the taken-for-granted content of the ethics at the roots of bioethics.

Yet, the medical humanities themselves remain conceptually underdetermined and lack a critical self-consciousness absent the philosophy of medicine connecting them to the internal morality of medicine. This is to recognize that philosophy is not just one among the humanities, but the cardinal element of the humanities. Were it not for philosophy's critical reflection on the internal goals of medicine, the place and the significance of the other humanities would remain unarticulated. Hence, the role of the philosophy of medicine in laying out what is involved in human vulnerability and in the limits to human flourishing. All this has been understood by Pellegrino and is reflected in the essays collected in this volume. The essays offer the reader an opportunity to relocate the usual concerns of bioethics in terms of neglected, cardinal themes bearing on foundational concepts in virtue ethics and the philosophy of medicine.

The Third Humanism and the Medical Humanities: The Significance of Pellegrino's Work

The essays in this volume are important in their own right: they are substantive contributions to the philosophy of medicine, medical humanities, and bioethics. They are also important in reflecting the work of a figure who made the medical humanities and bioethics possible. Along with Daniel Callahan, the founder of the Hastings Center, and André Hellegers, the first director of the Kennedy Institute, Edmund Pellegrino, through his work with the Institute on Human Values in Medicine and the Society for Health and Human Values, supported the development of medical humanities programs in medical schools across the United States.[2] Many of these programs in the end gave their major accent to bioethics. However,

Pellegrino's broader vision left an enduring mark that has generally given philosophy a prominence in such centers. The influence of his presence, his presentations, and his scholarship framed a broader appreciation of bioethics. Besides relocating bioethics in a wider context, Pellegrino helped lay out its roots in foundational issues within the philosophy of medicine. He accomplished this in particular through his role as the founding editor of the *Journal of Medicine and Philosophy*, a journal he directed to placing bioethics within the reflections of the philosophy of medicine.

Individuals and ideas change history. From the latter part of the nineteenth century there had been a hunger to place the growing power of the sciences and technologies within the context of the humanities. In the late nineteenth century and the first part of the twentieth century in the United States, there was the emergence of what came to be known as the New Humanism. It involved persons such as Irving Babbitt (1865–1933) and Paul E. More (1864–1937). The movement was in part a response to a sense of loss of meaning in the face of an industrial, urban, mass society increasingly structured by new technologies.[3] An analogous phenomenon became salient in Europe in the first half of the twentieth century: the Third Humanism. This movement included such persons as Ernst Robert Curtius (1886–1956) and Werner Jaeger (1888–1961). The latter had at least some influence on Edmund Pellegrino. The New Humanism and the Third Humanism emerged quickly in the wake of the so-called Second Humanism, in which Friedrich Immanuel Niethammer (1766–1848) played an important role.[4] It is no accident that the Second Humanism had taken shape following the Enlightenment, Napoleon's self-crowning (December 2, 1804), and the secularization of Europe.[5] In the face of profound developments in the sciences and technologies, as well as the emergence of new social structures after the Industrial Revolution, new cultural guidance was sought. Because the usual sources of guidance, in particular the church, were being progressively marginalized, a moral vacuum was created, engendering a hunger to find perspective.

This hunger for orientation was often passionate. There was a sense of a profound need for a cultural revival. As Curtius puts it, "If humanism is to live again in the second third of the twentieth century, it can only be a total humanism: one that is sensual and spiritual, philological and touched

Herman Hesse?

by the muses, philosophical and artistic, pious and political, all in one."[6]
Curtius' plea was joined by such as Werner Jaeger, who raised a call to return to serious study of the humanities and to avoid the danger of a mass
culture. He characterized the latter under the rubric "Americanization."
"The percentage of the population that has a truly internal share in the an-
cestral intellectual assets of our nation decreases from year to year as indicated by the factory-like mass production of popular science and the *still*
introduction of the cinema, radio, and pocket microscopes in the school."[7] *happening!*
There was a view that a return to the humanities would allow a connection with that which is most truly human. The humanities were understood as central to the possibility of human flourishing.

Directly and indirectly, Edmund Pellegrino should be counted as a
major figure in the latter part of these humanist movements that arose
in the late ninetennth and mid-twentieth centuries. His genius was to tie
the humanities to medicine. Remarkably, this possibility and need were
largely overlooked by Abraham Flexner, who made his name in spurring
the medical educational reforms of early twentieth-century America.[8]
Flexner saw the general importance of the humanities, but was not able
to connect them substantively to medicine. For example, in his 1928 Tay-
lorian lecture, where he argues that true humanism must be distinguished
from technical scholastic engagements in philology (a point made by Pellegrino in this volume), he also notes that "the assessment of values, in so
far as human beings are affected, constitutes the unique burden of humanism."[9] A robust connection between the humanities and medicine is not
achieved until it is realized by Pellegrino and others in the mid-twentieth
century.[10]

There are a number of reasons one can advance for the special recep-
tivity in America in the latter half of the twentieth century to acknowledging a connection between the humanities and medicine. Through a
complex set of social developments, American society was secularized
and the profession of medicine transformed from a guild to a trade, just as
medicine became effective, expensive, and productive of major cultural
and moral questions.[11] Pellegrino had the genius to recognize and respond
to the hunger for orientation that arose as traditional guides (wise physicians and moral theologians) were brought into question. His response
was to reconnect medicine with the humanities, and the humanities with

medicine. As Pellegrino puts it "medicine is the most humane of sciences, the most empiric of arts, and the most scientific of humanities."[12] Pellegrino acted to bridge the cultural gulf separating the discourse of the humanities and the world of medicine.

Although Pellegrino emphasizes the importance of the medical humanities, he recognizes as well that many have held uncritical and unrealistic expectations regarding what the humanities can offer.

> Medical humanism has achieved the status of a salvation theme, which can absolve the perceived "sins" of modern medicine. The list of those sins is long, varied, and often contradictory: overspecialization; technicism; overprofessionalization; insensitivity to personal and sociocultural values; too narrow a construal of the doctor's role; too much "curing" rather than "caring"; not enough emphasis on prevention, patient participation, and patient education; too much science; not enough liberal arts; not enough behavioral science; too much economic incentive; a "trade school" mentality; insensitivity to the poor and socially disadvantaged; overmedicalization of everyday life; inhumane treatment of medical students; overwork by house staff; deficiencies in verbal and nonverbal communication.[13]

Pellegrino's strong commitment to the humanities is balanced with a critical appreciation of their limits and of the unjustified expectations of many concerning the possible contributions that the humanities can make to medicine. His ability to locate and appreciate reflectively the strengths and limitations of the humanities is undoubtedly rooted in his concerns for the philosophy of medicine as a grounding perspective.

The Collection: An Overview

This volume opens with an exploration of the philosophical foundations of medicine and the medical profession under the rubric "Toward a Philosophy of Medicine." This section encompasses two areas. The first examines the philosophy of medicine. The three essays in the first subsection range from two that examine the conceptual foundations of the field ("What the Philosophy *of* Medicine *Is*" and "Philosophy of Medicine: Should It Be Teleologically or Socially Construed?") to one ("The Internal Morality of Clinical Medicine") that gives special accent to the internal morality of medicine as defining medicine and therefore to a major focus of the philosophy of medicine. In the opening essay, Pellegrino draws a careful distinction among (1) philosophy *and* medicine (i.e., an examination of the relationship of philosophy and medicine in which each maintains its identity and is simply in dialogue with each other), (2) philosophy *in* medicine (i.e., an examination of philosophical issues that surface in medicine, ranging from logic and metaphysics to axiology and ethics, none of which is peculiar to medicine), (3) medical philosophy (i.e., informal reflection regarding the conduct of medicine, as for example views concerning appropriate styles of clinical practice), and (4) the philosophy *of* medicine (i.e., a philosophically critical reflection on the concepts, presuppositions, and method peculiar to medicine as medicine). By employing a historical overview and conceptual analysis of philosophy's engagement with medicine, Pellegrino shows the integrity of the field, the philosophy of medicine. This he understands to be concerned with "the phenomena peculiar to the human encounter with health, illness, disease, death, and the desire for prevention and healing."

The second essay, "Philosophy of Medicine: Should It Be Teleologically or Socially Construed?", develops further Pellegrino's restriction of the philosophy of medicine to those conceptual, methodological, and other issues peculiar to medicine. In this piece he is responding to criticism by Kevin Wm. Wildes that Pellegrino construes the philosophy of medicine too narrowly by excluding medical logic, medical epistemology, and the examination of concepts of health and disease. This omission, as Pellegrino argues, is justified in that these issues are not peculiar to medicine and therefore do not specifically define a philosophy *of* medicine. Pellegrino responds as well to Wildes' criticism of the teleological character of Pellegrino's account of the philosophy of medicine.

In the last of the first three essays, "The Internal Morality of Clinical Medicine: A Paradigm for the Ethics of the Helping and Healing Professions," Pellegrino investigates the internal morality of clinical medicine and how it defines the character of medicine, the object of the philosophy of medicine. He begins by responding to calls for a new ethic of medicine.

Rather than attempting to establish such an ethic, Pellegrino instead draws the reader's attention to the internal value commitments of the practice of medicine itself, arguing that medicine has ends, which give it definition. Here Pellegrino begins an analysis of the good of the patient, which he develops further in other chapters in this volume, but especially in "Moral Choice, the Good of the Patient, and the Patient's Good." As he argues, the health care professions are defined by the end or *telos* of pursuing the good of a person vulnerable to disease, disability, and death.

The four essays in the second part of the section concerning the philosophy of medicine address the relationship between medicine and humanism, as well as the proper role of physicians. In "Humanistic Basis of Professional Ethics," Pellegrino argues that a "more reliable source for a more humanistic professional ethics resides in the existential nature of illness and in the inequality between physician and patient intrinsic to that state." That is, only when a truly humanistic relationship is established between physicians and patients will both physicians and patients be able to express their humanity fully. This theme is taken up with a special focus on the intrusion of the market and concerns for profit in the contemporary character of health care in "The Commodification of Medical and Health Care: The Moral Consequences of a Paradigm Shift from a Professional to a Market Ethic." Here Pellegrino in particular explores "the ethical consequences of commodification of health and medical care on the relations of physicians with patients, with each other, and with society." As a result of these factors, physicians and the profession of medicine face two quite different roads to the future, each leading to a different profession, a different understanding of the patient, and different possibilities for human flourishing. The question is whether the ethic of the marketplace or an ethic built primarily on the physician's commitment to the healing and care of the patient will define medicine.

These concerns are explored further, as Pellegrino addresses the goals of medicine in "Medicine Today: Its Identity, Its Role, and the Role of Physicians." In this essay, he examines the *telos* that defines the art of medicine. Drawing on Aristotle, Aquinas, and Leon Kass, he looks with care at the nature of the medical good, the patient's perception of that good, the good for humans, and the spiritual good. All of this he brings together in an investigation of the proper role of physicians, which he defines in terms of their relationship to patients and their mutual determination of the ends of medicine. As Pellegrino puts it, "physicians do not determine the ends of medicine; it is their task to realize these ends in a specific clinical encounter with a particular patient. Physicians are charged with ascertaining, together with the patient, the content of the end of healing. Note, the content of healing is not a social construction of the end, but it accepts healing as an end." In this relationship, physicians encounter the possibility for virtue as a professional.

This section closes with a quasi-autobiographical essay ("From Medical Ethics to a Moral Philosophy of the Professions") in which Pellegrino reviews his work from the 1940s to the present, tying his personal journey to the cultural developments that fed the need for a moral philosophy of the health care professions. As he shows, our current condition is characterized by the need "to 'recapture' the idea of professional commitment. Without a reconstruction of the moral foundations of the idea of a profession, [this effort] cannot be fully successful." As Pellegrino argues, "Professional ethics, its groundings, the sources of its moral authority, and the way they are justified are of concern to all of us. It is not the whole of bioethics to be sure. But it is through professionals that bioethics becomes a benefit or a danger for every human being in a technological society. A philosophy of the profession that grounds the ethics of the professions is therefore more than an idle academic exercise." This section, in short, ties the practice of medicine and the framing context of bioethics to the need to develop an adequate philosophy of the profession of medicine.

The section "Physician-Patient Relationship" focuses on the healing relationship. It opens with "Moral Choice, the Good of the Patient, and the Patient's Good." In this essay Pellegrino confronts the difficulty of defining the patient's good in a morally heterogeneous society. He distinguishes among four themes bearing on the nature of the good: (1) "the patient's concept of ultimate good," (2) "biomedical or techno-medical good," (3) "the patient's concept of his own good," and (4) "the good of the patient as a person." Pellegrino ties these relatively abstract concerns to the concrete issue of no-code orders and the limiting of cardio-pulmonary resuscitation. He draws as well from Aristotle's account of the good, thus establishing connections among the philosophical traditions, understandings of the good, and good clinical decision making.

The next essay in this section, "The Four Principles and the Doctor-Patient Relationship: The Need for a Better Linkage," brings Pellegrino's analysis one step further by critically reassessing Beauchamp and Childress's four principles of autonomy, beneficence, non-maleficence, and justice. This essay provides a careful analysis of the implications of different senses of autonomy for different models of the physician-patient relationship. In so doing, Pellegrino lays out cardinal conflicts between autonomy and beneficence, and between autonomy and justice. In the process, Beauchamp and Childress's principles are embedded in the realities of clinical decision making, as well as in the foundational scaffolding of the physician-patient relationship. "The obligations that arise from the nature of the relationship provide the theoretical grounding lacking in the approach through *prima facie* principles. Rather than principles, we can speak of obligations freely undertaken when we freely offer to help a sick person." All of this Pellegrino locates in terms of the primary context of medicine, the healing relationship.

The last essay in this section, "Patient and Physician Autonomy: Conflicting Rights and Obligations in the Physician-Patient Relationship," completes the analysis of the healing relationship, as well as of Pellegrino's critical recasting of the significance of Beauchamp and Childress's four principles. As Pellegrino notes, these principles mark points of strategic tension and ambiguity. They directly and indirectly indicate areas where further exploration is needed. Although the principle of beneficence is in tension with autonomy, the physician's autonomy receives little attention, and the autonomy of medical ethics has come under threat. Pellegrino's analysis of Beauchamp and Childress's principles brings him to five conclusions: (1) autonomy and beneficence, if rightly understood, turn out to be complementary, not contradictory; (2) in both theory and practice, autonomy is not merely a negative but a positive principle as well; (3) the actual content of the principles of beneficence and autonomy is defined in the context of specific actions and decisions; (4) the physician's autonomy both as a person and a professional must also be taken into consideration; and (5) medical ethics must maintain its autonomy over against political and socio-economic pressures.

The third section of this collection brings together three major essays in which Pellegrino examines the nature of virtue in general, its meaning in the medical profession in particular, and moral challenges to the conscience and integrity of physicians. The first essay, "Character, Virtue, and Self-Interest in the Ethics of the Professions," confronts the place of professional virtue and the difficulty of contemporary medical professionals recognizing the claims of virtue. Commercialization, competition, government regulation, malpractice suits, and advertising, as well as public and media hostility have engendered a profound professional malaise. Pellegrino argues that, though these forces are real and threatening, the major danger is posed by deficiencies in medical-professional character and virtue. Medical professionals, in order to maintain their integrity, will need to embrace an ethos of altruism and fidelity that will often be incongruent with the dominant, conventional morality. To do this, Pellegrino argues, medical professionals must recognize that professions are moral communities, able to sustain their members if their members sustain their professional moral communities. Success in establishing a sound foundation for the professional life requires recognizing (1) the vulnerability of patients, (2) the inequality between physicians and patients, (3) the special fiduciary character of the professional in such relationships, (4) the ways in which professional knowledge does not exist for its own sake, (5) the professional relationship as able to bring both help and harm, and (6) the professional relationship as dependent on the professional being a member of a moral community with its own internal morality.

The second of this trio of essays, "Toward a Virtue-Based Normative Ethics for the Health Professions," invites the reader to confront the meaning and foundations of virtue. As Pellegrino reminds us, the classical medieval synthesis understood virtue as excellence of character, as a trait appropriately oriented to defining ends and purposes, as an excellence of reason, not emotion, as centered in practical judgment, and as a trait acquired by practice. Pellegrino contrasts this account with Alasdair MacIntyre's account, which regards virtues as dispositions or acquired qualities necessary (1) to achieve the internal good of practices, (2) to sustain the communities in which individuals seek the higher good of their lives, and (3) to sustain traditions necessary for the flourishing of individual lives. Despite his defense of virtue ethics, Pellegrino frankly acknowledges the difficulties of virtue-based accounts: (1) virtue-based accounts tend to be circular (i.e., the good is defined in terms of what virtuous persons do, and the virtuous are those that do what is good), (2) virtue-based accounts tend to be thin on definitive moral guidelines, (3) virtue-based accounts have difficulty in distinguishing obligation from supererogation. All of this leads Pellegrino to underscore that virtue-based accounts cannot stand alone and must be lodged within a more comprehensive moral philosophy, which he acknowledges does not now exist. This problem is compounded in medicine, where the Hippocratic tradition is, at best, in disarray. The practice of medicine is marked by moral pluralism, relativism, and the privatization of morality. In the face of these challenges, Pellegrino calls physicians to an act of profession that can tie them to their engagement in healing, so that they can come to appreciate professional virtue in terms of the *telos* of the clinical encounter: the patient's good. Pellegrino lists among the virtues that should mark the good physician: fidelity to trust and promise, benevolence, effacement of self-interest, compassion and caring, intellectual honesty, justice, and prudence.

Having spoken to professional virtue in the clinical context, Pellegrino turns in the next essay to challenges to the physician's moral conscience. His focus is on the conflicts engendered as a result of practicing medicine in an often affirmatively secular culture. This tension is rooted in the circumstance that traditional Christians know things about medical morality unrecognized within secular society. In "The Physician's Conscience, Conscience Clauses, and Religious Belief: A Catholic Perspective," Pellegrino lays out a geography of some of the resulting moral conflicts, giving special attention to the rising reluctance of the state and others to confront honestly what should count as violations of conscience. For example, although religious exemption laws and conscience clauses have protected physicians from being directly coerced to engage in abortion or physician-assisted suicide, there is nevertheless often a requirement that they refer patients to others to do things the Christian physician knows to be immoral (that is, since abortion is equivalent to murder, then referring a woman to an abortionist is equivalent to referring someone to the services of a hit man, even if one will not engage directly in the murder oneself). In addition, there are growing constraints on religious institutions, once they receive tax funds, to provide services they would recognize as immoral, though their co-religionists have been forced to pay those very taxes. Among the failures in such public policy approaches is not appreciating that institutions, in order to maintain an integrity and commitment to virtue, must preserve the character of their commitments to the particular communities that brought them into existence and sustain them. It is through institutions such as sectarian hospitals that individuals realize their concrete lives in moral communities, with the result that the moral integrity of the individual is put at jeopardy if they are not able to protect and maintain the moral character and integrity of their institutions and their moral communities.

The last section offers Pellegrino's analysis of the ambiguities of humanism, the limitations of the Hippocratic Oath, and the challenges to framing a medical ethics for the future. The first subsection, "Humanities in Medicine," brings together essays exploring the role of humanism in medicine and medical education. The first essay, "The Most Humane of the Sciences, the Most Scientific of the Humanities," already partially quoted in this introduction, is an early manifesto that in many ways inspired the development of humanities teaching in medical schools. It includes Pellegrino's famous synopsis of the relationship of humanities and medicine: "Medicine is the most humane of sciences, the most empiric of arts, and the most scientific of humanities. Its subject matter is an ideal ground within which to develop the attitudes associated with the humanistic and liberally educated." Throughout this piece, Pellegrino is careful to acknowledge the often underexamined ambiguities in many of the ordinary usages of humanism, humanitarian, humanities, and liberal studies. As he stresses, the humanities have traditionally been recognized as quite different from the liberal arts. Pellegrino also stresses a point underscored by Abraham Flexner: "the pull toward specialization and scholarship" tends to transform the study of the humanities from the pursuit of wisdom to the pursuit of information and pedantry. The consequence is that the forest is lost in the trees.

The humanities should be lived. This point is developed further in the second essay, "The Humanities in Medical Education: Entering the Post-Evangelical Era," where Pellegrino again emphasizes that the liberal arts, from classical times, have compassed "the intellectual skills needed to be a free man . . . the liberal arts are the cognitive instruments needed in every truly human activity." The goal of humanities education, Pellegrino argues, is to liberate the mind and the imagination and to open persons to a better appreciation of the human condition. The humanities bring us to deeper insights into what it is to be human. "The humanities deal with the dramatic, the artistic, the meanings of language, symbol, and myth, and the history of men's ideas about reality and how men respond to . . . living." As Pellegrino stresses, the humanities are engaged "to free the mind, to free the imagination, and to enrich the experience of being human." This liberation of vision will not succeed in medicine unless one engages the humanities within the clinical context, embedding humanistic education in the experience of the medical student and the physician. The humanities must be made integral to the life of the medical student and the physician. In actual practice, medical students and physicians must see how the medical humanities support the physician's virtuous response to actual patients.

The next essay locates concerns regarding humanism and the virtue of the physician in the context of Roman Catholic perspectives on medical morality. In "Agape and Ethics: Some Reflections on Medical Morals from a Catholic Christian Perspective," Pellegrino reviews the recent Roman Catholic dialogue with "the dominant cultural ideas of the time" and the competing accounts of morality and ethics which this has produced. He selects for his focus what he terms an agapeistic ethic: a virtue-based ethic which affirms charity as the principle that should structure the relationship between physicians and patients. With charity taken as the ordering principle of discernment in moral choice, Pellegrino places the general concerns of the humanities and the liberal arts within the more concrete focus of a particular Roman Catholic understanding. In this fashion, he gives content to the meaning of the virtuous and humane physician. He suggests as well the importance of the tie between Christian belief and virtuous practice.

This section ends with an essay that locates the previous discussions in terms of the challenge of bringing bioethics to speak to the pressing issues of normative ethics: "Bioethics at Century's Turn: Can Normative Ethics Be Retrieved?" As Pellegrino recognizes, bioethics has fragmented under the pressure of a plurality of moral visions, a multiplicity of theoretical accounts, and a failure to justify a particular, content-rich, moral view. The default position in bioethics and health care policy tends to be procedural rather than substantive, because substance divides and engenders dispute. Bioethics is either multiple or empty. Quoting Gilbert Meilaender, Pellegrino concludes that bioethics has "lost its soul." As bioethics matures and goes "into the next century, it will need to retrieve its connection with philosophical and theological ethics as the source of normative principles, rules, guidelines, precepts, axioms, middle level principles, etc." Pellegrino calls for traditionalists, modernists, and postmodernists to join in the project of giving new substance to bioethics, so as to recall bioethics to the normative task it has either abandoned or never appropriately embraced.

The last subsection is a brace of papers exploring the Hippocratic tradition and its capacity to inform a bioethics for the future. The first essay, "Toward an Expanded Medical Ethics: The Hippocratic Ethic Revisited," begins by recognizing that "Good physicians are by the nature of their vocation called upon to practice their art within a framework of high moral sensitivity. For two millennia this sensitivity was provided by the oath and the other ethical writings of the Hippocratic corpus. No code has been more influential in heightening the moral reflexes of ordinary individuals. Every subsequent medical code is essentially a footnote to the Hippocratic precepts, which even to this day remain the paradigm of how good physicians should behave." Through an examination of *The Oath*, *The Physician*, *Decorum*, *Precepts*, and *Epidemics*, Pellegrino underscores the Hippocratic principle taken from the last work: *primum non nocere*. This Hippocratic ideal he shows to lie at the heart of the Hippocratic commitment to protecting the vulnerability of the patient. Pellegrino then examines the shortcomings of the Hippocratic Oath and its ethos in the service of pointing to the possibility of "the elaboration of a fuller and more comprehensive medical ethic suited to our profession as it nears the twenty-first century."

The final essay in this collection, "Medical Ethics: Entering the Post-Hippocratic Era," continues the critical appraisal of the Hippocratic ethos. Through a study directed primarily to the Oath, Pellegrino displays its limitations, while yet recognizing its importance for the history of medical ethics. As he appreciates, the Hippocratic tradition, despite its past influence, must be reappropriated through a moral philosophy of medicine that takes account of "the moral heterogeneity of modern societies and the cosmopolitan character of scientific medicine." This project will require elaborating a philosophy of medicine internal to medicine itself and not derived from any external, philosophical system. That is, Pellegrino argues that medicine's internal morality must be understood through a moral philosophy internal to medicine and prior to medical ethics. Only such a moral philosophy of medicine, when adequately developed, so Pellegrino claims, will be able to meet the challenges of the future. "The post-Hippocratic era need not be viewed as the end of medical morality but as the beginning of an era of more responsible, more adult, more open, and more morally responsive relations between the sick and those who offer to help and heal them." Pellegrino identifies the hunger for professional identity and moral purpose in a post-traditional age and points to the possibility of recovering a sense of professionalism and moral dedication.

Pellegrino and the Future

This volume both reflects a cultural crisis or rupture and indicates possible responses to the challenges this brings. This collection of essays recognizes medicine's break from its sense of possessing tradition, a sense of continuity repeatedly re-achieved over the centuries by means of an affirmation of that period's understanding of the Hippocratic ethos. Pellegrino attempts to find a surrogate ethos and sense of professionalism in the face of rapid cultural change by reaching to the humanities and a philosophically recast bioethics. These essays of Pellegrino show a deep appreciation for the search for orientation in the face of post-modernity's cacophony and the constant presence of the moral concerns integral to the physician-patient relationship. It recognizes as well that bioethics attempted to claim hegemony over medical ethics, though bioethics itself failed to realize a unified normative undertaking. Though bioethics arose to give guidance in a cultural vacuum consequent upon the secularization of American society and the marginalization of the traditional authority of physicians, bioethics has nevertheless failed to provide, much less justify, a canonical moral perspective that can supply the guidance sought.[14]

Pellegrino's response to these challenges is to turn medicine's attention through the humanities to a philosophy of medicine that takes the internal morality of medicine seriously, so as to recapture moral substance and direction. Again, he locates bioethics within a vision of the human enterprise, a core contribution of the humanities. He then places all of this within a philosophy of medicine that takes seriously that which is essential to the calling of physicians. Laying out this project is no mean contribution on Pellegrino's part. It offers an interesting proposal for rethinking the nature of the philosophy of medicine and its office in grounding and directing not just the medical humanities and bioethics, but medical ethics and medical professionalism.

Pellegrino has shaped the development of the philosophy of medicine, the medical humanities, bioethics, and medical ethics. The past would not have been the same in the absence of his scholarship and personal engagement. His scholarship reaches to the future and to the possibility of recapturing an authentic medical ethics, an ethics for the medical profession. Pellegrino's work offers a basis for approaching bioethics and the medical humanities afresh. By addressing core but underexamined issues in the philosophy of medicine, he indicates an avenue toward recovering a sense of commitment to virtue and service on the part of the medical profession. By recognizing the physician-patient relationship as the central, moral-epistemic context for medical ethics, he provides a teleological account of the practice of medicine in terms of its pursuit of the medical good of the patient. The project he has begun promises a deeper understanding of medicine, as well as an opportunity for recapturing a moral sense of medical-professional identity.

Pellegrino's work thus points to the possibility of recapturing an intellectually vigorous medical ethics that, by being focused on the conditions for rightly directed medical professionalism and identity, will not be grounded merely in the concerns of bioethics. The essays collected here in particular offer a better appreciation of how a philosophy of medicine can reorient physicians, the medical humanities, and bioethics to Hippocratic themes reshaped and sustained in a conceptual and moral framework that transcends the cultural context of Greece, which produced the Oath. Not only has Pellegrino creatively examined the foundations of a philosophy of medicine in the strict sense, but he has also shown how it can redirect the medical humanities and bioethics. In so doing, he has succeeded in articulating a vision of how medicine can meet the challenges of the future.

Notes

1. For an account of the interplay among concerns with realizing that which is truly human, acting humanely, and possessing the learning of the humanities, see H. T. Engelhardt, Jr., *Bioethics and Secular Humanism* (Philadelphia: Trinity Press International, 1991), pp. 43–86.

2. Thomas K. McElhinney (ed.), *Human Values Teaching Programs for Health Professionals* (Ardmore, PA: Whitmore Publishing, 1981).

3. For an overview of this movement, see David Hoeveler, Jr., *The New Humanism* (Charlottesville: University Press of Virginia, 1977).

4. Friedrich Immanuel Niethammer, *Der Streit des Philanthropinismus und Humanismus* (Jena: Frommann, 1808).

5. In the early part of the twentieth century, Western Europe was radically secularized by Josephism (the policy of confiscating monastery properties begun in 1780 by Emperor Joseph II of Austria), the French Revolution (especially after the founding of the Republic in 1793), and the German secularization that followed the extraordinary Reichsdeputation of August 24, 1802 (which led to the confiscation of Roman Catholic properties and the subsequent transfer of education and welfare services from the church to the state). For an overview of this last phenomenon, see Joseph Freiherr von Eichendorff, "Über die Folgen von der Aufhebung der Landeshoheit der Bischöfe und der Klöster in Deutschland," in *Werke und Schriften* (Stuttgart: Cotta'sche, 1958), vol. 4, pp. 1133–1184.

6. Ernst Robert Curtius, *Deutscher Geist in Gefahr* (Stuttgart: Deutsche Verlags-Anstalt, 1932), p. 129.

7. Werner Jaeger, *Antike und Humanismus* (Leipzig: Quelle & Meyer, 1925), pp. 5–6.

8. Abraham Flexner, *Medical Education in the United States and Canada, A Report to the Carnegie Foundation for the Advancement of Teaching*, Bulletin No. 4 (New York: Carnegie Foundation, 1910).

9. Abraham Flexner, *The Burden of Humanism* (Oxford: Clarendon Press, 1928), p. 22.

10. For an example of others who, with Pellegrino, recognized the importance of the humanities in medicine, see Maurice Vischer (ed.), *Humanistic Perspectives in Medical Ethics* (London: Pemberton, 1973).

11. For an overview of these social-cultural changes and the hunger they produced for moral, cultural, and metaphysical orientation, see H. Tristram Engelhardt, Jr., "The Ordination of Bioethicists as Secular Moral Experts," *Social Philosophy & Policy* 19 (Summer 2002), 59-82.

12. Edmund D. Pellegrino, *Humanism and the Physician* (Knoxville: University of Tennessee Press, 1979), p. 17. The chapter in that book is a modified version of the Sanger Lecture entitled "The Most Humane Science: Some Notes on Liberal

Education in Medicine and the University" and delivered at the Medical College of Virginia of Virginia Commonwealth University, Richmond, on April 10, 1970.

13. Pellegrino, *Humanism and the Physician* (Knoxville: University of Tennessee Press, 1979), p. 9.

14. May the reader be informed: the first editor of this volume recognizes that such substance and guidance can only be found by choosing a religion, and that care must be taken to choose the right religion. See H. T. Engelhardt, Jr., *The Foundations of Christian Bioethics* (Salem, MA: M & M Scrivener Press, 2000).

o

I

TOWARD A PHILOSOPHY OF MEDICINE

Philosophical Foundations of Medicine

ONE

What the Philosophy *of* Medicine *Is*

I will now turn to medicine, the subject of the present treatise, and set

forth the exposition of it. First I will define what I conceive medicine to be.

—Hippocrates, "The Art"

The philosopher is under obligation to study the nature of philosophy,

itself. . . ."

—R. G. Collingwood, *An Essay on Philosophical Method*

Introduction

Philosophical reflections about matters medical are as old as medicine and philosophy. In every era, critical thinkers, both in medicine and
philosophy, have sought levels of understanding about medicine and its
practice not attainable within the purview of the methodology of medicine itself. Only recently, however, has a debate arisen about whether or
not there is, or can be, a legitimate field of inquiry called the philosophy *of*
medicine. If there is such a field, in what does it consist? Can it be distinguished from the philosophy of science? What is its relationship to the

emergent field of bioethics? Does any practical consequence follow from these distinctions?

Fr. Giovanni Russo has invited me to set forth my current personal response to these questions based on my interest in this field as presented in my own work as well as my collaborative work with Dr. David Thomasma.[1,2,3] I will divide my responses into two parts. Part One deals with three perspectives on the present state of the question "Is there a philosophy of medicine, and, if so, in what does it consist?" Part Two compares, contrasts, and distinguishes four models for conducting philosophical inquiry into medicine, i.e., philosophy *and* medicine, philosophy *in* medicine, medical philosophy, and philosophy *of* medicine.

I shall argue, contra Caplan,[4] that there is a defensible and legitimate field of philosophical inquiry that can be termed properly the philosophy of medicine, that it can be distinguished from other forms of philosophical reflection about medicine, and that the distinctions are of more than heuristic value. In doing so, I shall expand on a set of distinctions I proposed more than twenty years ago, but which are even more cogent now than they were then.[5]

Part One: State of the Question: Three Perspectives — Negative, Expansive, and Specific

The history of philosophical reflections about medicine is long, complex, and parlous. I cannot possibly do justice to its historical development nor to the many versions in which it has appeared in the past and the present. Fortunately, there are several fulsome reviews of that history in the ancient and modern worlds, to which the reader may refer.[6,7,8,9,10] These reviews speak to the long duration of the dialogues between medicine and philosophy, the several forms they may take, and the range of topics that may fall within—and between—the domains of each discipline. While I will not repeat that history, I will draw upon it selectively to illustrate some of the distinctions and definitions I hope to make.

What is evident in that history is the apparent inevitability of the dialogue for both positive and negative reasons.[11] On the positive side, there is the fact that the preoccupations of medicine with humanity's complex and urgent problems—like life, death, suffering and disease—could hardly escape the inquiry of critical minds in any era. On the negative side, there is the obvious conflict of methodologies, the observational, empirical and experimental bent of medicine colliding with the analytical, speculative and abstract deliberations of philosophy. Attractions and repulsions notwithstanding, neither physicians nor philosophers could in fact desist from puzzling over such universal human experiences as the nature of illness and healing, the ethics of the professed healer, or the relationship of those phenomena to prevailing philosophical schools of thought.

Until recently, however, these reflections rarely met the criteria for formal, systematic, orderly analysis required to qualify them as a legitimate branch or sub-branch of philosophy. Today, however, physicians and philosophers have begun to speak seriously of the possibility of the philosophy *of* medicine as a field of inquiry, either to affirm or deny it. Today's interest in what Engelhardt and Erde have termed "a newly emerging field of philosophical study"[12] has several sources.

First is the mutuality of interest in the subject matter of medicine to which I have already referred. In every era, there were physicians who wanted to understand the phenomena they observed and the nature of the art they were practicing. In every era there were philosophers fascinated by the need for a deeper understanding of the phenomena than medicine could afford. To achieve these ends, the critical trans-medical perspective of philosophy has always seemed essential.

A second reason for the current interest in philosophy of medicine is the tremendous emphasis in the last twenty-five years on medical ethics and bioethics. As successive theories of medical ethics have surfaced, it has become apparent that there is need for a grounding for ethics in something beyond principles, virtues, casuistry, care, hermeneutics, etc. The first step in this grounding would have to be the articulation of a theory and philosophy of medicine. Such a theory is necessary if we are to put the competing ethical theories into some proper relationship to each other and resolve some of the contradictions between and among them. In short, we need to move from medical ethics or bioethics to a more comprehensive moral philosophy of medicine and the health professions.

A third factor fostering interest in a philosophy of medicine is the turn to Existential, Hermeneutic, Phenomenological, and Post-Modern approaches to ethics and philosophy. These philosophical perspectives are more open to lived experiences of patient and physician and to the particularities of moral choice, suffering, dying, finitude and compassion. These are phenomena of great interest to philosophers who seek to comprehend them in more concrete ways than is congenial in the analytical mode still dominant in contemporary Anglo-American philosophy. These are also the same phenomena physicians and patients confront experientially every day. Critical reflections on these lived experiences leads naturally to the kind of fundamental and comprehensive grasp that could qualify as philosophy of medicine. To be sure, a post-modern philosophy of medicine would reject ideologies, emancipatory narratives, and absolutism in favor of a diversity of language and concept. But it still would be a philosophy *of* medicine.

Currently, in response to these forces, three general positions are held regarding the nature and existence of the philosophy of medicine. For convenience of discussion, I will label these the negative, the broad, and the narrow positions.

The *negative* viewpoint is that of Arthur Caplan, who contends that there is at present no legitimate field of inquiry that warrants designation as philosophy of medicine.[13] Engelhardt and Erde,[14] Engelhardt and Schaffner,[15] and Engelhardt and Wildes,[16] on the other hand, recognize a very broad field of inquiry under the rubric of philosophy of medicine. Last is the narrower view of David Thomasma and myself, who hold to a more specific definition of a field we identify as philosophy *of* medicine *qua* medicine.[17,18,19] In our work, we go further and ground our philosophy of medicine in a theory of the healing relationship. Alfred Tauber builds a philosophy of medicine on the philosophy of Levinas.[20] Different combinations and versions of these three perspectives can be found in the issues of the *Journal of Medicine and Philosophy* and *Theoretical Medicine,* in the long series *Philosophy and Medicine,* and in recent books which have included philosophy of medicine in their titles. All qualify as philosophical reflection broadly speaking, but not all qualify as philosophy *of* medicine. They form a spectrum of philosophical reflections on the matter of medicine, and it is within this spectrum that I wish to locate philosophy of medicine as a distinguishable region of inquiry.

The Negative View: Philosophy of Medicine as Non-Existent

Caplan's line of argument is as follows: He sets forth the criteria he deems essential to define a legitimate field of inquiry. Then, he shows what he believes to be the failure of current definitions to meet those criteria. Caplan's own criteria include key books, articles, special journals, and a distinctive set of problems. He admits that, on first inspection, these criteria seem to be met by the field today. But, on further specifying his definition of the philosophy and medicine and the criteria that would give it intellectual stature, he concludes, regretfully, that there is no such field.

Caplan's evidence against the existence of a field of inquiry is as follows: First, he says, there is no agreed upon definition. He then offers his own definition, which he then proceeds to show is not met by any of the current fields of study. Caplan says philosophy of medicine is not to be equated with bioethics, which is normative, while philosophy of medicine should be metaphysical or epistemological. He likewise rejects identification of philosophy of medicine with humanities in medicine, health care policy, or medical aesthetics. He holds it as evidence against the existence of philosophy of medicine that there is not enough ". . . debate, anguish, posturing and mutual recrimination."[21]

Caplan offers his definition of philosophy of medicine as ". . . the study of the epistemological, metaphysical, and methodological dimensions of medicine; therapeutic and experimental; diagnostic, therapeutic, *[sic]* and palliative."[22] But, if this were in fact the case, he argues, philosophy of medicine would deal with "key problems" in the philosophy of science and thus be a subdiscipline of the philosophy of science—not a distinct discipline. Caplan's position is similar to that taken by Jerome Shaffer twenty years ago in the first volume of the Engelhardt and Spicker Series entitled *Philosophy and Medicine*[23] when the debates began, at least in the United States. It also accords well with the span of topics proposed by Sadegh-Zadeh and Lindahl as the domain of the philosophy of medicine which was the focus of the journal *Metamedicine,* later renamed *Theoretical Medicine.*[24,25]

Caplan admits the existence of a large literature and several organizations identified with philosophy of medicine. He even admits the possibility that there might be a "field" of inquiry but it is not one now because it is not part of a broader field, has no recognizable canon of books and no distinctive set of problems. Caplan laments the non-existence of the philosophy of medicine since he thinks a philosophy of medicine would be important as a foundation for bioethics, for the philosophy of applied science, and for certain special problems in genetics and similar fields.

The Broad View: Engelhardt Et Alia

Caplan's line of argument against the existence of the philosophy of medicine is circuitous, ambivalent, and based largely on simple assertion. Engelhardt and Erde, and Engelhardt and Schaffner are much more definitive in their assessment of the evidence for the existence of the philosophy of medicine. They define philosophy of medicine, not too differently than Caplan, as ". . . encompassing those issues in epistemology, axiology, logic, methodology and metaphysics generated by and related to medicine."[26] However, they specify several broad areas of inquiry they see as distinctive to the philosophy of medicine such as models of medicine, concepts of health and disease, the logic of diagnosis, prognosis, clinical trials, artificial intelligence, disease causation, etc. Engelhardt and his coauthors support their contention by a substantial bibliography of works drawn from many eras and countries, covering an extraordinarily wide range of topics at the juncture of medicine and philosophy. It is difficult to see how Caplan could dismiss such an extensive body of work as not constituting a field of inquiry.

The Engelhardt and Erde, and Engelhardt and Schaffner, definitions of philosophy of medicine are close to Caplan's. But, contra Caplan, their review supports the criteria for a "field," given the great range and number of books and articles they cite that deal with philosophy and medicine. For their part, however, they have cast their net too widely. Many of the works they cite are at the margin of their own definition. Some, however, are now so often cited as to constitute a beginning "canon." The Engelhardt, Erde, Schaffner, and Wildes definition embraces every conceivable intersection between philosophy, medicine, and physical and social science. While such studies are important, such a broad definition, which embraces such a wide spectrum of studies, dilutes the specificity of philosophy of medicine and weakens the identification of a definitive set of problems. Yet, this specificity is precisely what needs to be examined more closely if we are to determine whether an independent philosophy of medicine does, indeed, exist.

Much of what Engelhardt, Schaffner, and Erde cite as work in the philosophy *of* medicine could qualify, just as Caplan suspects, as the philosophy *of* science or biology or as sub-branches of extant fields of philosophical inquiry like metaphysics, epistemology, or axiology, or, in my terms, as philosophy *in* medicine. This would not diminish the importance of the questions studied. But it does obscure the outlines of a philosophy of medicine, a field whose focus would be more narrowly on the precepts, presuppositions, concepts, and values peculiar to medicine as medicine and not simply as examples of problems already pursued in science or philosophy.

It is interesting, and somewhat puzzling as well, that the philosophies *of* many disciplines other than medicine are recognized as legitimate fields of inquiry. The most recently published *Dictionary of Philosophy*,[27] for example, has no entry under "philosophy of medicine." Neither does the currently available but outdated *Encyclopedia of Philosophy*.[28] Yet both reference works have entries for philosophy of biology, economics, education, language, law, literature, logic, mathematics, mind, religion, psychology, science, and social science. Each of those philosophy of ". . ." articles speaks of the concepts, methods, theories, presuppositions, and justifications fundamental to the discipline in question. Thus, for every discipline, except medicine, a narrow, specific field of philosophical inquiry is recognized that deals with the "what is" question and the problems "internal" to the discipline but not susceptible to resolution by the method of the discipline itself.

Engelhardt and Schaffner's article embraces the whole range of philosophical reflection on medicine. Some of their citations would be classified as philosophy of science, much as philosophy *in* medicine or philosophy *and* medicine, and some as medical philosophy. To some extent, this is also the case with Van der Steen, who identifies philosophy of medicine with (a) questions "left over" from science, (b) normative questions, and (c) methodological questions.[29] Other authors also take the broad or expansive view of philosophy of medicine.[30,31] In the remainder of this paper, I shall attempt to define the various regions of philosophy of medicine more clearly, particularly that region of the spectrum I believe to be distinguishable as the philosophy *of* medicine.

Part Two: Four Modes of Philosophical Reflection on Medicine

In this section, I wish to compare, contrast, and distinguish these four regions in the spectrum of philosophical inquiry into medical matters. I shall not distinguish between different philosophical methodologies, e.g., Anglo-American, Analytic, Classical, Medieval, Phenomenological, Post-Modern, or Hermeneutical systems of thought. Any, or all, of those schools of philosophical thought can be applied to medicine or can examine problems specific to its own enterprise as it exists in the context of medicine. What is significant in defining the field of philosophy of medicine is not the school of philosophical thought but the end and purpose for which that philosophy is applied to medical topics.

Philosophy *and* Medicine

In this mode of philosophizing, philosophy and medicine each retains its identity and enters as a distinct discipline into independent and autonomous dialogue with the other. The subject of that dialogue is variable. It can be an effort at identification or at comparing and contrasting the way each discipline studies the phenomena peculiar to medicine. It can define similarities and differences in subject matter, method, or mutual influences of one on the other. In the Hippocratic writings, for example, the two treatises "The Art"[32] and "Ancient Medicine"[33] are devoted to establishing the independence of the method of medicine from that of philosophy. The Hippocratic authors affirm the importance of observation of individual cases and reasoning based in empirical evidence. They repudiate speculation and particularly speculation as practiced by certain philosophers and philosopher-physicians.

Socrates and Plato, for example, frequently used medicine as an example of a *techné* practiced within ethical constraints.[34] Plato, at one point, went so far as to liken the physician who was also a philosopher to a god. Galen, who practiced both medicine and philosophy, took this identity relationship seriously in his own work. On the other hand, in the *Symposium*, Plato chides the physician Eryximachus for his technicism, for his attempt to explain all human existence through his art.[35] Elsewhere, he has Nicias say that physicians should not presume to go beyond knowledge of the nature of health and disease.[36] Here, Plato clearly seems to disapprove of medicine extending its reach into philosophical problems.

Medicine, for its part, was equally ambivalent about philosophy. In the Hellenic Period, physicians and physician philosophers drew heavily on the teachings of the major philosophical schools—The Academy, the Peripatetic, and the Stoa—for their theories of disease and healing.[37,38,39] Each of the major schools of medicine—Methodists, Dogmatists and Empiricists—adopted and adapted the philosophical doctrines of the major schools of Greek philosophy. In a similar way, in later centuries, Stahl's theory of vitalism drew on the philosophy of Leibniz, while mechanistic theories of medicine drew on Descartes and J. O. de La Mettrie. Lester King provides a detailed account of how seventeenth- and eighteenth-century philosophical systems drew upon theories of medicine, especially for their metaphysical and logical content.[40]

This reliance on philosophy for theoretical understanding was a reversal of the stance of the Hippocratic School which had been explicit in distancing itself from philosophy. Thomas Sydenham and other eighteenth-century "Hippocratic" physicians repeated this rejection of philosophy:

> In writing the history of a disease, every philosophical hypothesis whatsoever, that has previously occupied the mind of the author should be in abeyance. This being done, the clear and natural phenomena of the disease should be noted—these and these only.[41]

To the contrary, others in later antiquity and the early Christian periods made medicine and philosophy identical with each other. Varro (BCE 116–27), for one, included medicine as one of the several liberal arts[42] and Cassiodorus (490–585) and Ennodius (473–521) identified *philosophus* and *medicus* as one and the same.[43] This intermingling became stronger in

the later sixteenth and in the seventeenth centuries when the growing influence of physical and experimental science on medicine became widely
manifest. Discovery of the telescope and microscope opened up new ways
of observation of nature and the possibility of subjecting philosophical
speculations to empirical verification.[44] On the other hand, these extant
observations were often interpreted in terms of newer philosophical systems. The philosophies of Descartes, Leibniz, Malebranche, Bacon and
others were closely interwoven with the new visions of reality uncovered
by the access the new instruments gave to both the microcosmos and
macrocosmos.

In the seventeenth century, the "natural philosophers" and the newer
philosophers of science were often interested in medicine as a science as a
branch of chemistry; physicians or mathematics. They exchanged ideas
and occasionally blows over the proper methodology for investigation of
nature. Medicine, because it is both a science and in many senses one of
the humanities, occupied a central place in these debates. Later, in the
eighteenth century, as experimentation and clinical investigations were
introduced into medicine, philosophical interest shifted to questions of
nosography, the logic of diagnosis and theories of health and therapeutics
as well as logic of statistical inference, and ideas of causality.[45]

In the last twenty-five years, philosophical reflection on medicine has
shifted again, this time to medicine as an ethical enterprise.[46] In the 1960s,
philosophers were attracted by the need for a more rigorous and sophisticated analysis of the dilemmas of medical progress than medicine itself
afforded. Physicians and philosophers drew on principles and concepts
developed in the great ethical traditions—the classical, medieval, the
Kantian, and the Utilitarian. Most recently, as philosophers explored the
practical issues, they also uncovered the need for a more substantial
grounding for medical ethics than ethical analysis, problems, dilemmas,
or cases could provide. As a result inquiry was directed to alternative theories as opposed to those based in principles. Ethical theories based in casuistry, philosophies of care, experience, or virtue became prominent. In
Europe, more attention was paid than in America, to hermeneutics, phenomenology, narrative and interpersonal relational theories as they were
exemplified in medical ethics and practice.[47,48,49]

Equally apparent today is the realization that medical ethics cannot
be pursued without a closer inquiry into the moral philosophy *of* medi-

cine.[50,51] Medical ethics requires clarity not just about the ethical concepts on which it depends, but clarity also about the ends and purposes of medicine as well. Healing, caring, suffering, finitude and a variety of other concepts have come to be legitimate objects of philosophical inquiry in their relation to the ends of medicine. As a result, need for mutual understandings of philosophy and medicine, or the science and praxis of medicine, and the healing relationship, have become active fields of research.

Philosophy *in* Medicine

By philosophy *in* medicine, I mean the application of specific, recognized branches of philosophy—e.g., logic, metaphysics, axiology, ethics, aesthetics to matters medical. This is essentially what Engelhardt and Schaffner would define as philosophy of medicine. Most of their attention is devoted to philosophical study of the scientific foundations of medicine. This is the sense in which most recent review articles and books now interpret philosophy of medicine. Also, on this view, theories of medical knowledge or ethics, for example, drawn from existing theories of epistemology or moral philosophy are applied to medical problems, concepts, or experiences.[52,53,54,55] Medical diagnosis, for example, is examined for its logic, and concepts of health and disease are examined for their ontological or epistemological status. In these cases, the starting point is a question of interest to philosophy as such. The concepts, methods, or presuppositions of science generally, or of the social sciences, statistics, logic, etc. are examined as they may be specified in the activities peculiar to medicine.[56]

Wulff et al., for example, draw on phenomenology, hermeneutics, and existentialism as well as on the philosophies of Kierkegaard, Heidegger, and Gadamer to gain insights into the phenomena of medicine.[57] Similarly, Natanson extrapolates the philosophy of Heidegger and *dasein* analysis to the data of classical psychiatry.[58] Sinha looks for insights into the concepts of health and disease and the ontological, axiological, and epistemological problems of medicine in the Asian philosophical tradition.[59,60] In the same spirit, Fleck undertakes the socio-cultural epistemology of medical fact,[61] and Foucault does so with the clinical "gaze" and the birth of the clinic.[62] Another example is Brody's use of Rawls' method of reflective equilibrium to study the placebo effect and the ethics of its use. Other examples of philosophy in medicine would be the treatises on medical logic.[63,64,65] Similarly, exploration of the themes of explanation and reasoning, and probability and normality, have employed philosophical modes of analysis. Current inquiries into the use of Bayesian logic, artificial intelligence, and decision analysis are further examples of philosophy's effect on medicine.

Obviously, philosophy *in* medicine has been, and is, fruitful for both medicine and philosophy. For philosophy, there is the discovery of subjects of intrinsic interest to the enterprise of philosophy itself. For medicine, there is the opening of the subject matter of medicine in ways not contained within the language and method of medicine itself.

The most fruitful example of the power of philosophy in medicine is the principle-based system of Beauchamp and Childress.[66] They have skillfully and wisely taken four principles of "the common morality" as *prima facie* guides to the resolution of practical medical ethical dilemmas. But the success of their system is now questioned because the *prima facie* principles are not grounded in a more general or fundamental moral philosophy.[67] While I believe principles are essential to any viable ethics of medicine, I have tried to ground them in a philosophy of medicine, one derived from the clinical phenomena of medicine itself.[68] In doing so, I hope to show that there is no essential conflict between philosophy *in* medicine and philosophy *of* medicine.

Medical Philosophy

Another category that needs definition is medical philosophy. This is the vaguest and most loosely defined of the current terms. I take it to mean any informal reflection on the practice of medicine—usually by physicians on clinical medicine based in their reflections on their own clinical experiences. Here, we might include "styles" of practice such as: therapeutic enthusiasm, nihilism, or minimalism; diagnostic enthusiasm which leaves no test unused; diagnostic artistry which pursues an elegant form of clinical epluchage, selecting just the right number and kind of tests; then there are those who want to be a friend to the patient; those who, on the contrary, feel a certain "distance" is more conducive to the healing relationship; those who favor formal or informal modes of address or dress; etc. These matters are rarely subjected to formal analysis but are argued as conducive to good or bad care of patients.

There is also a kind of medical philosophy, based in the clinical wisdom of reflective clinicians that has always been a source of inspiration and practical knowledge for conscientious clinicians. Among writers in English, one thinks of William Osler[69] and Francis Peabody,[70] or of Richard Cabot[71,72] and Lewis Thomas.[73] Their works are not philosophical in any formal sense, but in the more informal, traditional sense of the search for wisdom. In their cases, that wisdom emerges from reflective and meditative cogitation on years of learning by experience. They are examples of practical wisdom, the kind of reflective understanding beyond empiricism of how to practice a craft with perception contained in the Greek notion of *techné*.[74,75]

In contrast to this kind of informal medical philosophy, well-grounded in the received wisdom of experienced clinicians, are the grand theories and systems of medicine that emerged in the late seventeenth and eighteenth centuries.[76,77,78,79] These were attempts to classify, explain, and treat diseases according to mostly fanciful appropriations of quasi-philosophical notions. Some examples use Stahl's animism, John Brown's theory of stimuli, Hoffman's mechanism, Hahnemann's homeopathy as well as vitalism, mesmerism, and many other lesser known theories, all energetically debated. Some of those speculative medical philosophies were directly influenced by philosophical systems—e.g., Descartes' influence on J. O. de La Mettrie, Condillac's on Pinel, or Leibniz's on Hoffman.[80,81]

Descartes' flirtations with medicine illustrate how complex a serious philosopher's reflections on medicine may be. For one thing, Descartes wanted to draw ". . . rules for medicine . . . more firm than those which have been attained to present."[82] At the same time, he looked to medicine for a definition of the goals, ends, and purposes of human life and ethics. Finally, he wanted to ground medicine in infallible demonstrations and sought from it to extend his own life and health.[83] Descartes employs philosophy *in* medicine to develop rules for medicine, philosophy *of* medicine to develop the goals of life, and philosophy *and* medicine to mathematize medicine and make it a branch of his philosophy.

With these difficulties as illustrated in Descartes and other works cited above in mind, I will turn now to that portion of the spectrum of reflection I believe properly qualifies as a philosophy of medicine.

Philosophy *of* Medicine

The philosophy of medicine consists in a critical reflection on the matter of medicine—on the content, method, concepts, and presuppositions peculiar to medicine *as medicine*. To this end, philosophy of medicine, of necessity, must transcend the methods of medicine (i.e., the methods of science, clinical observation, and clinical judgment). Its purposes are different than the purposes of medicine *per se*. Philosophy of medicine makes the specific method and matter of medicine the subject of study by the method of philosophy. Philosophy of medicine seeks philosophical knowledge of medicine itself. It seeks to understand what medicine *is* and what sets it apart from other disciplines, and from philosophy itself. It seeks to show what medicine is, as did the Hippocratic physicians in their two treatises on the nature of medicine ("The Art" and "Ancient Medicine").[84,85] This is no trivial task or labor at the obvious. Lain-Entralgo, perhaps the most astute of the Hippocratic commentators, took this question to be among the most profound in the Hippocratic corpus.[86] Lester King had to admit that he abandoned his project of writing a history of Eighteenth Century medicine because he could not determine ". . . what medicine was."[87]

Philosophy of medicine has the same relationship with philosophy as the philosophies of history, art, law, literature, etc. have to those disciplines. In each case, critical reflection seeks something beyond the content of those disciplines, something beyond the methods of inquiry peculiar to each as a discipline. The philosophy of any discipline is a search for ultimacy, for a grasp of the reality of the things studied beyond what is discernible by the discipline studied.

It is impossible to define clearly what constitutes the philosophy of medicine without a definition of medicine itself. Indeed, the controversy about whether the philosophy of medicine is nothing more than the philosophy of science hinges on what we mean by medicine. If medicine is nothing more than a branch of science, i.e., if we equate it with the sciences basic to medicine (e.g., anatomy, physiology, biochemistry), then the philosophy of medicine is, indeed, only the philosophy of science. But if medicine embraces activities beyond those inherent in the pursuit of scientific knowledge, then a philosophy *of* medicine is a separate and separable entity from philosophy of science. Whether medicine is more than science is a question to be answered factually and phenomenologically in one sense, and by philosophy of medicine in another.

Obviously, medicine does rest, in part, on the sciences of human physiology and pathophysiology as well as pharmacology, microbiology, psychology, genetics, etc. Those are the realms of physical, chemical, and biological phenomena observable by the methods of science in studying the functioning and malfunctioning of human organisms. The end and purpose of the sciences basic to medicine is the pursuit of truth, a grasp of the realities of human bodily function and dysfunction to the extent that they are subject to observation, hypothesis formulation, and experimental manipulation. But medicine is more than a search for truth. It is a search for truth determined by a practical end which truth serves, namely health and healing of human beings.

Medicine *qua* medicine comes into existence in the clinical encounter or in public health when the knowledge of the sciences basic to medicine is employed for a specific end, i.e., for the cure, containment, ameliora-tion, or prevention of human illness in individuals or in human societies. Medicine *qua* medicine, therefore, is shaped not just by the ends and pur-poses of the sciences. Medicine uses scientific knowledge for its own spe-cific ends, which are healing, helping, curing, and preventing illness and disease and promoting health, i.e., the optimum well-functioning of the whole human organism or human society. Pursuing those ends with indi-vidual patients and families is the enterprise of clinical medicine; pursu-ing them with communities and societies is the enterprise of public health or social medicine.

Philosophy *of* medicine as medicine, then, has as its subject matter the problems of clinical and public health medicine that it examines with its own perspective—one different from the perspective of science and even from clinical or public health medicine themselves. Philosophy of medicine seeks to understand the nature and phenomena of the clinical encounter, i.e., the interaction between persons needing help of a specific kind relative to health and other persons who offer to help and are desig-nated by society to help.

Philosophy of medicine is concerned with the phenomena peculiar to the human encounter with health, illness, disease, death, and the desire for prevention and healing. It is rooted in concepts and conceptions like healing, helping, curing, health, illness, disease, care, the good of the patient, and the moral claims of the sick on the well, on society, and on the health professions. Concepts like causality, probability, taxonomy, logic, and mind-body relationships are studied as part of a philosophy of medicine to the extent that there is something in them that is peculiar to the human encounter with bodily and psychological well-being or dysfunction. Philosophy of medicine examines these ideas and phenomena as instantiations in the experiences of individual persons, in the relationships of physicians with patients or with physicians, patients, and society.

Medicine draws upon every discipline important to attaining its *telos*, a right and good healing decision and action for a given individual or society. Medicine uses all, shapes all, and studies pertinent branches of knowledge in terms of its *telos*. Indeed, medicine *qua* medicine comes into existence when it appropriates knowledge and skills, no matter what their origin, in order to further its healing purposes.[88,89]

Thus, medicine is not the arithmetic sum of the disciplines on which it draws—whether they are the humanities or the social, physical, or biological sciences. The philosophy of medicine, therefore, is not the sum of the philosophies of science, biology, the social sciences, literature, etc. Its special domain is the way the concepts, presuppositions, and methodologies of the disciplines it draws upon are differently nuanced by the complexities of the human relationships, as well as by the purposes of those relationships peculiar to medicine.

A philosophic study of causality, for example, could be approached in several ways. As a topic in the philosophy of science, it would be necessary to examine the concept in its most general form. This would require abstraction from the differences in the way causality operates in the medical relationship. This would be philosophy *in* medicine or philosophy of science *in* medicine. But, if the emphasis were on those things that make causality in illness and disease unique—if such exist—then we would deal with a philosophy of medicine. Here, attention would be directed to the phenomena peculiar to medicine as the particular kind of activity it is. Claude Bernard recognized these differences in nuance in the idea of causality in his epochal work on experimental medicine.[90]

Similarly, a study of Bayesian concepts could be examined as a problem in mathematical logic. However, it would become a problem for the philosophy of medicine when, and if, there were elements of application of Bayesian logic peculiar to the realities of medical observation and decision. Again, the philosophy of psychology would focus on understandings of the nature of the mind-body problem as a general phenomenon of human life. Examined as a question in philosophy of medicine, the focus would be on the uniqueness of the anxiety, dependence, suffering, vulnerability, and exploitability of a sick person seeking help from another person who has the power and the skill to help and heal, as well as to harm. Or, its focus could be the way mind may produce illness and dysfunction of body or body may cause emotional and psychic dysfunction.

Any topic examined as part of the philosophy of medicine should start with the realities, phenomena, and data of medicine itself. Such a study would derive from what medicine *is* as a phenomenon of the real world. In its turn, a philosophy of medicine would help to define what medicine is ontologically and morally. This is a narrower view than the more expansive definitions of philosophy *of* medicine, but it is more suited to the depth and levels of understanding and the reach for ultimacy that characterize philosophical reflection when it is directed to medicine as medicine.

The emphasis on medicine's realities and phenomena does not imply that physicians are the best, or the only, philosophers of medicine. For obvious reasons of inadequacy or lack of formal training in philosophy, personal identification with the phenomena as persons or professionals, and an inclination to scientific positivism, physicians may not be qualified at all. They may lack the emotional and intellectual distance that critical analysis of their own enterprise requires. Contrariwise, the putative possession of critical distance by philosophers need not necessarily authenticate them as philosophers of medicine. Philosopher or physician, the person who reflects philosophically on medical matters must respect simultaneously the phenomena of medicine and the canons of valid philosophical inquiry.

At this point, it might be objected that all of this is well and good, but the question remains: is not what I have described simply the sum total of the knowledge and skills pertinent to the sciences basic to medicine? To this I reply that the difference lies in the unifying perspective and integrative aspects of the conceptions of helping and healing that are specific to medicine and not to any of the contributing sciences. But the objection now might be that the microbiologist also seeks healing when she synthesizes an antibiotic for the specific purpose of killing a specific bacterium, virus, or fungus. In doing so, does microbiology become medicine, or the microbiologist a physician?

They do, in a limited sense, in that now microbiology becomes a science basic to medicine and, thus, different from the study, let us say, of bacterial or viral genetics with no therapeutic purpose in view. But, even so, this is not medicine in the fullest sense, since to be medicine, the fruits of microbiological science must be integrated into the life of particular patients or societies by and through an interpersonal relationship. Microbiological knowledge is essential to curing an infection but not sufficient to "heal" the patient. Healing requires a much fuller grasp of the patient as a person, of the place of *this* illness in his life at *this* time, and, in the future, of the ethical dimension and inter-relationships between the patient and his environment—the persons, places, jobs, etc. in her life story. None of the sciences of medicine—clinical, basic, epidemiological, etc.—even the psychological—fully encompass all these dimensions as they relate to healing and helping. In ways still only vaguely grasped, the interpersonal relationship between healers and patients conditions the healing process not only in "psychological" disorders, but in "physiological" disorders as well. Psyche and soma, soma and psyche, are inseparable in health as in illness, for both individuals and societies. Like individuals, societies have physiologies as well as pathologies. Like individuals, they can be healed and harmed. Both involve a relationship of persons to a specified purpose not contained in science as science.

Medicine must be concerned with the "good" of the patient. As David Thomasma and I have emphasized elsewhere, the patient's good is a compound notion. It is not synonymous with the patient's medical good. Healing means "to make whole again." Therefore, ascertaining and enhancing all four realms of the patient's good are involved in healing—the patient's biomedical good, his own conception of the good for him as an individual, his good as a member of the human species (i.e., the good for humans), and his good as a spiritual being (i.e., the good for the soul).[91,92] The concept of wholeness, together with its asymptotic attainment through relationships between, and among, persons is the specific end of medicine. It is not an end proper to any of the sciences basic to medicine. But without a concept of healing, medicine as such does not exist.

In short, medicine embraces a wide range of physical and social sciences as well as the humanities. Its distinction lies in its organizing principle of healing, in its centering on human inter-relationships, on its reach beyond a simple addition of disparate pieces of information from a wide variety of sources and its need simultaneously to engage the ethical as well as the technical dimensions of illness and healing.

Again, it is important to emphasize that medicine embraces insights from the humanities as well as the physical and social sciences. Healing is an experience as are illness and suffering. Literature, history, philosophy, language, and theology are all full of rich insights into these human experiences and, in this sense, medicine is a "humanistic discipline." But medicine is also distinct from other humanistic disciplines since its specific *telos* is helping and healing. One may use the humanities as one uses the sciences, to assist in healing, but healing is not the defining characteristic of literature, let us say, that it is for medicine in the fullest sense. A philosophy of medicine would relate philosophy, theology, science, etc. to medicine conceptually, but it would not conflate them.

Medicine is also an ethical enterprise since it is aimed at the good of patients not their harm, and, therefore, it must discern what is right and good, what *ought* to be done as well as what *can* be done. A philosophy of medicine would concentrate on the ethics "internal" to medicine[93]—to those ethical issues arising in the kind of activity medicine is—one based in a healing relationship and one founded in the phenomena of that relationship as well as competence in knowledge and skill appropriate to a healing relationship.[94,95,96,97,98]

Medicine has been called a "science of particulars."[99] This is a useful, but not a precise, description. It is useful in placing emphasis on the necessity of taking into account the existential particularities of the experience of illness and the requirements for curing, caring, or healing in particular patients. But medicine-*qua*-medicine is also interested in, and capable of, generalized principles, that is to say, of a theory of medicine. The sciences, for their part, are also deeply concerned with particularities. It is out of particular instances and specified experimental or observational conditions that general scientific laws are derived by induction or applied by deduction. In its practice, science draws validity from the richness and reliability of its particulars. Solution chemistry must deal with particulars—temperature, ionic strength, ionization constants, ionic sizes, hydration envelopes, equilibrium conditions, etc. It is as much a science of particulars as medicine. But the theory of solutions must abstract from these particulars to a general set of laws governing all types of solution.

Like a chemical theory of solutions, a philosophy of medicine begins in the particularities, in phenomena determined by the kind of activity medicine is, and the phenomena it must consider in pursuit of its healing purposes for individuals and societies. The practice, the ethics, and the social role of medicine depend on the philosophy of medicine to which we commit ourselves. So, too, do answers to such issues as: the ends of medicine and how and by whom they are determined; the dependence or independence of medical ethics *vis-à-vis* politics, law, or economics; the place of bioethics; the resolution of cross-cultural conflicts in a world society; etc. These are the contributions a philosophy of medicine can make to those who actually use medicine—one of Caplan's criteria for a legitimate field of inquiry.[100] Our responses to this challenge must wait for another time.[101] For the moment, I have confined myself to an attempt to show that philosophy of medicine does, indeed, exist as a legitimate field of study.

Conclusion

Philosophical reflection on matters medical is a very old enterprise. Given the projects of medicine and philosophy, the dialogue between them is inevitable. Four ways in which philosophical reflection may take place are: (1) philosophy *and* medicine, (2) philosophy *in* medicine, (3) medical philosophy, and (4) philosophy *of* medicine. Three opinions exist on the nature of philosophy *of* medicine: that it does not exist as a valid field of inquiry, that it includes all forms of philosophical reflection, and that it is a definable field of its own, a specific form of philosophical reflection.

I have argued: (1) that the philosophy of medicine is a definable field with its own specific perspective on the subject matter of medicine; (2) that its subject matter and *telos* are different in kind from those of the sciences basic to medicine; (3) that the practice of medicine draws upon the physical, biological, and social sciences and the humanities, but medicine is not a sub-branch of any of those disciplines. Rather, the disciplines pertinent to medicine become part of medicine when they are used to advance the healing, helping, caring, and curing purposes of the patient-physician and medicine-society relationships. It is the critical, reflective, systematic study of the concepts and presuppositions of the healing encounter between human persons as individuals or societies that is the domain of a philosophy of medicine, philosophically considered.

Notes

1. E. D. Pellegrino and D. C. Thomasma, *A Philosophical Basis of Medical Practice: Toward a Philosophy and Ethic of the Healing Professions* (New York: Oxford University Press, 1981).

2. E. D. Pellegrino and D. C. Thomasma, *For the Patient's Good: The Restoration of Beneficence in Health Care* (New York: Oxford University Press, 1988).

3. E. D. Pellegrino and D. C. Thomasma, *The Virtues in Medical Practice* (New York: Oxford University Press, 1993).

4. A. L. Caplan, "Does the Philosophy of Medicine Exist?" *Theoretical Medicine* 13 (1992): 67–77.

5. E. D. Pellegrino, "Philosophy of Medicine: Problematic and Potential," *Journal of Medicine and Philosophy* 1(1) (1976): 5–31.

6. H. T. Engelhardt, Jr., and E. Erde, "Philosophy of Medicine," in *A Guide to the Culture of Science, Technology, and Medicine,* ed. P. T. Durbin (New York: Free Press, 1984), pp. 364–461 and 675–677.

7. W. Szumowski, "La Philosophie de la Médecine: Son Histoire, Son Essence, Sa Dénomination, et Sa Définition," *Archives Internationales d'Histoire des Sciences* 2(9) (October 1949): 1097–1139.

8. O. Temkin, "On the Inter-relationship of the History and Philosophy of Medicine," *Bulletin of the History of Medicine* 30 (1956): 241–251.

9. See also articles by J. Doroszewski; D. Lamb et al.; R. Qiu; and D. N. Walton in *Metamedicine* 1982 (vol. 3) for philosophy of medicine in Poland, United Kingdom, China, and Canada. For philosophy of medicine in Austria, Germany, Scandinavia, The Netherlands, and the U.S.A., see articles by T. Kennen; M. Kottow; B. B. Lindahl; H. Ten Have et al.; and D. C. Thomasma in *Theoretical Medicine* 1985 (vol. 6).

10. H. T. Engelhardt and K. Wm. Wildes, "Philosophy of Medicine," *Encyclopedia of Bioethics,* 2nd ed., ed. W. T. Reich (New York: MacMillan Publishing Company, 1995), vol. 3, pp. 1680–1684.

11. E. D. Pellegrino, "Medicine and Philosophy: Some Notes on the Flirtations of Minerva and Aesculapius," *Annual Oration of the Society for Health and Human Values,* November 1973 (Philadelphia: Society for Health and Human Values, 1974).

12. Engelhardt and Erde, "Philosophy of Medicine," p. 364.

13. Caplan, "Does the Philosophy of Medicine Exist?"

14. Engelhardt and Erde, "Philosophy of Medicine."

15. H. T. Engelhardt, Jr., and K. F. Schaffner, "Philosophy of Medicine," in *Encyclopedia of Philosophy* (London: Routledge and Kegan Paul, 1996).

16. Engelhardt and Wildes, "Philosophy of Medicine."

17. Pellegrino and Thomasma, A Philosophical Basis of Medical Practice.

18. Pellegrino and Thomasma, *For the Patient's Good.*

19. Pellegrino and Thomasma, The Virtues in Medical Practice.

20. A. I. Tauber, "From the Self to the Other: Building a Philosophy of Medicine," in *Meta Medical Ethics: The Philosophical Foundations of Bioethics,* ed. M. A. Grodin (Dordrecht and Boston: Kluwer Academic Publishers, 1995), pp. 158–195.

21. Caplan, "Does the Philosophy of Medicine Exist?" p. 70.

22. Ibid., p. 69.

23. H. T. Engelhardt, Jr., and S. F. Spicker, eds., "Round Table Discussion," *Evaluation and Explanation in the Biomedical Sciences, Philosophy and Medicine I* (Dordrecht, Holland: D. Reidel Publishers 1975), pp. 215–219.

24. K. Sadegh-Zadeh, "Toward Metamedicine" (editorial), *Metamedicine* 1 (1980): 3–10.

25. B. Lindahl and B. Gemar, "Editorial," *Theoretical Medicine* 11 (1990): 1–3.

26. Engelhardt and Schaffner, "Philosophy of Medicine."

27. R. Audi, ed., *The Cambridge Dictionary of Philosophy* (Boston: Cambridge University Press, 1995).

28. P. Edwards, ed., *Encyclopedia of Philosophy* (New York: MacMillan Publishing Company, 1967).

29. W. J. van der Steen and P. J. Thung, *Faces of Medicine: A Philosophical Study* (Dordrecht: Kluwer Academic Publishers, 1988).

30. A. K. Sinha, *Philosophy of Health and Medical Sciences* (India: Associated Publishers, 1983).

31. Department of Philosophy of Medicine and Science, Institute of History of Medicine, *Philosophy of Medicine and Science: Problems and Perspectives* (New Delhi, India: Institute of History of Medicine and Medical Research, 1972).

32. Hippocrates, "The Art," *Hippocrates II,* Loeb Classical Library 148, trans. W. H. S. Jones (Cambridge, MA: Harvard University Press, 1981), pp. 185–218.

33. Hippocrates, "Ancient Medicine," *Hippocrates I,* Loeb Classical Library 147, trans. W. H. S. Jones (Cambridge, MA: Harvard University Press, 1972), pp. 1–64.

34. W. Jaeger, *Paideia: The Ideals of Greek Culture*, vol. III, trans. G. Highet (New York: Oxford University Press, 1944), pp. 3–45.

35. S. Rosen, *Plato's Symposium* (New Haven, CT: Yale University Press, 1968), p. 119.

36. Plato, "Laches," in *The Collected Dialogues of Plato*, Bolligen Series LXXI, ed. E. Hamilton and H. Cairns (Princeton, NJ: Princeton University Press, 1982), 195C, p. 139.

37. R. O. Moon, *The Relation of Medicine to Philosophy* (New York: Longmans, Green and Co., 1909).

38. O. Temkin, *Hippocrates in a World of Pagans and Christians* (Baltimore: Johns Hopkins University Press, 1991).

39. Pellegrino, "Medicine and Philosophy."

40. L. King, *The Philosophy of Medicine: The Early Eighteenth Century* (Cambridge, MA.: Harvard University Press, 1978).

41. T. Sydenham, "Medical Observations Concerning the History and Cure of Acute Diseases," (3rd ed., 1676) in *The Works of Thomas Sydenham*, vol. I, trans. R. G. Latham (London: The Sydenham Society, 1848), pp. 11–21, reprinted in L. King, ed., *A History of Medicine* (New York: Penguin, 1971), p. 118.

42. H. T. Peek, ed., *Harper's Dictionary of Classical Antiquity* (New York: Cooper Square Publishing Company, 1965), p. 952.

43. P. Riché, *Education and Culture in the Barbarian West, from the Sixth to the Eighth Century*, trans. J. J. Contreni (Columbia, SC: University of South Carolina Press, 1978), p. 46, n. 206.

44. C. Wilson, *The Invisible World, Early Modern Philosophy and the Invention of the Microscope* (Princeton, NJ: Princeton University Press, 1995).

45. Engelhardt and Schaffner, "Philosophy of Medicine."

46. E. D. Pellegrino, "The Metamorphosis of Medical Ethics: A 30-Year Retrospective," *Journal of the American Medical Association* 269(9) (March 3, 1993): 1158–1163.

47. P. Sundström, *Icons of Disease* (Linköping, Sweden: Linköping University, 1987).

48. Van der Steen and Thung, *Faces of Medicine*.

49. H. R. Wulff, S. A. Pedersen, and R. Rosenberg, eds., *Philosophy of Medicine: An Introduction* (Boston: Blackwell Scientific Publications, 1986).

50. M. A. Grodin, *Meta Medical Ethics: The Philosophical Foundations of Bioethics*, Boston Studies in the Philosophy of Science, vol. 171 (Dordrecht: Kluwer Academic Publishers, 1995).

51. R. Gillon, *Philosophical Medical Ethics* (New York: John Wiley and Sons, 1986).

52. Ibid.

53. C. M. Culver and B. Gert, *Philosophy in Medicine: Conceptual and Ethical Issues in Medicine and Psychiatry* (New York: Oxford University Press, 1982).

54. M. Baldini, *Epistemologia Contemporanea e Clinica Medica* (Firenze: Città di Vita, 1975).

55. L. Reznek, *The Nature of Disease* (New York: Routledge & Kegan Paul, 1987).

56. L. King, *Medical Thinking: A Historical Preface* (Princeton, NJ: Princeton University Press, 1982).

57. Wulff, Pedersen, and Rosenberg, eds., *Philosophy of Medicine.*

58. M. Natanson, "Philosophy and Psychiatry," in *Psychiatry and Philosophy,* ed. E. W. Straus, M. Natanson, and H. Ey (New York: Springer Verlag, 1969), pp. 85–110.

59. Sinha, Philosophy of Health and Medical Sciences, p. 10.

60. Department of Philosophy of Medicine and Science, Institute of History of Medicine, *Philosophy of Medicine and Science.*

61. L. Fleck, *Genesis and Development of a Scientific Fact* (Chicago: University of Chicago Press, 1979).

62. M. Foucault, *The Birth of the Clinic: An Archaeology of Medical Perception* (New York: Pantheon Books, 1973).

63. G. Blane, *Elements of Medical Logick* (London: Underwood, 1819).

64. F. Oesterlen, *Medical Logic,* ed. and trans. G. Whitney (London: Synderham Society, 1855).

65. E. Murphy, *The Logic of Medicine* (Baltimore: Johns Hopkins University Press, 1976).

66. T. L. Beauchamp and J. F. Childress, *Principles of Biomedical Ethics,* 4th ed. (New York: Oxford University Press, 1994).

67. K. D. Clouser and B. Gert, "A Critique of Principlism," *Journal of Medicine and Philosophy* 15(2) (1990): 219–236.

68. E. D. Pellegrino, "The Four Principles and the Doctor-Patient Relationship: The Need for a Better Understanding," in *Principles of Health Care Ethics,* ed. R. Gillon (Chichester, England: John Wiley & Sons, 1994), pp. 353–366.

69. W. Osler, *Aequanimitas with Other Addresses to Medical Students, Nurses, and Practitioners of Medicine* (Philadelphia: P. Blakiston's Son and Company, 1905).

70. F. Peabody, Doctor and Patient: Papers on the Relationship of the Physician to Men and Institutions (New York: MacMillan, 1930).

71. R. C. Cabot, "Introduction," *Differential Diagnosis,* 3rd ed. (Philadelphia and London: W. B. Saunders Company, 1916), 1:17–23.

72. R. C. Cabot, *What Men Live By: Work, Play, Love, Worship* (Boston and New York: Houghton Mifflin Company, 1914).

73. L. Thomas, *The Youngest Science: Notes of a Medicine Watcher* (New York: Viking Press, 1983).

74. Plato, "Gorgias," in *The Collected Dialogues of Plato,* Bolligen Series LXXI, ed. E. Hamilton and H. Cairns (Princeton, NJ: Princeton University Press, 1982), 501A, pp. 283–284.

75. Plato, "Phaedrus," in *The Collected Dialogues of Plato,* Bolligen Series LXXI, ed. E. Hamilton and H. Cairns (Princeton, NJ: Princeton University Press, 1982), 268b–d and 270b–c, pp. 513–516.

76. A. Castiglione, *A History of Medicine* (New York: Alfred Knopf and Company, 1941).

77. F. H. Garrison, *An Introduction to the History of Medicine,* 4th ed. (Philadelphia: W. B. Saunders, 1966).

78. L. King, *The Philosophy of Medicine.*

79. R. French and A. Wear, eds., *The Medical Revolution of the Seventeenth Century* (Cambridge: Cambridge University Press, 1989).

80. Castiglione, *History of Medicine,* pp. 582–593.

81. Garrison, An Introduction to the History of Medicine, pp. 310–319.

82. R. Descartes, "Discourse on Method," in *Oeuvres,* vol. III, p. 78, ll. 8–13 as cited in R. B. Carter, *Descartes' Medical Philosophy: The Organic Solution to the Mind-Body Problem* (Baltimore: Johns Hopkins University Press, 1983), p. 4.

83. E. Gilson, *The Unity of Philosophical Experience* (New York: Charles Scribner's Sons, 1937), pp. 147–148.

84. Hippocrates, "The Art."

85. Hippocrates, "Ancient Medicine."

86. P. Lain-Entralgo, *Quaestiones Hippocraticae: Disputatae Tres* in *La Collection Hippocratique et Son Role Dans L'Histoire de la Médicine,* Colloque de Strasbourg (Leiden: E. J. Brill, 1975), pp. 23–27.

87. King, *The Philosophy of Medicine,* p. v.

88. E. D. Pellegrino, "Toward a Reconstruction of Medical Morality: The Primacy of the Act of Profession and the Fact of Illness," *Journal of Medicine and Philosophy* 4(1) (March 1979): 32–56.

89. E. D. Pellegrino, "The Healing Relationship: The Architectonics of Clinical Medicine," in *The Clinical Encounter: The Moral Fabric of the Patient-Physician Relationship,* ed. Earl Shelp (Dordrecht: D. Reidel, 1983), pp. 153–172.

90. W. A. Wallace, *Causality and Scientific Explanation,* vol. 2, *Classical and Contemporary Science* (Ann Arbor: University of Michigan Press, 1974), pp. 141–154.

91. Pellegrino and Thomasma, *For the Patient's Good.*

92. Pellegrino and Thomasma, *The Virtues in Medical Practice.*

93. J. Ladd, "The Contract Model of the Doctor-Patient Relationship: A Critique and an Alternative Ethics of Responsibility," *Mount Sinai Journal of Medicine* 60(1) (January 1993): 6–10.

94. Pellegrino and Thomasma, *For the Patient's Good.*

95. Pellegrino and Thomasma, *A Philosophical Basis of Medical Practice.*

96. Pellegrino and Thomasma, *The Virtues in Medical Practice.*

97. E. D. Pellegrino and D. C. Thomasma, *Helping and Healing* (Washington, DC: Georgetown University Press, 1996).

98. E. D. Pellegrino and D. C. Thomasma, *The Christian Virtues in Medical Practice* (Washington, DC: Georgetown University Press, 1996).

99. S. Gorovitz and A. MacIntyre, "Toward a Philosophy of Medical Fallibility," *Journal of Medicine and Philosophy* 1 (1976): 51–71.

100. Caplan, "Does the Philosophy of Medicine Exist?" p. 70.

101. E. D. Pellegrino and D. C. Thomasma, *A Moral Philosophy for Medicine* (forthcoming).

TWO

Philosophy of Medicine

Should It Be Teleologically or Socially Construed?

I am grateful to the editor of the *Kennedy Institute of Ethics Journal* for the invitation to respond to Kevin Wildes's comments on my philosophy of medicine in the March 2001 issue of the *Journal*. The philosophy I espouse has been developed with my coauthor and colleague David Thomasma (Pellegrino and Thomasma 1981, 1988, 1993). However, on this occasion I will respond in my own name. Thomasma and I are preparing a revision of our book *A Philosophical Basis for Medical Practice* in which our joint response to Wildes and other critics will be available. Thomasma is, therefore, not responsible for any logical improprieties I may commit in the present essay.

Let me begin with my points of agreement with Fr. Wildes. First, we both believe, contra Caplan, that there is a legitimate field of philosophical enquiry properly termed "philosophy of medicine." Indeed, we also agree that the criteria demanded for legitimacy by Caplan in 1992 have been fulfilled. Finally, we agree that bioethics today is in need of a philosophy of medicine and that many of bioethics' most fundamental questions are unresolvable without such a philosophy.

We disagree, however, on several major points related to the nature and scope of a philosophy of medicine and particularly on how it is to be derived and by what method of philosophical enquiry it is best pursued.

For his part, Wildes holds that I construe philosophy of medicine too narrowly, that I slight its social context, that I overemphasize the healing relationship, and that I use an outmoded method of philosophical enquiry rather than the method he prefers, namely, social construction.

49

I will confine my present response to these major criticisms. I have many other points of disagreement with Wildes's line of argument, but I shall consider these only briefly as *obiter dicta*. I appreciate Wildes taking my ideas seriously, and I am grateful for the opportunity to clarify my position and counter some misunderstandings of that position.

Toward a Teleologically-Based Medical Ethic

I shall begin with the method of philosophical enquiry by which I have derived a philosophy of medicine. My interest in a theory of medicine dates to the 1970s (Pellegrino 1979). This is a time when the moral precepts of traditional medical ethics first came under serious philosophical scrutiny. Generally speaking, that scrutiny consisted in the application of existing systems of ethics, like utilitarianism, deonotology, or prima facie principles, to the ethical dilemmas then emerging from a combination of scientific progress and changes in social and political mores.

It soon became evident that no convincing case could be made for universal agreement on the ethics of medicine. A multiplicity of theological and philosophical viewpoints resulted. This was not entirely disadvantageous, for it brought to light questions previously unrecognized or neglected. It did, however, create practical problems when ethical dilemmas in professional ethics or in clinical decisions had to be made in complex and urgent circumstances. Further, the resultant difficulties of agreeing on the right and the good created a tendency toward procedural rather than normative ethics. This tendency is now so far advanced that it is a critical issue for the evolution of bioethics (Pellegrino 2000).

It seemed to me then, and it seems to me now, that some of the difficulties derived from the lack of a consistent philosophy or theory of medicine, which, with its associated ethics, could provide something of a moral philosophy for medicine, some foundation for moral judgment. Moreover, if the project were to aim at medical ethics, it was important to distinguish the ethics of the profession of healers—doctors, nurses, dentists, psychologists, and so forth—from the ethical issues of particular dilemmas like euthanasia, withdrawing treatment, reproductive technologies and the like. There seemed more likelihood of agreement on the former than the latter.

This did not mean that such a distinction was total, but rather that it was important to develop a theory of medicine based in what medicine is in reality. This meant a concentration on the central realistic phenomena of healing, which I took to be the end, the telos, and purpose of the clinical encounter. This did not mean that the ethics of medicine was independent of general ethical theory. It did assert that the realities of clinical medicine as a personal encounter should be central to any theory of medicine and hence to any ethic of the healing professions.

When there is as sharp a dissonance as I perceived in medical ethics, one tries to begin the discussion with what, conceivably, most might accept. This I took to be the realities of being ill, being healed, and the profession to heal (Pellegrino 1983). Whatever else had to be decided in medical ethics ultimately would confront these realities. This was my starting point and it meant that I first must ask what is the end of medicine? I asked this in the classical sense of the end as that from which an activity exists, and that which when attained would constitute a good (Pellegrino 2001a). I do not use teleology in the modern consequentialist sense.

It is here that Wildes and I part company. I adopted what Wildes correctly diagnoses as a teleological, realist, phenomenological approach that sought to discern the ends of medicine by reflecting on the medical relationship of healing and helping. Clearly, this relationship was not the whole of medicine, but it is still in my opinion that which makes it a distinct human activity. My aim was, and is, to build a comprehensive theory of medicine based in a grasp of the ends of medicine taken in a classical sense (Aristotle, NE 1094a1–18). If the ends of medicine could be discerned, then the good of medical relationships would be known. The virtues of the practitioner could be grounded in this good and second-order obligations of professional ethics could be defined (Pellegrino 1999).

Clearly, this was a conscious step away from the dominant modes of philosophical reflection, like linguistic analysis, a priori assertions, prima facie principles, and of course from the social constructionism that Wildes favors. There was nothing in the realist position intrinsically at odds with particular conclusions that might derive from other theories of medicine. There was, and is, the distinct stand that whatever difference there might be would ultimately have to meet the test of the ends of medicine realistically ascertained (Pellegrino and Thomasma 1993).

This is not the place to replay the tensions between classical philo-sophical reflection and the modern forms of reflection. I did eschew the modernist bias toward subjectivity, goals rather than ends, and dialogue and societal convention in favor of the intrinsic moral requirement inter-nal to a practice. There is enough disagreement and confusion in nonreal-ist postmodern constructionist philosophies to keep the older tradition alive as a philosophical counterpoint at the very least.

But there are stronger reasons for a classical approach than maintain-ing a dialectical balance. It is now clear that traditional essentialist percep-tions are still alive in the modern day philosophies of natural kinds (Kripke 1971) or in the nomic universals of Nelson (1966–68). Distinguished and respected modern philosophers like MacIntyre (1990, pp. 127–148; 1999) have called for a serious re-engagement of contemporary philosophy with the Aristotelian-Thomistic synthesis, especially in ethics and moral phi-losophy. We are also seeing an updating of natural law theories in ethics in terms more congenial to the contemporary analytical temper (Lisska 1996, pp. 151–152; Rhonheimer 2000). The dialogue between postmodernist phi-losophy and the metaphysics and ethics of Aristotelian-Thomists holds the promise of new insights into the way out of the contemporary meta-physical wasteland (Reichberg 1997; Asselin 1997; Pellegrino 2000; John Paul II 1998).

I am not so naive as to predict the end of the ages-old debates about the nature of philosophy. Nor do I expect some irenic compromise or ca-pitulation between opposing positions. But I do believe that the approach I take cannot be disposed of as quickly as Wildes suggests. To label it as outmoded or not in conformity with current notions of philosophy is hardly a refutation of a world-view with a long history and such promis-ing reexamination as now seem possible (Seifert 1997).

Moreover, the underlying metaphysical questions so easily classified as "meaningless" and closed to logical discussion are still very much alive. Concepts like *ends, persons, freedom, good, right, unity, dignity,* and *norm* are present in every ethical and philosophical disquisition. Every argu-ment in which they appear depends on how their meaning is construed, on what they mean ontologically. Metaphysics can be ridiculed, ignored, and denied, but it will not "go away."

A philosophy of medicine and an ethics of medicine grounded in such a philosophy are not balkanized provinces forcibly detached from the body of philosophy as Wildes seems to suggest. It remains in dialogue and dialectics with current and accepted theories like principlism, caring, and deontological or virtue theories. It may arrive at certain conclusions in agreement with other theories like principlism, but it will ground them in something more fundamental than common morality (Pellegrino 1994).

A teleologically oriented philosophy of medicine is certainly not a doctor- or a patient-defined entity. The very notion of a reality-based philosophy of medicine contravenes any idea that physicians or patients determine what medicine is (Pellegrino 1998). Rather, physicians do what they do and patients act as they do because both are pursuing an end in which they are joined by the realities of being ill, being healed, and professing to heal. The moral pursuit of these relationships is what determines what is right and good. The "good" as we have pointed out in detail elsewhere is a compound notion in which medicine, the patients, and the good of humans and for humans are closely interrelated (Pellegrino and Thomasma 1988).

A philosophy and ethic of medicine defined by the doctor or the medical profession would in fact not be teleologically grounded. Doctors may have many subsidiary ends in their pursuit of medicine, but none of them defines medicine's primary end, which is healing and helping and which supercedes the doctor's self-interests. Indeed, a doctor-defined medicine would be a social convention closer to Wildes' preferred social construction theory of ethics than to mine.

A teleologically based ethic of medicine is the only tenable basis for an ethics of the healing professions as a whole in an era of widespread moral and social pluralism like ours. It is also the only basis for its moral authority. Authority derives from an understanding of the ends and purposes for which the health professions were established. A professional society can act responsibly by assuming authority for enforcing a code, but the moral authority for the code itself does not derive from the profession's affirmation or annunciation of a code. Rather, professional societies are stewards of moral truths. It is these truths they are committed to protect (Pellegrino 2001b).

The Social Context of a Philosophy of Medicine

The second major criticism Wildes offers is that I neglect the social context of medicine. By this he means the team and cooperative nature of modern-day health care, the supporting social structures for medical institutions and practices and research, the statistical nature of much of clinical knowledge, the importance of public policy, the gatekeeper role of the physician, the need for a social definition of medicine itself, and the like.

My recognition of these and many more social issues is evident in my published work, which I will not detail here. There, one will find articles on ethics and education for team care, the relationships of ethics and economics, the ethics of collective moral agency in hospitals, the profession as a moral community, the ethics of a good health care system, and the doctor's social responsibility. In my book with Thomasma now under revision, one can find chapters on the social ethic of primary care, on the hospital as a moral agent, and so forth.

I agree that we have not developed this dimension of our philosophy of medicine as fully as our philosophy of the physician-patient or healing relationship. This is because we consider it essential to begin with the "good" health professional and then proceed to the "good" institution and society that are needed to sustain the good health professional. In this we follow the order of Aristotle's progression from the *Nicomachean Ethics* to the *Politics*—i.e., from the individual virtues to the virtuous society.

There is, however, no warrant for Wildes' assertion that I believe that the other health professions ought not to be present or that their presence ought not to define the character of medicine (Wildes 2001, p. 79). Medicine is indisputably a team effort. Health professionals move in and out of the healing relationship depending on the kind and severity of the patient's needs. My point is that each of the health professionals has a specific set of obligations that derive from the ends each profession serves. Nevertheless, those ends are analogous and often overlapping, both with each other and with physicians' ends and purposes.

In team care, as in individualized professional care, the ethics of each profession is based in the philosophy of that professional's encounter with the patient. Each is defined by the same phenomena of being ill, being healed, and professing to heal. Each profession is governed by the virtues essential to attaining the ends of healing relationships—e.g., fidelity to trust, suppression of self-interest, attending to the best interests of the patient, confidentiality, courage, and so forth. All team members share in these virtues to the degree that they become involved with the personal lives and needs of those they presume to help. Health professionals thus share certain personal virtues entailed by the act of healing. Their obligations, however, may differ considerably since each profession satisfies different needs of patients and involves different techniques of healing.

Each health professional, even when acting in the team, bears moral accountability for his or her actions. But when acting as a team member, or as an institutional review board member, each professional also shares in the collective responsibility for the group's actions. The ethics of collective responsibility is a particularly complex issue that still needs to be explored adequately (Pellegrino 1982).

It is true that I have focused on the physician-patient relationship. I have done so because it is in many ways paradigmatic and illustrative of a relationship pertinent for other health professionals as well. The physician-patient relationship has the longest history. The ultimate responsibility legally as well as morally usually will rest with the physician. This is not to belittle other health professionals, their absolute necessity, nor the gravity of their responsibilities. There is a philosophy *of* nursing as there is of the other health professions, each defined in terms of its ends and the nature of its relationship with the sick person.

The philosophy of each health profession, and parenthetically of other professions like law, ministry, or teaching as well, must take into account the social context within which it resides. I deliberately started my reflections on a philosophy of medicine, but this is clearly not the whole of a philosophy of healing professions, nor was it ever intended to be such.

The social and historical context of illness and the way patients respond to its presence are variable. There is a commonality in the experience, however, that transcends time, culture, and geography. One need only compare the common threads of ethical obligation running across centuries and cultures to appreciate that they are a response to a universal human experience. Codes of ethics from India, China, Japan, Ancient

Greece and Rome, the Middle Ages, the Enlightenment, eighteenth-century England, and nineteenth-century America have a common body of precepts. All focus on the ethical primacy of the welfare of the sick person.

This fact is not the result of a historical collusion between and among physicians. Codes have no validity by themselves unless they reflect the realities of the clinical encounter. The departure of contemporary physicians from the moral precepts of the Hippocratic ethic do not invalidate its moral precepts. Only if medical ethics and a theory of medicine were social constructs could they be changed at the will of society, physicians, or patients.

My notion of a philosophy of medicine is not a unique, nor an idiosyncratic, use of philosophical reflection. There is already a credible history of philosophical enquiry into a wide range of human activities, like philosophy of law, of history, of literature, of art, physics, biology, aesthetics, education, and the like (*Oxford Companion to Philosophy* 1995, p. 678; *Cambridge Dictionary of Philosophy* 1995, pp. 681–687). Each is an enquiry into the nature of the field in question. In classical terms, these are enquiries into the formal object and the distinguishing perspective each discipline brings to the subject, namely that which sets it apart from the others. All, for example, study man but each from a different point of view–i.e., art from the aesthetic, biology from the physiological, and medicine from the therapeutic viewpoint.

I do not deny that the topics Wildes, Engelhardt, and Erde embrace in their wider view of philosophy of medicine are important. But such things as medical logic, epistemology, aesthetics, causality, and concepts of health and disease are more properly placed under my rubric of philosophy *in* medicine. These are particular problems within already well-established branches of philosophy. They are not peculiar to medicine, but only the philosophy *of* medicine studies what medicine is, ontologically and formally.

There is nothing in my viewpoint to suggest a lack of humility about the powers of philosophy, nor the limits of human knowledge. It does suppose however that philosophy strives for something more than clarification of ideas, uncovering assumptions, or creating "intellectual roadmaps." The minimalist view of philosophy espoused by Wildes is less an exercise of philosophical humility than an expansion of philosophy of medicine into already occupied territory.

Social Construction

Wildes rejects any attempt to "discover" the *nature* of medicine in any classical sense. Instead, Erde and Engelhardt propose a philosophy of medicine built on the social construction of medicine. As Wildes argues the case, it has two major pediments: One is the negative argument that the capacities of philosophy are limited and that any attempt to "discover" the nature of medicine through its agency is doomed to failure. I have responded to this criticism in the first part of this paper.

Wildes's second argument for social construction of medicine is the positive assertion that medicine exists within a social context, shaped by social forces, practiced in a social milieu with implications that are social as well as individual. One may admit all of this, as I do here and in other writings, without coming to the conclusion that its nature is socially constructed. There is no inevitable logical relationship between the existential fact that medicine is practiced in a social context and the conclusion that the only way to know what it is is to define it by social construction.

I shall pass over the fact that in making this argument Wildes is relying on an empirical observation about the state of medicine and "discovering" the fact that it is practiced in a social context. Thus Wildes uses the very method I have proposed of discovering something about medicine by observing its actualities. But accepting his observational fact in no way entails acceptance of his conclusion that social construction is the way to understand what medicine is by its nature. I too agree that medicine is practiced in a social context, but deny that this entails social construction as the method for defining the ends or goals of medicine.

Wildes does not state specifically what he means by social construction. I will take it to mean the doctrine that our concepts of knowledge, reality, or moral good and right are the resultant of human relationships, practices, and consensus. A variety of methods can be used to arrive at a social construction, for example, hermeneutics, praxis, theories of intersubjectivity, dialogue, reflective equilibrium, and the like. What is common is the blurring of subjective and objective distinctions. What things are depends on our common perception of them, rather than on anything intrinsic to them as ontological entities (Hacking 1999).

On this view, medicine becomes what a particular society wishes it to be. This is a popular approach in an era of moral and epistemological pluralism and in democratic societies as well. It is the approach of the Hastings Center study of the goals of medicine (Hanson and Callahan 1999). It denies the search for universals, essences, or the nature of things, and it is content with what "reasonable" people say they are. In its extreme forms, it is a modern reincarnation of nominalism, namely the belief that things that share the same name share nothing but the fact that they have the same name.

Social construction allows for no permanent theory of medicine and therefore allows no permanent or stable ethics of the profession. These can become the victim of a socially aberrant society as was the case under German national Socialism, Maoist China, Stalinist Russia or Imperial Japan. In each case, medicine was redefined as an instrument of social and political purpose, and the physician was made a social functionary. Medical ethics itself became the ethic of social purpose.

Wildes thinks this does not follow because he supposes that moral boundaries beyond medicine would act as deterrents. He fails to note that these "moral boundaries" would themselves be socially constructed and thus subject to the same pathologies that distorted medicine and its ethics in the first place. We cannot have it both ways. Either social construction is a valid way to arrive at the truth of things or it is not. If it is, then all moral boundaries are subject to its workings.

There is already a move among some ethicists, economists, and policymakers to redirect physicians from a person-centered to a society-centered ethic. The purpose is to preserve resources by relieving the physician of her traditional primary commitment to act for the welfare of her patient. Medical ethics in this way would become socially constructed in accord with the canons of economics rather than the personal obligation of doctors to their patients. The primacy of the sick person is thus to be displaced by the needs of distant, unidentified, possible future patients according to some schema of social worth.

A socially constructed philosophy of medicine, and the ethic derived from it, would be entirely extrinsic to the ends of medicine. It would redefine those ends in such a way as to undermine the covenant of trust that should guide the healing relationship. The choice between a philosophy of medicine based in the special nature of medicine and a philosophy based in social construction is of the utmost significance for the kind of society we choose to be.

Summary

The philosophy of medicine has matured sufficiently to become a legitimate field of scholarly endeavor. It is a fundamental and requisite component of any moral philosophy of medicine that seeks to ground medical ethics in something more than a technical ethic of conflict resolution. Indeed, many of the present and coming problems crucial to the evolution of bioethics are rooted in the philosophy of medicine.

Fr. Kevin Wildes and I are agreed on the existence of the field and its importance. We differ on what topics it should engage and most seriously on how it should be derived. Wildes opts for a broad interpretation embracing questions that I take to be more proper to existing fields of philosophy. Wildes also opts for social construction as the determinant of the shape of a philosophy of medicine while I propose a teleological, phenomenological, realist methodology. Clearly, the ethic that emerges from these contrasting models is different and that difference makes the separation in our conceptions of importance to bioethics as it is evolving today.

My hope has been to clarify my position in response to Wildes's well considered critique. I hope our dialogue will stimulate others to engage the issues we have both raised.

References

Asselin, Don. 1997. "Catholic Philosophy: Realism and the Postmodern Dilemma." In *Postmodernism and Christian Philosophy,* ed. Roman T. Ciapalo, pp. 23–37. Washington, DC: Catholic University of America Press.

Cambridge Dictionary of Philosophy. 1995. Ed. Robert Audi. New York: Cambridge University Press.

Hacking, Ian. 1999. *The Social Construction of What?* Cambridge: Harvard University Press.

Hanson, Mark, and Callahan, Daniel. 1999. *The Goals of Medicine. The Forgotten Issues in Health Care Reform*. Washington, DC: Georgetown University Press.

John Paul II. 1998. Encyclical Letter, *Fides et Ratio*.

Kripke, Saul. 1971. "Identity and Necessity." In *Identity and Individuation*, ed. Milton K. Munitz, pp. 135–164. New York: NYU Press.

Lisska, Anthony J. 1996. *Aquinas's Theory of Natural Law*. Oxford: Clarendon Press.

MacIntyre, Alasdair. 1990. *Three Rival Versions of Moral Enquiry*. Notre Dame, IN: University of Notre Dame Press.

———. 1999. *Dependent Rational Animals: Why Human Beings Need the Virtues*. Chicago, IL: Open Court.

Nelson, Everett J. 1966–68. "The Metaphysical Presuppositions of Induction." In *Proceedings and Addresses of the American Philosophical Association*, pp. 19–33. Yellow Springs, OH.

Oxford Companion to Philosophy. 1995. Ed. Ted Honderich. Oxford: Oxford University Press.

Pellegrino, Edmund D. 1979. "Toward a Reconstruction of Medical Morality: The Primacy of the Act of Profession and the Fact of Illness." *Journal of Medicine and Philosophy* 11: 9–16.

———. 1982. "The Ethics of Collective Judgement in Health Care." *Journal of Medicine and Philosophy* 7: 3–10.

———. 1983. "The Healing Relationship: The Architectonics of Clinical Medicine." In *The Clinical Encounter*, ed. Earl Shelp, pp. 153–172. Dordrecht: D. Reidel.

———. 1994. "The Four Principles and the Doctor-Patient Relationship: The Need for a Better Linkage." In *Principles of Health Care Ethics*, ed. Raanan Gillan, pp. 353–367. New York: Wiley.

———. 1998. "What the Philosophy of Medicine Is." *Theoretical Medicine* 19: 315–336.

———. 1999. "The Goals and Ends of Medicine: How Are They Defined?" In *The Goals of Medicine: The Forgotten Issues in Health Care Reform*, ed. Mark J. Hanson and Daniel Callahan, pp. 55–68. Washington, DC: Georgetown University Press.

———. 2000. "Bioethics at Century's Turn: Can Normative Ethics Be Retrieved?" *Journal of Medicine and Philosophy* 25: 655–675.

———. 2001a. *The Telos of Medicine and the Good of the Patient*. University of Padua Lanza Foundation.

———. 2001b. "The Use and Abuse of Professional Codes in Bioethical Discourse." In *Methods of Bioethics*, ed. Jeremy Sugarman and Daniel Sulmasy. Washington, DC: Georgetown University Press.

———, and Thomasma, David C. 1981. *A Philosophical Basis for Medical Practice*. New York: Oxford University Press.

———. 1988. *For the Patient's Good: The Restoration of Beneficence in Health Care*. New York: Oxford University Press.

———. 1993. *The Virtues in Medical Practice.* New York: Oxford University Press.

Reichberg, Gregory M. 1997. "Contextualizing Theoretical Reason." In *Postmodernism and Christian Philosophy,* ed. Roman T. Ciapalo, pp. 173–204. Washington, DC: Catholic University of America Press.

Rhonheimer, Martin. 2000. *A Thomistic View of Moral Autonomy.* New York: Fordham University Press.

Seifert, Josef. 1997. *Back to Things in Themselves.* New York: Routledge and Kegan Paul.

Wildes, Keven. 2001. "The Cries of Medicine: Philosophy and the Social Construction of Medicine." *Kennedy Institute of Ethics Journal* 11: 71–86.

The Internal Morality of Clinical Medicine

A Paradigm for the Ethics of the Helping and Healing Professions

Every art and every inquiry, and similarly every action and pursuit, is thought to aim at some good; and for this reason the good has rightly been declared to be that at which all things aim.

—Aristotle, *Nicomachean Ethics,* 1094a1–3

And the medical art is a good, and it is for the sake of health that the medical art has received the friendship, and health is a good is it not?

—Plato, *Lysis,* 219

Introduction

In response to the unprecedented changes effected in medical practice by scientific and social change, many people are calling for a new ethic of medicine. By this they usually mean a revision of medicine's traditional ethic in a way more congenial to contemporary mores. They look, too, to a continuing evolution of the goals and purposes of medicine by a process of social and historical construction or dialogue. An ethics thus conceived is an ethic external to medicine. It denies that there is something essentially in the nature of medicine as a kind of human activity which determines its ends and its ethics internally.

In this essay, I shall argue for the internal morality of medicine and the other healing and helping professions. By this, I mean that the ethics of these professions has its source in the nature of these professions, in what is distinctive about them and the good at which they aim. I shall use medicine as the paradigm case but I will extend the same argument by analogy to the other healing and helping professions, i.e., those which purport to meet certain fundamental needs of humans like health, justice, knowledge, and spiritual consolation.

My argument is teleologically constructed taking "teleology" in its Aristotelian/Thomist sense and not in its modern consequentialist or socially constructed sense. It is also essentialist and realist. I recognize the disfavor and even scorn these terms invoke, but I believe they deserve serious consideration when the question of the goals, purposes, and ends of medicine and other professions is as problematic as it is today (Hanson and Callahan 1999).

This essay is a continuation of my interest in developing a philosophy of medicine as the basis for the ethics of medicine (Pellegrino and Thomasma 1981; Pellegrino 1998). My approach has been to derive a philosophy of medicine from the phenomena of the clinical encounter, the confrontation of doctors and patients whose lived worlds intersect in the moment of clinical truth (Pellegrino 2001b). This is the omega point upon which the actions of individual doctors as well as the whole health care system converge—that moment when some human being in distress seeks help from a physician within the context of a system of care.

In this essay, I will not attempt to reply to specific criticisms of the notion of an internal morality as offered by the other contributors. Rather, my aim is to clarify the notion of an internal morality and to facilitate further discussion. Unavoidably, since my perspective on the topic of internal morality is the subject of considerable commentary in this issue, I will be using more citations to my own work than would otherwise be seemly. Many of the ideas I shall use are the result of years of collaborative effort with my colleague David C. Thomasma (Pellegrino and Thomasma 1981, 1993). This essay, however, expresses my personal views, many of which

David Thomasma would share. He, however, bears no responsibility for any errors of fact or logic I might commit.

This essay addresses five questions: (1) The origins of the contemporary concept of an internal morality; (2) An outline of some distinctions about what an internal morality is and is not; (3) The need for a philosophy of medicine grounded in the good of the patient as the telos of medical activity; (4) The implications of an internal morality for professions beyond medicine; (5) The relations of a teleological ethic to other sources of morality, especially principle- and virtue-based theories.

Contemporary Origins of the Concept

In 1983, John Ladd modified the concept of an internal morality that Fuller had used in his philosophy of law and applied it to medical ethics (Ladd 1983; Fuller 1969). He called it an internal morality of medicine, by which he meant to designate a body of norms binding on physicians by virtue of membership in the profession of medicine (Ladd 1983, p. 209). He related these norms to the special features of the physician-patient relationship. Ladd distinguished these *internal* norms from *external* norms like the right to refuse treatment, telling the truth, etc., because the latter norms might not always coincide with the good of the patient.

Ladd advanced his idea tentatively and proposed that it be examined further as a way to resolve the question of the aims of medicine (Ladd 1983, p. 228). His argument was largely descriptive, noting what he termed as the *esoteric* service and goals served by medicine and peculiar to it among professions. Ladd did not derive the ends of medicine from the nature of medicine teleologically. Rather, he used a "problems approach," which sought to find the deep structures of certain specific problems encountered in medical practice. In this, he paralleled Fuller's grounding of the internal medicine of law in the preconditions necessary for a valid system of law to function successfully.

Leon Kass had earlier taken a different approach to the definition of the ends of medicine (Kass 1975, 1981). His analysis was distinctly Aristotelian and end oriented. Kass defined the end of medicine as health, i.e., the well working of the human organism as a whole; "an activity of the human body in accordance with a specific excellence" (Kass 1981, p. 29). For Kass, the morality of medicine depended on the advancement of the aims and ends of medicine. Ladd rejected this view and a similar one advanced by Curran as too general to be useful (Curran 1980).

Kass's analysis is closest to the conception of an internal morality, as I shall argue it here. Since 1976, I have focused on the clinical encounter as the central moral defining phenomenon of a clinical philosophy of medicine. The phenomena which characterize this real world relationship form the basis for the moral obligations the physician assumes when he or she offers to heal, help, care for, or comfort a sick person. These compromise the good of the patient as the end of medicine. This morality is internal since it is derived from the nature of medicine itself and not from the application of pre-existing moral systems to medicine.

A powerful influence on the concept of an internal morality is the notion of a practice articulated by Alasdair MacIntyre is his seminal work *After Virtue* (MacIntyre 1981). In that work, MacIntyre attempted a resuscitation of Aristotle's view on ends with his idea of a *practice* as a socially generated form of human activity with certain goods *internal* to that activity. MacIntyre's notion of a practice is complex and rich in its relevance to the identity and virtues of the professions but different from the essentialist teleological position I am taking.

What is relevant to my inquiry is MacIntyre's distinction between goods internal to and external to a practice. Internal goods are those realized when trying to achieve the standard of excellence definitive of that practice. External goods are those which do not contribute directly to attainment of the aims characteristic of a practice. A profession like medicine can be viewed as a practice in MacIntyre's sense. Excellence in healing is, then, a good internal to that practice; making money is a good external to that practice.

MacIntyre places emphasis on societal context and construction in the absence of which the activity in question would not come into existence. Certain societal decisions are necessary to sustain the virtues essential in practices. A profession is a particularly distinctive activity from a social point of view since it is related to the common good and is embedded in an institutional matrix. MacIntyre's notion implies that those within a practice (or profession) function within a community with

defined standards, skills and virtues, which are not individually determined by its practitioners.

Many valuable facets of MacIntyre's notion of a profession as a practice are congruent with the idea of an internal morality. MacIntyre, however, places much emphasis on a societal construction of the profession
and its goods and virtues. In my view, these are external to clinical medicine. Medicine exists because being ill and being healed are universal
human experiences, not because society has created medicine as a practice. Rather than a social construct, the nature of medicine, its internal
goods and virtues, are defined by the ends of medicine itself, and therefore, ontologically internal from the outset. In the same way, Fuller's eight
preconditions for law would have to be derived from something essential
to the idea of "law." If they were to be an internal morality of law, their validity would be self-justified (Fuller 1969). The preconditions for successful law are stipulated because law exists; law does not exist because of the
preconditions.

The Case of Clinical Medicine

What It Is

I will confine this inquiry to clinical medicine and not "medicine" generically. By clinical medicine I mean the use of medical knowledge for
healing and helping sick persons here and now, in the individual physician-patient encounter. This clinical, face-to-face encounter is the starting
point for a philosophy of medicine and is the root of its internal morality
(Pellegrino 1976). Clinical medicine is the activity that defines physicians
qua physicians, and sets them apart from other persons who may have
medical knowledge but do not use it specifically in clinical encounters
with individual patients. Clinical medicine is the physician's *locus ethicus*
whose end is a right and good healing action and decision (Pellegrino
1979). Moreover, clinical medicine is the final pathway through which
public policies ultimately come to affect the lives of sick persons. Finally,
no matter how broad or socially oriented we make medicine, illness remains a universal human experience, and its impact on individual human

persons remains the reason why medicine and physicians exist in the first place (Hippocrates, *On the Art*).

All the members of the health care team who confront patients directly are also clinicians. Each is engaged in a special kind of human relationship with humans in distress, which defines their profession as a specific kind of activity, e.g., nursing, clinical psychology, dentistry, allied health, etc. Each aims at health as a good, ultimately, and at a specific need essential to health. They may overlap with each other and with medicine yet remain distinct. Each shares with medicine a generic set of obligations as healers and helpers in addition to other obligations specific to the nature of their profession.

To use clinical medicine as a paradigm case is not to neglect the other branches of medicine, each of which has its own distinctive end. Thus, for basic scientists, the end is the acquisition of fundamental biological knowledge of health and illness. This knowledge becomes a part of clinical medicine specifically when it is applied to the needs of a particular human being here and now. Similarly, *preventive medicine* has as its defining end the cultivation of health and avoidance of illness. *Social medicine* has its end in the health of the community or the whole body politic. When the knowledge and skills of any of the other branches of medicine are used in the healing of a particular person, then the ends of that branch fuse with the ends of clinical medicine. Each end is a good in Aristotle's sense.

The terms "telos" and "teleological ethics" are used here in their classical sense. They are not to be equated with any form of consequentialism or its most popular expression in utilitarianism. Nor are they equivalent to the simplistic biological teleology so disfavored and ridiculed by contemporary science. Nor are ends to be confused with goals, purposes, or values. These latter are defined externally by social, economic, or political convention. They are not what make clinical medicine the kind of activity it is or aims at. Goals and purposes are thus external to medicine.

An end-oriented internal morality of medicine is an ethic based in the notion of the good as the end which characterizes moral acts. The *good* is defined in terms of the aim of the activity for which that activity exists. This is an ethic consistent with the notion of the good contained in the quotations from Aristotle and Plato in the epigraph for this paper.

Such an ethic is the antithesis of an ethic based in a social construction of the goals and purposes of medicine. This latter is an external morality with perilous implications for the patient's good (Pellegrino 2001a).

What It Is Not

An internal morality of medicine is not a morality defined or authenticated by physicians or the profession of medicine. The moral authority of an internal morality of medicine is independent of whether or not physicians accept or reject it. Adoption of the precepts of an internal morality in a professional code or oath is not a warrant for its moral authority. That authority arises from an objective order of morality that transcends the self-defined goals of a profession.

An internal morality of medicine or any other profession is not a morality divorced from all ethical theories. It is not a self-justifying body of norms. Rather, it is consistent with a virtue- or principle-based ethics. It is not closed to insights from other ethical methodologies like casuistry or a caring system of ethics. The generic notions of the right and the good, truth, and logical consistency still function within an internal morality in the judgment about the way the good end of medicine is defined and actualized.

An internal morality is not closed to insights from literature, history, or the social and physical sciences. Indeed, these disciplines are valuable sources for detailed existential accounts of the moral life. These disciplines facilitate the realist assessment of the telos of medicine. An internal morality draws on all these disciplines to the extent that they enhance our grasp of the existential phenomena of the clinical phenomena of being ill, being healed and professing to heal. It looks, however, beyond cultural and historical contexts to what is common to the human predicament of being ill and being healed.

The internal morality of medicine, which I develop here, is not intended to be a complete morality for all the ways medical knowledge can be used. As stated above its present development will focus on clinical medicine, on the doctor-patient relationship. There is a good, an end, and an internal morality for the other usages of medicine and medical knowledge, but unpacking them is the work of another day.

A Philosophy of Medicine and the Good of the Patient

A Philosophy of Medicine

The first principle of medical ethics, the end to which it is directed, is the good of the patient:

> I will follow that system or regimen which according to my ability and judgment I consider for the benefit of my patient and abstain from whatever is deleterious and mischievous. (Hippocrates, *The Oath*)

All other moral precepts of the Oath and the other deontological books of the Hippocratic corpus are elaborations of this first principle, which also defines the end of medicine in the Aristotelian teleological sense. The well being of the patient is the good end of medicine and of the physician's art and action.

Today, this first principle is under serious attack from a variety of sources. Some historians claim that the idea of a Hippocratic tradition accepted by all physicians is a myth (Baker 1993). Some ethicists, philosophers, and policymakers are urging a reorientation of the physician's beneficence from an exclusive focus on the good of individual patients to a focus on societal good. Physicians, sociologists, and the general public are asking—What is a physician? What is so special about medical ethics? What should physicians be? Are they primary healers of sick persons, servants of the patient's or society's wishes and demands, businessmen, entrepreneurs, bureaucrats, scientists, instruments of social or political purpose?

These questions bear on the ends of medicine and the conception of the good it should aim at. What happens when ends, purposes, and goals are in conflict? How do we establish some hierarchy among the many purposes medical knowledge and physicians may serve (Nordin 1999)? These conflicts can only be resolved by reference to a primary defining good, which takes priority over other goods.

The current debate and confusion about the nature of medicine and the ends the physician should serve are a culmination of the erosion of the

Aristotelian notion of ends, their relation to the good and the relation between the idea of the good and the idea of ethics itself. If the end of medicine is to be re-defined, the ancient concept of ends must be retrieved from its extradition to moral limbo by contemporary philosophy. A moral philosophy of medicine depends on a philosophy of medicine built upon the personal relationship of the clinical encounter.

Aristotle based his treatise on Ethics on the proposition that the good is the end of human activity, the telos of human nature. Ethics was concerned primarily with attainment of this telos. Ends, as Hans Jonas pointed out, answer the question, "What for?" (Jonas 1984, p. 52). We do not impute ends to things and activities. They are not good because we desire them. We desire them because they are good. We can put medical knowledge to the goals and purposes we contrive. But whether these goals are morally good or bad uses of medical knowledge depends upon whether they fulfill the ends for which medicine exists and which define it qua medicine.

Aristotle uses medicine as an example of a techné whose end is health. He likens it to other examples of techné like navigation whose end is to guide a ship to its port of destination. Aristotle uses bridle making and lyre playing as other examples of activities with definable ends. These activities are structured by their very nature to specific ends and those ends when attained are the good for that activity. When attained with excellence they become virtuous activities.

Aristotle, and Aquinas in a similar fashion, treated the good for humans as the end or telos of human activity. Both structured their moral philosophies on the good, as the end of human life. For Aristotle this end was a life consistent with the intellectual and moral virtues, which led to happiness, flourishing, and well being. For Aquinas, it was a life lived in accord with both the natural and spiritual virtues, which led to the beatific vision and fulfillment of the spiritual nature of humans.

Thus, in determining the ends and good of human life, generally and in everyday life, ends and the good are intimately related. Of course, there are unresolved questions: the apparent contradiction in Aristotle between the primacy of intellect or will in perception of the good; whether the good is determined because we choose it, or we choose it because it is good (Plato, *Euthyphro*, 391); and whether telos and end are coextensive in

Aristotle (Hardie 1967, pp. 254–257). Those are important questions, but their answers are still cast within the teleological tradition.

However, from the late thirteenth and fourteenth centuries to our times, the foundations for a teleological ethic have been seriously eroded. The Nominalists began the process by rejecting the ideas of universals or of essence in the nature of things, thus disarticulating the connections between ends and the good. This process accelerated in the eighteenth century and has continued to the present (MacIntyre 1966; Murdoch 1998). Four conceptual shifts over the centuries are deemed particularly relevant: (1) the rupture between ethics and metaphysics in Kant's insistence on locating the good in the will and ethics in reason alone; (2) Hume's denial of any logical connection between *is* and *ought,* between fact and value, and his preference for affect over reason in ethics; (3) G. E. Moore's declaration that the good is an indefinable quality; and (4) the post-modern discrediting of any stable foundation for moral philosophy as well as extreme skepticism about the possibility that moral truth is ascertainable by the use of human reason.

The upshot of all of this has been profound for moral philosophy, and particularly for Anglo-American ethical theory. Ethics has shifted from a search for the good, to rights, values, and social convention. Morality, itself, is increasingly seen as the creation of our choices and the mores of a liberal society. Iris Murdoch puts it this way:

> The philosopher is no longer to speak of the good as something real and transcendent but to analyze the familiar activity of endowing things with value. If we want to place the definitive breach with metaphysical ethics at any point, we can place it here. (Murdoch 1997, pp. 59ff.)

On the modernist view, especially in Anglo-American philosophy, moral choices are simply our preferences among the sentiments dominant in our society at a particular time. Our differences are differences of language or interpretation in light of certain facts. This is the "foundation" for the now-dominant coherence and social construction theories of morals. These theories are a direct antithesis of the natural law tradition which recognizes a transcendent moral reality which the moral person can discover by the use of reason (Lisska 1996).

Aristotle and Aquinas both define the end of medicine, generically, as health; Plato says the same thing (*Lysis,* 219). Kass defines this end more specifically as the well functioning of the human body. These definitions are general enough to encompass clinical medicine as well as the basic sciences related to medicine, including social and preventive medicine. But they need to be specified further for our project, which is to define the ends of clinical medicine.

Clinical medicine centers on the clinical encounter, the personal interaction between someone who is ill and someone who professes to be a healer. Certainly, health is the ultimate end for healing, but often the fullest functioning of the human body and mind are not attainable. A more proximate and immediate end toward restoration of the physiology and psychology disrupted by illness is to make a right and good decision for *this* patient. That is, the immediate good expected by the patient as the end of his visit with the physician. Often, the meaning of the word health, namely "making whole again," cannot be achieved, but much can still be done to restore harmony or physiological and psychological function. To care, comfort, be present, help with coping, and to alleviate pain and suffering are healing acts as well as cure. In this sense, healing can occur when the patient is dying even when cure is impossible. Palliative care is a healing act adjusted to the good possible even in the face of the realities of an incurable illness. Cure may be futile but care is never futile.

The optimal end of healing is the good of the whole person—physical, emotional, and spiritual. The physician, manifestly, is no expert in every dimension. He or she, however, should be alert to the patient's needs in each sphere, do what is within his or her capabilities and work with others in the health care team to come as close as clinical reality permits to meeting the several levels contained in the idea of the good of the patient.

The Good of the Patient — Four Components

The Medical Good

The medical good is that which relates most directly to the aim of the art of medicine, that part which is based in the knowledge, science and technique of medicine. The medical good aims at the return of physiological function of mind and body, the relief of pain and suffering, by medication, surgical interventions, psychotherapy, etc. At this level, the patient's good depends on the right use of the physician's knowledge and skill, those which are intrinsically part of the medical techné.

But the medical good must be brought into proper relationship with the other levels of the patient's good. Otherwise, it may become harmful. What is medically "good" simply on grounds of physiological effectiveness may not be "good," if it violates higher levels of good, like the patient's good as he perceives that good. This perceived good is the second level of patient good.

The Patient's Perception of the Good

The medical good serves the many, complex facets of what the patient perceives as his own good. Here, we are concerned with the patient's personal preferences, choices, and values, and the kind of life he wants to live, the balance he strikes between the benefit and burdens of the proposed intervention. These qualities and values are unique for each patient and cannot be defined by the physician, the family, or anyone else. They are determined by the inter-relationships between and among the factors of age, gender, station in life, occupation, etc. To serve the good as perceived by the patient, the medical good must be placed within the context of *this* patient's life plans and life situations.

The Good for Humans

Medical good and the patient's perception of the good life must be related to the good for humans as humans. This was the good Aristotle and Aquinas sought to define as the telos of human life. At this level, we are concerned with the good peculiar to humans, like preservation of dignity of the human person, respect for his rationality as a creature who is an end in himself and not a mere means, whose value is inherent and not determined by wealth, education, position in life, etc. The patient is a fellow human with the physician to whom he is bound by solidarity and mutual respect.

It is at this level that some of the familiar principles of medical ethics are philosophically rooted, like autonomy, beneficence, non-maleficence, and justice. In American bioethics, these principles are taken to be *prima facie* principles grounded in a "common morality." This suggests that they could be changed if the common morality were to change. In the more classical view, the good for humans is not subject to social construction. It lies within human nature and is a requirement of the natural law.

In the clinical encounter, the medical good and the personal good must, in their turn, be consistent with, and protect, the good for human beings as humans. Physicians who ignore the patient's notion of the good violate the good of the patient as a self-determining rational being. Denial of care to the poor violates their dignity and value as human beings. Devaluing the lives of the handicapped does the same. Putting patients at risks that outweigh potential benefits, even with patient consent, violates the duty of beneficence and avoidance of evil.

Spiritual Good

The highest level of good which must be served in the clinical encounter is the good of the patient as a spiritual being, i.e., as one who, in his own way, acknowledges some end to life beyond material well-being. This may, or may not, be expressed in religious terms. But all, except the most absolute mechanistic materialists, acknowledge a realm of "spirit," however differently they may define it.

This realm of spirit gives ultimate meaning to human lives. It is that for which humans will often make the greatest sacrifices of other good things. For many people, the realm of the spirit is religion. They would be guided by a set of specific beliefs or doctrines that carry ultimate weight in their decisions. From the perspective of natural law, the spiritual destiny of man is his highest and ultimate good. Indeed, the dictates of the natural law are, themselves, that portion of divine law ascertainable by human reason (Lisska 1996).

Whatever the origin and content of one's spiritual beliefs, the three lower levels of good I have described must accommodate to the spiritual good. For example, blood transfusion might be medically "indicated" for the Jehovah's Witness, abortion of a genetically impaired fetus for a Catholic, or discontinuance of life support for an Orthodox Jew. But in these cases, the mere medical good could never be a healing act since it would violate the patient's highest good. Similarly, the Muslim, the Buddhist, the Hindu, or the humanist patient has his own spiritual good, which must be encompassed within a clinical decision if it is to serve the "good" of the patient.

Some Complexities

In many clinical encounters it may not be possible to assess each of the four levels of patient good and establish the order of priorities among them. This is the case with infants, children below the age for responsible decision-making, the intellectually retarded, the elderly, or those in permanent vegetative states. In these circumstances knowledge about the patient's personal preferences or spiritual beliefs may be lacking. Yet clinical ethics imposes the duty to come as close as circumstances permit for an estimate of the patient's good as a whole.

In such cases, two levels of the good are still accessible, i.e., the medical good, and the good of the patient as a human being. In the case of infants it is impossible to know about personal preferences, etc. In the case of adults, surrogates and others must be relied upon to represent the particularities of the other two levels from prior knowledge of the patient. How these are best balanced against medical good is a matter for more extended analysis than permissible here. Suffice it to say, that surrogates must be without significant conflicts of interest to be morally valid representatives. In the end, the physician is still responsible for the orders written and must therefore remain a guardian of the welfare of the most vulnerable patients.

In a pluralist society, another issue centers on the degree to which a particular patient's preferences, world-views, and religious practices impinge on the physician's own beliefs about what is good for the patient. The good as perceived by the patient and the physician himself must be respected as well. The dictum of the primacy of the good of the patient includes the physician's judgment of what is good medicine, what he thinks of the human life issues, and the spiritual destiny of himself and his patient. The total good—that is, the summation of the four levels of good—must not be equated with the patient's perception of the total good.

The most common misunderstanding of the notion of the internal morality of medicine based in the good of the patient is the assumption that the physician is bound to do whatever the patient defines as good. This is to make the second level of the good of the patient dominant over all other goods. It would make patient preference morally and lexically superior to the medical good, the good for humans, and the spiritual good.

Some would argue that the patient's good should include all that medicine can do provided the patient sees it as "good." The list of medically possible treatments is enormous. The possibility that a patient may choose as good that which is morally dubious is a real one. What the patient describes as good for himself—cloning, let us say, or self-mutilation, human embryo research, euthanasia—may violate the good for humans or the spiritual good. The good perceived as good by the patient is not to be a moral law in itself. It too must meet the tests of moral defensibility, established by a more fundamental source of the good than the patient's preferences.

To give supremacy to the patient's definition of his own good over the other levels of good is to absolutize the patient's autonomy and to violate the autonomy of the physician. It asks the physician to lay aside his own moral integrity and to become *value neutral* (Blustein and Fishman 1995; Miller and Brody 1995). This is a psychological impossibility as well as an abandonment of moral integrity by the physician. The physician, like the patient, therefore cannot be used as a mere means. The physician is entitled to respect for his autonomy, religious beliefs, and scientific integrity. Ethical conflicts between and among patients, physicians, families, and other health workers are a growing problem in clinical ethics. But the existence of complexities cannot be used to justify a utilitarian, legalistic, or libertarian definition of the ends of medicine or the physician's or patient's good. Nor can it reduce ethics to simple conflict resolution.

Emphasis on the good of the patient as central to medical ethics does not mean that physicians must always treat vigorously until the patient's last breath. The principle of beneficence in the Hippocratic Oath and ethos requires cessation of futile efforts (Hippocrates 1981). Historically, it is clear that clinicians have recognized the clinical fact of futility for thousands of years (Pellegrino 1999). Ethically, to continue futile treatment is to violate canons of the medical good since it is unnecessary treatment. Futile treatment may, in fact, be maleficent if it is burdensome physically, fiscally, or emotionally for the patient or the family. From the moral point of view there is no obligation to provide futile or disproportionately burdensome treatments.

This paper confines itself to a definition of the ends of medicine and the good of the patient. It does not engage the issues of the ends of investigative medicine or social medicine. These are realms in which medical knowledge and physicians are involved for ends different from the immediate ends of clinical encounters. However, even in research and social medicine, the quadripartite conception of the good that I have developed in this essay will be relevant. The good is of a piece, and its unity must be intact even though, in practice, there may be tensions between and among its components.

Implications for the Other Helping Professions

The conceptual schema proposed in this essay to redefine the ends of medicine in terms of the good of the patient has applicability beyond medicine. With proper redefinition of the ends peculiar to each profession, this schema can be used to define the good of the lawyer's client, the teacher's student, and the minister's penitent or parishioner. As with medicine, the ends of these other helping professions are linked to a particular activity specific to each profession.

Those who seek out helping professionals share a certain common phenomenological ground. They all deal with a human being in compromised existential states. The persons they serve are dependent, anxious, in distress, and lacking something essential to human flourishing; that lack in medicine is health; in law, justice; in education, knowledge; and in ministry, union with God. Humans in these compromised existential states are eminently vulnerable and exploitable. Persons in that state are invited to trust the professional and, indeed, *must* trust him in order to be helped or healed. In each instance, the untrustworthy professional could exploit the patient's vulnerability for personal power, profit, or prestige. In each case, the character of the professional is the final safeguard. In each case, the end of professional activity is the good of the person in need of help.

As with the medical relationship, the "good" in each of the other three helping professions is a quadripartite concept: (1) the level of technical good; (2) the good perceived by the person served; (3) the good for the person as a human being; and (4) the spiritual good. Each profession operates most directly on one or other of the four levels. But, regardless of its specific focus, each profession must also attend to the totality of the good of the person served by that profession.

For example, the lawyer focuses on obtaining justice for his client. Justice is a good of the client as a human being necessary to fulfillment of his human nature. But the lawyer cannot attain that end unless he is also concerned with the first level of the good—the legal good, i.e., he must be competent in legal practice. He must be fully competent in legal procedures and in those techniques necessary to press his case in court, negotiations, or depositions. These are necessary for a right verdict but not entirely sufficient for a good verdict. The lawyer must also be aware of the other levels of the client's good.

Thus, at the second level: What does the client deem justice to be in his case? To what degree does he wish to risk gain or loss, to confess, to settle out of court, to demand retribution? At the third level, the lawyer's success or failure is attendant on the degree to which he can gain for his client the human right of justice, freedom, vindication, or, if his client is guilty, a fair sentence. Finally, at the fourth level, to the extent that his client's religious or spiritual beliefs shape his plea for justice, they must be taken into account. For example, the client may be willing to forego certain of his claims in the name of charity for his opponent. Thus, as in medicine, all four levels of the good must be factored into the outcome or ends of the morally valid lawyer-client relationship.

Teaching may be similarly treated. Knowledge and truth are goods essential to human flourishing and fulfillment. To help others to achieve those goods, the teacher must, at the first level, possess the knowledge and skill he purports to teach. He must have mastery of the teaching methods, sources, and technical apparatus without which the end of knowledge transmission cannot be attained. At the second level, teachers must also adapt, to some significant degree, to the interests, learning modes, work habits, and preferences of the student. In the interests of the good of the student, teachers also may have to modify, restrain, or replace values that interfere with the end of learning. At the third level, that of the good for humans, teachers are required to respect their students with the dignity owed to persons, to treat them fairly, honestly, etc. Finally, at the fourth level, spiritual beliefs must be respected, allowed to flourish, and integrated with the more technical or academic dimensions of the student's education. Education, like medicine, strives to engage the whole person and achieve harmony among the intellectual, spiritual and personal ends.

Finally, the priest-petitioner relationship has its moral dimension most specifically at level four, the level of the spiritual good. I shall use the priest-penitent's relationship as an example of the relationship of the minister as spiritual healer. There is no conventional noun parallel to doctor-patient, lawyer-client, or teacher-student relationship. Priest-penitent stands here as symbol for the personal moral relationship of any minister of religion to the person who seeks his help. This is what the penitent seeks from the minister: i.e., counsel in his relationship with God; how to be reconciled with God after sin; how to grow in the spiritual life; how to decide moral questions in light of revelation or church teaching; how to adapt to death, hardship, etc., in accordance with Divine Will. To attend to the spiritual good takes precedence over the other levels of good. But the other levels cannot, by that fact, be ignored since they are part of the integral good of the person served.

At the first level, therefore, priests must be skilled in the ends of the activities specific to the priestly vocation, i.e., mastery of the theological or pastoral skills required to make their counsel serve the good of the penitent. At the second level, they must take into account the penitent's unique values, the uniqueness of his spiritual predicament, his station in life, preferences for spiritual charisma, styles of prayer, life situation, etc. At the third level, the priest must protect the good of the penitent as a human being, i.e., maintain the seal of the confessional, help the penitent to integrate his spiritual and his temporal good, appreciate his dignity as a child of God, etc.

In each profession, the four components of the patient's good are arranged in lexical and hierarchical order. The spiritual good takes precedence over all, followed, in descending order, by the good for humans, the personal evaluation of the good, and, at the lowest level, the technical good specific to each profession. Moral decisions in the course of professional activities are *right* if they conform to the techné of each profession at the first level. But to be *good*, they must conform at the other three levels as well.

Relationships with Other Sources of Morality

Thus, there is another facet of professional conduct common to all helping professions, the fusion of a technically right and morally good decision and act on behalf of a vulnerable human being. This fusion requires certain virtues or character traits in the practitioners of all the healing professions. David Thomasma and I have examined the question of virtue in general and specific virtues in the health professions elsewhere (Pellegrino and Thomasma 1993, 1996), so I will only enumerate the professional virtues here.

We understand virtues as Aristotle did when he said, "the virtue of man also will be the state of character which makes a man good and makes him do his own work well" (*NE* 1106a22–25). In the professions, the virtues are, therefore, those traits that dispose the professional—doctor, lawyer, minister, teacher—habitually to be a good person and do his work well, that is to say, to achieve the ends to which his work is directed. To be *good,* the professional must predictably exhibit certain dispositions, those that enable his "work to be done well."

The end of professional activity, i.e., the good of the person served, entails the virtues of the professions. Some of the most essential virtues would be: (1) fidelity to trust, which is ineradicable in healing relationships; (2) some suppression of self-interest, since the person served is in a vulnerable state and dependent on the power of the professional; (3) intellectual honesty, since professional practice beyond one's expertise is injurious; (4) compassion, since understanding and feeling something of the unique predicament of the person's need is essential to healing; (5) courage to pursue the good in the face of today's commercialization, depersonalization, and industrialization of professional life; and (6) prudence in every act so that the measures chosen are best suited to the technical and moral good of the person served.

Finally, a clear perception of the good of the patient, client, student, or penitent can provide a moral grounding for the commonly employed "principles" of medical ethics. The good of the person served is linked ontologically to the end of the professional activity. It is not subject to change at will. With the good as the end of professional activity, autonomy becomes mandatory since to violate autonomy is to violate the dignity and humanity of the person. Justice, which is both a virtue and a principle, is tied to the good for humans *qua* humans and is critical to every professional act for individuals and human society. Beneficence becomes the *primum principium* of all ethics, professional as well as general, since its primary end is doing good and avoiding harm. These connections have been developed in more detail elsewhere.

In summary, the four helping and healing professions have a common end—the good of the vulnerable persons in need of professional help and expertise. Each profession deals with humans in vulnerable states; each confronts the most personal, intimate recesses of the lives of other humans; each is permitted access to the inner life of another human being; each promises to help and invites trust; each is judged by the degree to which the good of the person served is attained by their professional activities. Although each profession functions most directly at one or another of the four levels of human good, each professional also must, in its own way, serve the other levels as well.

We are speaking, here, of a "common devotion" (Cushing 1926) shared by each helping profession to the good of the persons served. That good is the end of all professional activity. Subsidiary ends may be different for each profession depending upon which level of the good is its major focus. Whatever that subsidiary end, however, certain virtues and principles are necessary, and they are defined in terms of the good of the person being served.

Conclusion

Do good and avoid evil is the *primum principium* of all ethics. All ethical systems, medical ethics included, must begin with this dictum, which means that the good must be the focal point and the end of any theory or professional action claiming to be morally justifiable.

This paper attempts to define the good of the patient in concrete terms related to the phenomenology of the clinical encounter. The good of the patients is found to be a quadripartite good, a complex interrelationship between medical, personal, human, and spiritual good, hierarchically arranged. This concept generates the duties of the clinician. The complexities of its application in medical practice are described. A theory of the good of the patient also has applicability for the ethics of the other healing and helping professions and the virtues and principles pertinent to their practitioners as well.

Note

This is a revised version of a paper delivered in Padua, Italy at the LANZA Foundation Conference in 1998.

References

Baker, R. 1993. "The History of Medical Ethics." In *Companion Encyclopedia of the History of Medicine,* ed. W. F. Bynum and R. Porter, p. 852. New York: Routledge.

Barnes, J. (ed.) 1984. *The Complete Works of Aristotle: The Revised Oxford Edition,* p. 1729. Princeton, NJ: Princeton University Press.

Blustein, J., and Fishman, A. R. 1995. "The Pro-life Maternal-Fetal Physician." *The Hastings Center Report* 21: 22–26.

Cicero. 1999. *De finibus bonorum et malorum.* With an English translation by H. Rackham. Cambridge, MA: Harvard University Press.

Curran, W. J. 1980. "The Ethics of Medical Participation in Capital Punishment by Intravenous Drug Injections." *New England Journal of Medicine* 302: 326–330.

Cushing, Harvey. 1926. "Consecratio Medici." Graduation Address, Jefferson Medical College, Philadelphia, June 5, 1926.

Fuller, L. 1969. *The Morality of Law.* New Haven, CT: Yale University Press.

Hanson, M. J., and Callahan, D. 1999. *The Goals of Medicine: The Forgotten Issue in Health Care Reform.* Washington DC: Georgetown University Press.

Hardie, W. F. R. 1967. "The Final Good in Aristotle's Ethics." In *Aristotle: A Collection of Critical Essays,* ed. J. M. E. Moravcsik, pp. 254–257. Garden City, NY: Anchor Doubleday.

Hippocrates. 1972. *The Oath.* With an English translation by W. H. S. Jones, p. 291. Cambridge, MA: Harvard University Press.

Hippocrates. 1981. *On the Art.* With an English translation by W. H. S. Jones, p. 193. Cambridge, MA: Harvard University Press.

Jonas, H. 1984. *The Imperative of Responsibility: In Search of an Ethics for the Technological Age,* H. Jonas (Trans.) and D. Herr (Collaborator), p. 52. Chicago: University of Chicago Press.

Kass, L. R. 1975/1981. "Regarding the End of Medicine and the Pursuit of Health." *The Public Interest* 40: 11–42. Reprinted in A. L. Kaplan, H. T. Engelhardt, Jr., and J. McCartney (Eds.), *Concepts of Health and Disease* (pp. 3–30). Reading, MA: Addison-Wesley.

Ladd, J. 1983. "The Internal Morality of Medicine: An Essential Dimension of the Physician-Patient Relationship." In *The Clinical Encounter: The Moral Fabric of the Physician-Patient Relationship,* ed. E. Shelp, pp. 209–231. Dordrecht: D. Reidel.

Lisska, A. J. 1996. *Aquinas's Theory of Natural Law: An Analytic Reconstruction.* Oxford: Clarendon Press.

MacIntyre, A. 1966. *A Short History of Ethics.* New York: Macmillan.

MacIntyre, A. 1981. *After Virtue: A Study in Moral Theory.* Notre Dame, IN: University of Notre Dame Press.

Miller, F., and Brody, H. 1995. "Professional Integrity and Physician-Assisted Death." *The Hastings Center Report* 25: 8–17.

Murdoch, I. 1992. *Metaphysics as a Guide to Morals.* London: Penguin.

Murdoch, I. 1998. *Existentialists and Mystics: Writings on Philosophy and Literature,* ed. P. Conradi. New York: Penguin.

Nordin, I. 1999. "The Limits of Medical Practice." *Theoretical Medicine* 20: 105–123.

Pellegrino, E., and Thomasma, D. 1981. *A Philosophical Basis of Medical Practice: Toward a Philosophy and Ethic of the Healing Profession.* New York: Oxford University Press.

Pellegrino, E. D. 1983. "The Healing Relationship: The Architectonics of Clinical Medicine in the Clinical Encounter." In *The Clinical Encounter: The Moral Fabric of the Physician-Patient Relationship,* ed. E. Shelp, pp. 153–172. Dordrecht: D. Reidel.

Pellegrino, E. D., and Thomasma, D. C. 1993. *The Virtues in Medical Practice.* Oxford: Oxford University Press.

Pellegrino, E. D. 1994. "The Four Principles and the Doctor-Patient Relationship: The Need for a Better Linkage." In *Principles of Health Care Ethics,* ed. R. Gillon, pp. 353–367. New York: John Wiley.

Pellegrino, E. D., and Thomasma, D. C. 1996. *The Christian Virtues in Medical Practice.* Washington, DC: Georgetown University Press.

Pellegrino, E. D. 1976. "Philosophy of Medicine: Problematic and Potential." *Journal of Medicine and Philosophy* 1: 5–31.

Pellegrino, E. D. 1979. *Humanism and the Physician.* Knoxville: University of Tennessee Press.

Pellegrino, E. D. 1998. "What the Philosophy of Medicine Is." *Theoretical Medicine and Bioethics* 19: 315–336.

Pellegrino, E. D. 1999. "The Goals and Ends of Medicine: How Are They to Be Defined?" In *The Goals of Medicine: The Forgotten Issue in Health Care Reform,* ed. M. J. Hanson and D. Callahan, pp. 55–68. Washington, DC: Georgetown University Press.

Pellegrino, E. D. 2000. "Decisions at the End of Life: The Use and Abuse of the Concept of Futility." In *The Dignity of the Dying Person,* ed. J. deDios Vial Correa and E. Sgreccia, pp. 219–241. Vatican City: Libreria Editrice Vaticano.

Pellegrino, E. D. 2001a. "Philosophy of Medicine: Should It Be Teleologically or Socially Construed?" *Kennedy Institute of Ethics Journal* 11(2): 169–180.

Pellegrino, E. D. 2001b. "The Lived World of Doctor and Patient." In *Handbook of the Philosophy of Medicine,* ed. G. Khushf. Dordrecht: Kluwer.

Plato. 1961. *Lysis.* In *The Collected Dialogues of Plato, Including the Letters,* Bollingen Series LXXI, ed. E. Hamilton and H. Cairns, p. 163. Princeton, NJ: Princeton University Press.

Seifert, J. 1987. *Back to Things in Themselves.* Studies in Classical and Phenomenological Realism. New York: Routledge and Kegan Paul.

Veatch, H. 1981. "Telos and Teleology in Aristotelian Ethics." In *Studies in Aristotle,* ed. D. O'Meara, pp. 279–296. Washington, DC: Catholic University Press.

Von Hildebrand, D. 1973. *What Is Philosophy?* London: Routledge.

The Medical Profession

FOUR

Humanistic Basis of Professional Ethics

Too much is taken for granted about the way physicians conduct themselves. There is a need to reexamine the sources of the normative principles which should govern the behavior of physicians in the ordinary medical encounter—i.e., the situation in which one human in distress seeks out another who professes to have the knowledge and skill to help or heal.

The traditional view of professional ethics is derived from overemphasis on what physicians are and on what they ought to do for their patients as a consequence of their special position in society. The whole of these obligations is rooted in an image and a professional ethos which have served well but which require serious reappraisal in contemporary society. Beyond this, the more reliable source for a more humanistic professional ethics resides in the existential nature of illness and in the inequality between physician and patient intrinsic to that state. The ethical imperatives binding physicians are reducible to a meeting of the requirements of an impaired humanity which sickness implies. (Although I am speaking almost exclusively to and about physicians, what I say applies to other health professionals whose ethical conduct is similarly determined.)

What is at stake, I believe, is a fundamental recasting of the traditional image of physicians, one with profound implications for their social situation as well as their education and image of themselves. The need for this recasting is implicit in the disquietude expressed by many patients who call for a more "humanistic profession." Without such a redefinition of professional obligations, it will be impossible to close the widening gap between what physicians conceive themselves to be and what increasingly larger segments of the public expect them to be.

Anyone today who uses the noun *humanism* or the adjective *humanistic* is compelled at the outset to give at least an operational definition. The terms have become veritable shibboleths. They are used as a challenge, a claim, or an ideal, justifying all sorts of diverse and contradictory human activities. They are linked to every sort of political or social ideology, so that we hear of democratic, socialist, communist, and even totalitarian *humanisms*—all espousing the cause of man but on vastly differing suppositions. *Humanism* is piously affirmed by each professional or bureaucracy as precisely what *it* aims to be, but finds missing in others.

I will take the term in the loose sense, that applied by most people today to the health professions and other professions as well. *Humanism* encompasses a spirit of sincere concern for the centrality of human values in every aspect of professional activity. This concern focuses on respect for the freedom, dignity, worth, and belief systems of the individual person, and it implies a sensitive, nonhumiliating, and empathetic way of helping with some problem or need.

I shall not use the term *humanism* in its more pristine meaning as a literary or educational ideal, or as dependent upon an in-depth education in the classics or the humanities. These older interpretations are admittedly more precise and, of course, still valid and important. But it is essential to distinguish them from the more popular usage for two reasons: first, to be clear about the domain we are exploring and, second, to be sure that we do not link an intellectual, cognitive, and educational ideal too exclusively with what many people see lacking in the profession today.

With this operational definition of humanism serving as a benchmark, we can now consider what might be the most compelling derivation of a specifically humanistic professional ethics. Our inquiry will proceed from an examination of the more traditional source in the image and ethos of the physician to a source in the specifically human dimensions of being ill and in distress. I will argue that a more sensitive and compelling guide to the care of the sick is to be found in the fact of illness as a human experience than in the assigned role of the profession. Without supplanting traditional professional ethics, the intrinsic dehumanizing nature of illness imposes additional obligations of greater sensitivity—precisely those so often found wanting by the critics of medicine today.

The Traditional Source of Professional Ethics

For most of its history, the relationship of physician and patient has been dominated by the physician's point of view. Ethical codes have been established more on the basis of the obligation physicians feel than those patients may impose. The image of physicians that dominates the profession and society is still based in the Hippocratic ideal. Physicians are, in this tradition, represented as learned and noble men, members of a select brotherhood, which is largely self-regulating and autonomous. I have already noted some of the central precepts which formed and sustained the image of the Hippocratic physician (*Humanism and the Physician* 1979, chapter 6). They were Christianized in the Middle Ages, adapted to the spirit of eighteenth-century England by Thomas Percival, and have been modernized in the successive codes of ethics of the American Medical Association and similar codes in other countries. They remain the lineament of the ideal physician as interpreted by many in the profession. Indeed, this image has attained a quasi-scriptural stature. Only in the last several decades has there been any challenge to this traditional image. During that time the additional and often competing image of the physician as scientist has appeared. The benefactions of science and technology in medicine have given credence to an image of physicians quite at odds with older medical value systems. The public is genuinely ambivalent toward this new image. It recognizes the power of scientific medicine but simultaneously fears the loss of the virtue inherent in the older image. Physicians and patients have yet to amalgamate the older hieratic and the newer scientific conceptions of the physician.

This uncertain process of amalgamation is complicated by sharp changes in the social, political, and economic climate within which physicians now function. We no longer have consensus as a nation about what we expect from physicians and from medicine. Our attitudes about the authority, privileges, and superiority of professional groups have changed drastically. In a democratic society, we expect everyone to participate in decisions which will affect them.

Clearly, the easy congruence between the values of physician and patient commonplace in the past is rarely attainable in a democratic society which tolerates, and guarantees, plurality of values. Sharp differences of opinion now separate physician from physician, and patient from patient, in such matters as euthanasia, abortion, sterilization, prolongation of life, and the like. In an educated and liberalized society, the values of patients and physicians are as likely to be divergent as convergent.

Part of the problem also arises from the position of physicians as technical experts. We are all fearful of the potential tyranny of anyone with esoteric knowledge that can alter our lives in ways, and by means, we cannot fully understand. Physicians are constantly portrayed as the most powerful of modern thaumaturges. Their power is no longer related to their unique contact with the world of spirit, with which they might negotiate in behalf of their patients. Instead, their power is linked to mastery of impersonal instruments, tests, procedures, and medications which can too easily be used in injurious ways, or to advance professional rather than public interest.

Everywhere there are efforts to restrain not only this new magic, but also the old Aesculapian power and authority. The list of mechanisms being invoked is a long one: legislative control of quality, costs, and distribution of medical care, as well as the education of physicians and other health workers; demands for consumer participation in the management, accreditation, and licensing of medical institutions; the declaration of a patient's "bill of rights" to guarantee the elementary human rights of confidentiality and consent in medical transactions; and the growing tendency consciously to limit the growth of high technology and research. The most extreme reactions call for removing the larger part of medicine from the hands of physicians and returning it to the patient [1], or seeking redress in malpractice suits for every real, potential, or imagined injustice in the patient-physician encounter.

There is clearly an overt public disquietude with a large part of the spectrum of medical activity. Almost every serious ethical responsibility which had heretofore been delegated solely to the profession is today being at least partially withdrawn, or critically scrutinized. The traditional ideal of a self-regulating elite and of a trusted profession to whom society cedes moral and technical authority has been undergoing serious erosion.

The ancient source of professional ethics, in the responsibilities assumed by physicians as members of a select group, has become insufficient in the eyes of many.

Before looking to an alternate source out of which we might develop more authentic and more lasting normative guidelines, it is useful to review briefly some of the social, cultural, and political forces which have irrevocably transformed the relationship of physicians with individual patients and with society. Such a survey is essential to understanding that the traditional view of the physician and of medicine is not likely to be resuscitated.

To begin with, the capabilities of modern medicine are now so expanded that physicians' decisions can have a profound effect on the quality of the individual's life. The right clinical decisions and their competent implementation can make the difference between life, health, and relief on the one hand and death, disability, or pain on the other. The quality of human existence is genuinely often in doctors' hands today, whereas it was only figuratively so in the past.

Moreover, the acts of modern physicians collectively can alter the quality of life for the whole of mankind. Already painfully obvious are the cumulative effects of such acts as prolonging life of the aged or the incapacitated, expansion of high technology to cover previously incurable disorders, and genetic manipulations and behavioral modification. Today separating the ethical impact of individual and social medical decisions is becoming more difficult. Medical progress and practice must of necessity answer questions of social purpose and value, questions which transcend the privileges any expert group might arrogate to itself.

In a democratic society we face, in addition, the crucial issues of how to enable people to participate as free individuals in the choices that affect them. These decisions cannot be delegated to the expert, whether a nuclear engineer, military expert, or physician. The community must generate the mandate under which experts can practice their technology as means toward ends society must define.

In a democracy too there must be some protection for pluralism of values about such fundamental matters as the value of life, the rights of the fetus, and the use or rejection of medical treatments. Values in these matters are no longer held in common, nor can they be established solely by the profession as they were of old. Many things forbidden in the

Hippocratic Oath have already been challenged in modern society—abortion, the proscription against euthanasia, and the use of dangerous medications, for example. These are instances where contemporary social values have taken precedence over professional ethical values previously held inviolate.

Complexities in the physician-patient relationship, introduced by the capabilities of medicine and the pluralism of values in a democratic society, are accentuated by the depersonalization inherent in the growing institutionalization and bureaucratization of the medical encounter. Authority is now diffused and partitioned among members of ever-larger teams of health workers, administrators, and other functionaries. The authority of the individual physician is increasingly transferred to institutional structures. This means standardization, reducing performance to an average uniformity and assuring outcomes by adherence to procedures and regulations, rather than depending on the initiatives of individual physicians.

Thus, at a time when medicine has begun seriously to threaten human values and therefore when the premium on humanizing medical care should be at its highest, the organization of medical practice is tending to the contrary. Patients not only have lost the person to whom they might make some assignment of moral values held in common, but they have also lost their personal advocate, who now recedes into the "system."

The final touch is added when, as in recent years, the profession subscribes to some of the economic values in its society. While legitimate for other professions or occupations, these are questionable in medicine. I refer to the growing tendency of physicians to adopt shorter work days and weeks, longer and more frequent vacations, and more regular hours. Many now take a unionist stance with respect to their "rights" and compensation. Whatever justification they might have, strikes or slow-downs by segments of the profession have seriously damaged the image of medicine as a profession dedicated to service above its own interests. One of the distinguishing features of the profession of medicine has thus been compromised by physicians themselves. Those who choose to pursue their self-interest, as union members may, cannot at the same time demand a superior moral position in society.

Factors like those just reviewed impart a vastly different quality to the relationship between physicians and patients. Its former hieratic quality has been challenged by the demands of a democratic society and diminished by contemporary patterns of medical organizations and practice. Physicians can no longer assume a moral stance for their patients or presume to derive moral authority from a unique position in society. In short, traditional professional ethics, as derived from the unique responsibilities the profession imposed on itself, have been damaged beyond rehabilitation. We must look elsewhere for a humanistic medical ethics.

The Humanistic Source of Medical Ethics

A more authentically humanistic basis for professional ethics is clearly needed, one more suited to contemporary society and less dependent on changing interpretations physicians or society may place on the role of medicine. This means we must derive physicians' obligations from the specific situation of the person seeking assistance in the state of illness. The most certain source of a humanistic ethics is the unique impact of illness (that is, the impact of *being* ill on the humanity of the person) because it is a source which gives meaning to the whole of the physician's activities. It is the need to repair specific damage done to patients' humanity by illness that imposes obligations on physicians.

To this state of "wounded" humanity we now turn—first to define its concrete features and then to delineate the ethical imperatives which stem from it. These imperatives cannot constitute anything but "humanistic" ethics because they are tied to a specifically human experience, not to a social or historical role for the profession.

The essence of humanistic ethics is this: particular features of illness diminish and obstruct a patient's capacity to live a specifically human existence to its fullest. These features create a relationship of inherent inequality between two human beings: one a physician, the other a patient. That inequality must be removed as fully as possible before the humanity of the patient can be restored. The obligation to restore the patient's humanity is intrinsic in the relationship physicians assume when they "profess" medicine. Specific obligations are derived from the "profession"—an active assumption by the physician as a free person entering a relationship with another person. These obligations transcend any responsibilities, rights, or privileges physicians may feel were conferred upon them by the degrees they possess.

I can now turn to a partial exemplification of this line of reasoning by first identifying the deficits in the patient's humanity imposed by illness, and then the obligation of physicians to repair them. It is the sum of the obligations which constitute an authentic, humanistic, professional medical ethics.

Those who are ill (that is, those who have experienced some event—a symptom, an injury, a disability—they regard as "ill-ness") suffer insult to their whole being. They experience a series of intimate insults to the aspects of their existence most integral to being human. Because of the event of illness, these patients lose their freedom to act; they lack the knowledge upon which to make rational choices or to regain their freedom to act; they must place themselves in the power of another human, as petitioners, to regain their humanity; their integrity (i.e., self-image) is shattered, or at least threatened.

In short, those patients who have just experienced illness as an acute event or who have lived with it as a chronic accompaniment of life are deprived in varying degrees of those things which distinguish humanity from other forms of existence. A closer inspection of these deficiencies will clarify the meaning of the state of "wounded" humanity and the resultant state of inequality that characterizes the relationship between physician and patient.

When we are ill, the body is no longer a ready instrument of the will; we lack the knowledge and the skill to make the choices which will restore it; we come necessarily under the power of others; and consequently the integrated image (our embodied selves) that gives meaning to our lives is shattered. The deficiencies in the humanity of those who are sick, therefore, can be examined under four headings: freedom of action, freedom to make rational choices, freedom from the power of others, and integrity of self-image, the latter of which gives meaning to the first three. A brief inquiry into each of these deficiencies and the obligations derived from them will illustrate what I mean by humanistically based professional ethics.

Freedom of Action. Certainly, one essential attribute of being human is the ability to use the body as a ready instrument of our own purposes—to attain goals which transcend the needs of the body itself. The body is man's instrument for work, play, esthetic or physical pleasure, and creative activity of every kind. The bodies of plants, in contrast, are rooted and passive; those of animals are responsive largely to needs which do not transcend the body itself, though locomotion permits a more active pursuit of those bodily needs. In the human, the body is the agent for highly individualizing and personalizing activities, which serve purposes beyond the body's own needs.

Illness compromises the span of trans-bodily goals a person may set for himself, or attain. Pain, disability, or malaise make the body the center and end of existence rather than its means. Instead of being commanded, the body commands attention, and by that fact the patient moves closer to an animal or even a vegetative existence. Pursuit of the "good" life, however we define it, must stop until the body can be restored as the ready vehicle for that pursuit.

Freedom to Make Choices. The second deficiency in humanity caused by the fact of illness is the lack of the information and skill necessary to restore the body to its former state. The sick person lacks almost all the information needed to make rational choices and decisions of the utmost importance to his life. He does not know what is wrong; how he became ill or why; how serious his problem may be, whether he can recover; what treatments are available and whether they are effective; and what risk, cost, pain, or loss of dignity they may impose.

The freedom to make informed choices in matters affecting our well-being, one of the most fundamental of human prerogatives, is lost or seriously impaired in illness.

The freedom to make choices and take action in terms of one's own value system is impaired. In addition, the pain and discomfort of being ill make the patient susceptible to easier assent than would ordinarily be the case. Organic or functional disturbances of the brain add to this susceptibility or may even obviate completely free, informed consent or choice. In short, lacking knowledge to make decisions deprives the patient of his prime and intrinsic characteristics as a human agent.

Lack of information for rational decision making is common in a technological society. Even in ordinary daily affairs, it is manifestly impossible to comprehend all the alternatives. Dependence upon others is a practical necessity. In matters of health, however, the decisions penetrate too deeply into personal values and identities to be treated casually. Increasing numbers of patients perceive this difference and are expressing their dissatisfaction in a spate of patients' "bills of rights." The central thrust of these bills of rights is a plea for genuine participation in the process of medical decision making.

Freedom from the Power of Others. A consistent aim of a democratic and humanistic social order is to insure the widest individual self-determination consistent with the good of all. Each person wishes to be free of the power of others and to enter into personal associations on the basis of equality as much as possible. In illness this freedom, like the others, is seriously compromised. Even the most powerful, the most wealthy, and the best educated must become petitioners. Dependence on professionals, institutions, administrators, technicians—indeed the whole human apparatus of hospitals and clinics—is imposed of necessity upon the sick person. While the dependence is not as absolute as that of a passenger in an airliner landing in the fog, it is nonetheless of the same kind and lasts much longer.

The power of others to harm and to help is intermixed in every medical transaction. The patient is at the mercy of the integrity, competence, or motivation of others, most of whom are strangers. In today's complicated, technologic medicine a "team" is often necessary for vital aspects of a patient's care. The patient never sees many team members, others only fleetingly. The dangers of impersonalized use of power by team members are grave.

The fact of being ill, therefore, not only limits our freedom to act and to make free, rational choices, but places us in the most vulnerable position conceivable before those who have the power to make up these deficiencies.

Threats to Our Self-Image. Finally, these impediments to ordinary human freedoms occur within a context where the patient's image of himself is overtly or covertly threatened. Every illness is an assault on the integrity of the person. The assaults are of the most direct kind—the threat or actuality of death or disability, pain, discomfort, and limitations. The patient's idea of a satisfying life is threatened by the possibility of or need to adapt to chronic illness or repetition of acute episodes.

A lifelong construction of a personal image to balance abilities and limitations is eroded by the fact of illness. The challenge of rebuilding, the weakening of self-confidence, and the simple fact of vulnerability must be faced and a new image constructed. Some patients succeed completely or partially, and some fail. But, all in some measure or other must confront the test of an assault on the integrity of the person—and at the same time the other human freedoms enjoyed by the well have been lost or circumscribed.

Moral Obligations of the Professional

It is the undeniable fact of these specific disabilities in the humanity of the sick person that must be the infrangible base for the obligations of the physicians and all others who profess to heal. These obligations when codified and explicated constitute the substance of professional medical ethics. Professional ethics derived from the existential situation of the patient are more authentic and more human than the traditional ethics derived from the self-declared duties of the profession. If we accept this distinction, then we have the basis for a humanistic medical ethics—one rationally and humanely justifiable.

Obligations to the wounded humanity of the patient fall squarely upon the professional because inequalities in the relationship place all the power on his side. If the professional does not consciously remedy the four deficiencies which impair the patient's expression of humanity, his "profession" is inauthentic.

Clearly the body must be healed. This duty is the one most easily assumed by the health professional. The primary reason for the highest degree of competence then is a moral imperative, not professional satisfaction.

But in making his competence available, the physician must also attend to the other deficiencies created by illness. His technical decisions must be congruent with the patient's needs to participate in choices as freely and rationally as education, time, and circumstances permit. The facts of the illness; the degree of its gravity; the alternatives open; their relative effectiveness, costs, and dangers; the physician's own experience and skill in comparison with others; and the likelihood of success or failure must all be disclosed. Only when the information gap is closed can patients approach truly valid consent, one which permits participation as a human and enables the patient to incorporate the decision into his own value system.

Every clinical decision involves technical and value choices. These must to the most careful degree be dissected from each other to avoid imposing the physician's values. The professional can make a valid claim for technical authority, but no longer for moral authority. In a pluralistic society, the patient has the right to his own moral agency if he wishes to exercise it. The physician has the moral obligation to ascertain the degree to which the patient wishes to exercise his moral prerogatives and to provide the fullest exposition which will enable the privilege to be exercised.

Obviously, these obligations are conditioned by the acuteness of the clinical situation, the physiological state of the patient. But before excusing himself from them, the physician has the obligation to assure that he has exerted the care necessary to assure patient participation. A "humanistic basis" for professional ethics has to include the most careful management of the intersections of values that medical care so frequently entails.

This obligation extends beyond the patient to his surrogate in those circumstances when the patient cannot act for himself. Parents in the case of children, guardians in the case of the incompetent, and family or friends in the case of unconscious adults—all share with the physician the obligation to make decisions which will protect the patient's values to the extent they are known. The implications are obvious in such common clinical decisions as initiation and termination of life-support techniques, selection of treatment for incurable fatal disorders, or abortion whether for social, medical, or genetic reasons. An ever-present, subtle temptation for the physician and other health professionals is to impose their own values. The meaning of life, death, and quality of life; the exact content of a healthy existence; the relationship of spiritual to temporal concerns—each is a matter closely identified with our integrity as persons. Decisions affecting them cannot be humane unless they allow for individuals to express their values meaningfully.

The physician too has a set of values to which he owes allegiance. He has a double obligation: to protect those of the patient and to be faithful to his own. Conflicts will, of necessity, occur from time to time. To deal with them humanely, the physician must know enough about his own beliefs to decide when he can compromise, when he cannot, and when he must give the patient an opportunity to transfer his care to another physician whose values more closely coincide. A truly "humanistic" relationship allows the physician as well as the patient to express his humanity as fully as possible.

This is essential also in dealing with the threatened self-image of the person who is ill. He must consciously be assisted in integrating the experience of illness with his life. To do so requires his active participation in the decisions that affect him. Patient and physician must together reconstruct a meaning in the events of illness, even when it requires drastic alteration of the patient's conception of himself.

The moral obligations which arise from the fact of illness bear not only on the individual physician but on the institutions which "pro-fess" to provide medical care. Hospitals share the moral responsibility to repair the injuries to the patient's humanity. The responsibility is a corporate one, vested in the board of trustees, but it is not less binding. This responsibility cannot be delegated to the physician totally. When the physician uses a hospital, he is in a decision-making context that is no longer isolated. The degree to which he fulfills the moral requirements of a humanistic medical ethics must be a corporate concern as well. I am suggesting that the hospital too must be a moral agent. Ethical concerns involving this institution have yet to be adequately explored, and they lie in the realm of social ethics, one which I believe will increasingly require critical scrutiny in the years ahead [2].

Notes

Presented in part as the Jubilee Lecture, Memorial University of Newfoundland, St. John's, May 13, 1975, and at the 170th Annual Meeting of the Medical Society of the State of New York, New York City, General Sessions, November 8, 1976. Also published under the title "Humanistic Base for Professional Ethics in Medicine" in the *New York State Journal of Medicine,* vol. 77, no. 9, August 1977, pp. 1456–62.

1. Ivan D. Illich, *Medical Nemesis: The Expropriation of Health* (New York: Pantheon, 1975).

2. E. D. Pellegrino, "Hospitals as Moral Agents: Some Notes on Institutional Ethics," The Harvey M. Weiss Annual Lecture, 1976. *Proceedings of the Third Annual Board of Trustees/Medical Staff Executive Committee Conference* (Saint Paul, MN: Sisters of Saint Joseph of Carondelet, March 26, 1977), pp. 10–27.

FIVE

The Commodification of Medical and Health Care

The Moral Consequences of a Paradigm Shift from a Professional to a Market Ethic

Introduction

In Book I of the *Republic,* Socrates asks Thrasymachus, his pragmatic young interlocutor, this question:

> But tell me, your physician in the precise sense of whom you were just speaking, is he a moneymaker, an earner of fees or a healer of the sick? And remember to speak of the physician who really is such . . . (Plato, *Republic* 341c)

Even the cynical Thrasymachus, who denies the viability of justice in a world dominated by powerful people, admits that physicians are healers first. Were Socrates's question to be asked in today's health care environment, the answer would be different. We would be told that physicians should be encouraged—indeed, impelled—by financial incentives and disincentives to become money-makers for themselves and money-savers for their corporate employers or investors. Physicians, in short, are asked to be primarily purveyors of a commodity and not the healers Plato said they should be if they were to be *true* physicians.

In this essay, I wish to examine the ethical consequences of commodification of health and medical care on the relations of physicians with patients, with each other, and with society. I will do so by posing three questions and offering three conclusions.

The questions are these: (1) is health care a commodity like any other, subject to distribution by the operations of the competitive marketplace? (2) what is the ethical impact of commodification on professional ethics and the care of the sick? (3) does commodification work? (4) if health care is not a commodity, then what is it, and how should it be treated in a just society?

To each question, I shall reply, in turn, as follows: (1) health and medical care are not, cannot be, and should not be commodities; (2) the ethical consequences of commodification are ethically unsustainable and deleterious to patients, physicians, and society; (3) commodification does not fulfill its economic promises; and (4) health care is a universal human need and a common good that a good society should provide in some measure to its citizens.

Is Health Care a Commodity?

It is a fundamental dictum of managed care that health care should be treated like any other commodity, i.e., its cost, price, availability, and distribution should be left to the free workings of a free marketplace constrained by a minimum of governmental regulation (Hertzlinger 1997; Enthoven 1980). Through the usual mechanisms of competition a "quality product" should emerge since providers will compete with each other in quality, price, and satisfaction of consumers to keep their market-share and/or profits.

For their part, "consumers" and "purchasers" will be free to choose among providers selecting the best "buy" suited to their individual needs. Costs will decline, and quality will be maintained or will improve. More care will be accessible to more people on their terms, not the doctor's. The laws of competition will reduce waste, overuse, and error to everyone's advantage. Medicine will be demystified, physicians will become employees, and physicians' decisions will be shaped to conserve society's resources.

In this view, these desirable ends can be facilitated by turning the physician's self-interests to the advantage of the competitive system. By controlling clinicians' expenditures, employing financial and other rewards and penalties, costs will be kept down, unnecessary care eliminated, and quality outcomes optimized. In this view, there is no objection to physicians being money-makers so long as this activity is confined to a managed environment and their "product" is traded on the open market. The fundamental question is a deeper one than we can examine here, namely, the issue of the proper relations of ethics to economics (Friedman 1967; Piderit 1993; Sen 1987).

The underlying ethos of managed care is the theory of Adam Smith's *Wealth of Nations* (1909) and *Theory of Moral Sentiments* (1817). If, as Smith taught, everyone pursues his or her own interests, the interests of all will be served. The profit motive as adduced by Smith ultimately works to social benefit. But, for Smith, profit is not the primary end of the market ethos. Rather, it is the best means of attaining the primary end which is ". . . a plentiful revenue of subsistence for the people" (Worland 1983, p. 8). As I shall note later in this essay, Smith also felt that some things could not be left to the fortuitous workings of the marketplace and could only be assured by government intervention (Worland 1983, p. 8). For some economists, this reservation would inhibit the liberty only an unrestrained market can provide (Friedman 1967).

In its most aggressive form, managed care expresses the market ethos in tightly restrained risk selection, high-powered marketing and advertising, strict rules about denial or approval of care, competitive price-cutting, and putting substantial portions of the physician's income at risk. Reward and penalty for doctors depend negatively on the clinical costs they incur and positively on meeting marketing goals and patient satisfaction (Kuttner 1998; Anders 1996). Gaining the benefits of market competition for health care when treated as a commodity will, of necessity, lead to a loss of professionalism (McArthur and Moore 1997).

Before discussing the ethical problems consequent on treating health care as a commodity, there is ample reason to question the validity of this line of reasoning even from the purely economic point of view. There is, today, an intense and growing reaction to managed care as it is now practiced. This is of sufficient proportions to cast doubt on the economic theory behind managed care. There is evidence that costs are again rising, services being reduced, young and healthy subscribers being favored over old and sick ones, emergency rooms being closed, etc. (Kassirer 1997; Smith 1997; Flocke 1997; Anders 1996; Pear 1998; Larson 1996). Restrictive legislation is currently before the Congress (Patient Access and Responsibility Act 1997), class action suits are beginning to surface, and legislation has been proposed to remove the protections of managed care organizations against liability provided by the Employee Retirement Security Act.

Economists, health care planners, governmental budget officers, industry investors, young and healthy persons who have not made use of the system, and entrepreneurial physicians, nurses, and administrators regard these as transient problems curable by fine-tuning the system. Their faith in democratic capitalism is not without reasonable foundation. After all, they argue, the free market concept has brought America to its position of preeminence and affluence among nations, it has contributed to the superiority of American medicine, and it accords with the spirit of enterprise, freedom, and self-determination Americans rightly cherish. Indeed, the dismal failure of government-operated enterprises and centrally regulated economies in Eastern Europe sharply underlines the superiority of free markets for most commodities.

Much more important than the economic short-comings of the managed care line of reasoning and operation are the ethical issues encompassed in the paradigm shift from a profession to a market ethic. Before examining these, it is necessary to see whether health and medical care are, in fact, commodities. If they are, then the managed care line of reasoning is essentially correct, and the present shortcomings should yield to instrumental manipulation. But, if they are not commodities, then instrumental manipulation will not cure the present ills. Attention will have to turn to the ends and purposes of medicine, to healing as a special kind of human activity governed by an ethic that serves those ends and not the self-interests of physicians, insurance plans, or investors.

The legitimacy of the marketplace, competition, and democratic capitalism, therefore, are not at issue. Rather, the ethical question commodification raises is whether the marketplace is the proper instrument for the distribution of health care. Specifically, is health care sufficiently different from pantyhose, ocean-front condominiums, or television sets to set it apart from other consumer goods? The answer to this question rests on what we mean by a "commodity" (Zoloth-Dorfman and Rubin 1995; Anderson 1990; Immersheim and Lestes 1996; Reynolds 1995; Anderson 1996).

The *Oxford English Dictionary* gives a wide range of meanings to the word "commodity" (*OED* Vol. II, 1961, p. 687). The definition most relevant to this discussion is the way the word is used in commerce, i.e., a thing produced for sale valued for its usefulness to the consumer or its satisfaction of his preferences. Implicit in this definition is the idea of fungibility, namely, that one health care encounter is like any other, just like any bag of beans of same weight and quality is like any other bag of beans. It follows also on this view that, providing they are equally competent, any physician is like any other, and any patient like any other. Hospitals, laboratories, and nursing homes are all interchangeable as well.

If health care is a commodity, then it is something we possess and can sell, trade, or give away at our free will. This implies that, like any commodity, ownership of medical knowledge upon which health care depends resides with health professionals or those who employ or invest in them (Nozick 1974, p. 160; Engelhardt 1996, p. 381). No one else can lay claim to their medical knowledge or skill unless they were acquired unjustly. In this view, there would be no duty of stewardship over medical knowledge which would require its use on behalf of those who need it but cannot pay for it. Nor can there be any valid moral claim by the sick on society for its allocation or distribution. Whether health care is a commodity in this sense will be discussed below as will the moral implications for the justice of moral claims in the allocation of resources.

The commodification question centers on "health care," not on the facilities, medications, instruments, dressings, and other disposable items used in or necessary to health care. These are, in one sense, commodities, since they can be owned, consumed, bought, traded, and donated. They are in a different category from commodities unrelated to health care. To a large extent, they must be subject to market forces. But in the interests of the common good, they become the subject of ethical and public concern when their scarcity threatens human well-being. The sale of body parts, kidneys, or blood is another instance of commodification with serious ethical implications (Titmuss 1997; Brecher 1991). Granted the importance of all the objects that are essential in health care, the central ethical issue is the quality and nature of personal relationships involved. The materials used are means to the end of healing and helping sick persons.

By "health care," therefore, I mean the provision of assistance to persons in need of care, cure, education, prevention, or help related to trauma, illness, disease, disability or dysfunction by other persons knowledgeable and skillful in providing such assistance. The central feature of health care is the personal relationship between a health professional and a person seeking help (Ray 1987; Pellegrino and Thomasma 1988). Commodities may be used in the process of providing care, but the totality of health care itself is not a commodity.

The most common assertion of those who see no objection against classifying health and medical care as commodities is that there is nothing unique about them as human activities. It is an assertion made usually by healthy people, the young and those who have not thought much about their own vulnerability and finitude. To be fair, there are undoubtedly a few people who steadfastly hold to this view despite everything, even when they themselves, or members of their families, become ill. Still, even they might reexamine that position at the moment when some dear family member is denied access to life-saving or life-enhancing treatments because of the fortuitous operations of the marketplace.

This is happening, today, in communities where hospitals are closing emergency rooms, burn units, premature baby care centers, and neonatal intensive care units to cut losses or to enhance profits. As a result, important care is not available or is so inconvenient or delayed that danger or death might occur. Acute care of this type is a need that may occur anywhere, anytime, and to anyone. If there is a first priority, this surely is one since other needs become insignificant until the emergency is over.

The same can be said for less dramatic medical and health care services. Human flourishing can and does occur in the presence of chronic illness, but it is certainly more easily attained when one is healthy. Chronic illness, pain, discomfort, or disability can constrain the most determined and best-adjusted person. For most people, it is difficult or impossible to do the things they want to do or enjoy when they are afflicted by illness. Health is a fundamental requirement for the fulfillment of the human potential and freedom to act and direct one's life. To lack health and to need treatment is to be in a diminished state of human existence—a state quite unlike other deprivations which can be borne if one is healthy.

Serious illness changes our perceptions of ourselves as persons. It forces us to confront the fragility of our own existence. Human finitude is no longer a distinct abstraction, but something illness forces us to confront as a possible present reality. Regardless of whether the illness is serious, if we wish to be treated, we are forced to seek help, to invite and authorize a stranger—the health professional—to probe the secret places of body, mind, and soul. Without this scrutiny, we cannot be helped. To be sure, lawyers are permitted access to some intimate secrets, tax advisors to others, and ministers to still others. But only the physician may need access to the widest range of secrets, since being ill is not confined to the body. It is a disturbance in the whole life-world of the patient.

What the sick person needs is healing, i.e., a restoration of what has been "lost," a reestablishment of the equilibrium that existed before the onset of illness. This "restoration" is not just a return of biological equilibrium (Gadamer 1996). It is rather a restructuring of our whole life world—one with its unique history, set of relationships, and social milieu. In that restoration, there is a meshing of the life and lived worlds of both the doctor and the patient (Pellegrino 2000). Healing is achieved by a combination of the physician's biological interventions (drugs, surgery, manipulations) with the healing power of the patient's own body. In the end, where self-healing and medical healing begin and end may be highly problematic, but in either case, the assistance of knowledgeable health professionals is indispensable.

Given the special nature of illness and healing, health care cannot be a commodity. Health care is not a product which the patient consumes and which the doctor produces out of materials of one kind or another. The sick person "consumes" medication and supplies, and expends money for them, but he does not consume health "care" as he would a bag of beans or a six-pack of beer. Health or amelioration of disease may be the end of medicine but health, itself, is not a weighable commodity.

In a commodity transaction, like buying bread, the persons who buy and who sell have no personal interest in each other beyond the transaction. They are focused on the object or product, on the commodity to be traded. Their relationship does not extend beyond the sale or the consumption of that commodity. The medical relationship, in contrast, is intensely personal. Confidence and trust are crucial as is a continuing relationship, at least in general medicine if not in the subspecialties.

There are other intimate professional relationships as well as medicine. But, even in such intimate services as legal or ministerial advice, the sheer totality of engagement with the biological as well as the psychosocial and spiritual, which occurs in medicine, is lacking. This is not to depreciate these other crucial human services. They, too, respond to fundamental human needs: the lawyer to the need for justice; the minister to the need for spiritual reconciliation. Those are human needs of such fundamental significance for human flourishing that they, too, cannot be classified as commodities. However, the universality, unpredictability, inevitability, and intimate nature of the assault of illness on our humanity, the impediments it generates to human flourishing, and the intimate and personal nature of healing give health care a special place even among the helping professions.

Another feature of a commodity is that it is proprietary. Commodities are produced by someone who makes something new out of preexisting materials. The seller herself, or her agent, owns the goods or commodities she offers for sale. For a price, she transfers ownership to the buyer who consumes the product as he wishes. This is not, and cannot be, the nature of the case with medical or health care. Physicians, nurses, and other health professionals are not the sole owners of their medical knowledge for several good reasons.

For one thing, the physician's knowledge comes from many years—and in some cases, centuries—of clinical observations recorded by his or her predecessors. All health professionals have free access to that record across national boundaries. In addition, the most reliable, clinically pertinent medical knowledge comes from autopsies or controlled experiments on other human beings. A research "break-through" often results in response to previous work. The investigator uses instruments and methods discovered by others. No research exists in a vacuum. The fruits of research also result from the willingness of our fellow citizens to be research subjects so that others might benefit. Biomedical research is funded by public agencies or by private philanthropies to which all contribute by paying taxes or purchasing products from whose profits the funds for philanthropy derive.

Moreover, the doctor's education depends upon the acquisition of a kind of knowledge and experience which is ethically possible only with society's sanction (Pellegrino 1995). In their first years, for example, medical students dissect human cadavers for which they would be criminally prosecuted without social sanction. Later, they are allowed to participate in the care of patients when they are incompletely trained, albeit under supervision of licensed practitioners. Students can only learn procedures and operations by "practice," again, under supervision. They participate in clinical care when, clearly, their skills are rudimentary. They continue to enjoy this privilege in their post-graduate years as residents or fellows.

Society sanctions these practices because the only way future physicians can be trained properly is by "hands-on" experience. Physicians in practice continue to enjoy these privileges in continuing education which is designed to maintain their skills or teach them new procedures. Surgeons develop and maintain their skills by continuing "practice," at first under supervision and, later, independently.

The argument has been made that medical knowledge is proprietary because it has been paid for by tuition and continuing education fees and by the many years of study and demanding work required for a thorough medical education (Sade 1971). But even this cannot make medical knowledge proprietary. There is no fee that could buy the privileges or waive the legal penalties that would be imposed if medical students, residents, and fellows did not have social sanction for what they are allowed to do. Moreover, these privileges are accorded not primarily so that doctors or nurses may have a means of livelihood or an "edge" in competing with their fellows. The privileges of medical and nursing education are permitted in exchange for the benefits society accrues from the assurance of a continuing supply of well-trained physicians and other health professionals.

As a result, when they accept the privilege of a medical education, medical and nursing students enter implicitly into a covenant with society to use their knowledge for the benefit of the sick. By entering this covenant, they become stewards rather than proprietors of the knowledge they acquire. Their fees and labor entitle them to charge for their personal services—not because they own the knowledge they employ, but because of the effort and time they invest and the danger they may incur in applying that knowledge to particular persons. They are entitled to compensation for their effort. But, to paraphrase Plato, they are *true* physicians when they are *healers* first, and *money-makers* second (Plato, *Republic* 341c).

Commodification, Market Ethics, Professional Ethics

Clearly, health and medical care do not fit the conceptual mode of commodities. They center too much on universal human needs which are much more fundamental to human flourishing than any commodity *per se*. They depend on highly intimate personal inter-relationships to be effective. They are not objects fashioned and owned by health professionals, nor are they consumed by patients like other commodities. Stewardship is a better metaphor than proprietorship for medical knowledge and skill.

All of this might be granted and still some might hold that, even if health and medical care are not commodities in the usual sense, they should be treated as such. In this view, the market is the best mechanism in a free society for the distribution of health care, like all human goods. It is the best guarantor of those special aspects of health and medical care we have insisted must be preserved. When consumers are free to choose and providers compete, the interests of all will be better served, especially when costs are high, quality among providers is variable, and resources are scarce.

Let us examine the consequences of such assertions from the point of view of their ethical meaning for persons who are ill and for society in general.

The most immediate and urgent ethical consequences of commodification occur at the bedside at the moment of actual decision-making. Here the major issues are divided loyalty, conflicts of interest, conflicts with the traditional ethic of medicine, and challenges to the personal integrity of physicians and nurses. These conflicts have been examined in some detail elsewhere (Pellegrino 1997; Rodwin 1995; Rodwin 1996; and McArthur and Moore 1997). The focus here will be on commodification and commercialization of the healing relationship and the supplanting of the traditional professional ethic by the ethic of the market and of business.

First of all, the commodification of health and medical care means that the transaction between physicians and patients has become a commercial relationship. That relationship, therefore, will be primarily or solely regulated by the rules of commerce and the laws of torts and contracts rather than the precepts of professional ethics. Profit-making and pursuit of self-interest will be legitimated. Inequalities in distribution of services and treatments are not the concerns of free markets. Denial of care for patients who could not pay was not unknown in the past. But this was not legitimated as it is in a free market system where patients are expected to suffer the consequences of a poor choice in health care plans, or a decision to go uninsured or to pay only for a plan with lesser levels of coverage. In this view, inequities are unfortunate but not unjust (Engelhardt 1996). Some simply are losers in the natural and social lottery (Nozick 1974). The market ethos does not *per se* foreclose altruism, but neither does it impose a moral duty to help, especially if helping impinges on the proprietary rights of others without their consent.

In a market-driven economy, commodities are fungible, i.e., any one of them can be substituted for any other similar commodity, provided quality and price are the same. In this view of health care, physicians and patients become commodities, too (Zoloth-Dorfman and Rubin 1995; Greenberg et al. 1989; Starr 1982, p. 217). The identity of physicians, hospitals, clinic locations, and laboratories makes no difference unless a clear quality gap or danger is demonstrated. Patients, too, become fungible. They are "insured lives." They can be traded and bargained for, back and forth, in mergers, network formation, or sales of hospitals and clinics. They are "profit" or "loss" centers, assets when they stay well and pay premiums, and debits if they become ill and need too many services (Greenberg et al. 1989). The "quality" of any group of patients is then measured by their profitability and this can be a "deal breaker" in mega-mergers, etc., when both doctor and patient become faceless counters in business mega-deals (Blecher 1998).

When both doctors and patients are fungible, choice of physician has no ultimate weight despite repeated surveys showing it is the most important factor in the therapeutic relationship. Physicians no longer look on patients as "theirs" in the sense that they feel a continuing responsibility for a given patient's welfare. Without this attachment of particular doctors to particular patients, it is easy to justify a strict 9-5 workday, signing out to another doctor on short notice, or being "unavailable" for all those personal concerns and worries that beset patients even with non-life-threatening illnesses. Even short-term continuity of care is difficult to come by and, in any case, reckoned as not essential for care to be "delivered" (Flocke et al. 1997). Similarly, necessary communications between primary care physicians and specialists are hampered, further aggravating the discontinuity (Roulidis and Schulman 1994).

To remedy this, patients are urged by the corporate ethos and the fungibility of physicians to regard the managed care organization as their "doctor." The corporation will provide. The organization will deliver the commodity and make certain that "someone" is there to deliver it. Many physicians are already socialized into this corporate way of thinking. They place less emphasis on continuity, personal commitment, and personalized relationships with patients than in the past. Physicians who are corporate employees become encultured in an ethic alien to the professional (McArthur and Moore 1997). The ethic of the marketplace and the ethic of the employee begin to displace the more demanding ethic of a profession. The ethic of individual patient welfare based on principles has moved towards greater dependence on the institutions providing care (Emanuel 1995).

There is no room in a free market for the non-player, the person who can't "buy in"—the poor, the uninsured, the uninsurable. The special needs of the chronically ill, the disabled, infirm, aged, and the emotionally distressed are no longer valid claims to special attention. Rather, they are the occasion for higher premiums, more deductibles, or exclusion from enrollment. There is no economic justification for the extra time required to explain, counsel, comfort, and educate these patients and their families since these cost more than they return in revenue. Despite the boast about prevention under a managed care system, the time required for genuine behavioral change—the essential ingredient in true prevention—is not recompensed. To be sure, immunizations, diet sheets, smoking cessation clinics might be offered. They are not as costly nor as effective as the constant effort required for genuine behavior modification with reference to diet, exercise, stress control, and the like. Effective prevention requires education and counseling, and these are personnel-intensive and rarely profit-making.

The business ethos puts its emphasis on the bottom line, on profit, on an excess of revenue over expenses. The aim of business is to maximize returns to investors (Friedman 1970). For-profit organizations return those profits to investors, executives, and board members. The care they provide turns out to be more expensive as well (Woolhandler and Himmelstein 1997). Non-profit organizations use profits to expand services or to "survive" the intense competition that characterizes the health care "industry" today. But in both for-profit and non-profit systems, health professionals who contribute to the bottom line are valued; those who do not are devalued or let go (Kuttner 1998, pp. 1562–1563).

In a commodity transaction, the ethics of business replaces professional ethics. Business ethics is not to be depreciated. Many businesspeople genuinely seek to be "ethical." A whole literature and a whole new set of experts in business ethics give testimony to a genuine interest in ethical business conduct in general and in health care in particular (Bowie and Duska 1990; Blair 1995; Evans 1988; Shortell et al. 1996). Emphasis on worth creation rather than profit maximization and better representation of patient interest are promoted by ethically sensitive corporations.

The question, however, is not the validity of a business ethics, but whether it is appropriate for health and medical care. If there is any weight to the arguments for the special character of health care, then a business ethics is inappropriate and insufficient as a guide for health professionals. Revisions of business ethics are admirable, especially if they ameliorate some of the crasser aspects of for-profit plans. But the problems are of a more fundamental sort not susceptible to cure by changes in management ideology.

The contrasts between business and professional ethics are striking. Business ethics accepts health care as a commodity, its primary principle is non-maleficence, it is investor- or corporate-oriented, its attitude is pragmatic, and it legitimates self-interest, competitive edge, and unequal treatment based on unequal ability to pay. Professional ethics, on the other hand, sees health care not as a commodity but as a necessary human good, its primary principle is beneficence, and it is patient-oriented. It requires a certain degree of altruism and even effacement of self-interest.

When humans are at their most vulnerable and exploitable, they need much more secure protection than a business ethics can afford. Buying an automobile, for example, is a tricky business, to be sure. Much faith must be placed in the manufacturer and the salesperson (a slender reed, indeed).

One hopes for an ethical dealer. But the vulnerability of the auto purchaser pales to insignificance when compared to entering an emergency room with a pain in the chest or a fractured skull.

The corrupting power of industrial and business metaphors has been commented upon elsewhere (Pellegrino 1994). Suffice it to say that substituting words like "consumers" for patients, "providers" for physicians, "commodities" for healing relationships, or speaking of health care as an "industry," or of "product-lines" or "investment opportunities" inevitably distorts the nature of healing and helping. Euphemisms, if repeated often enough, eventually will shape behavior as though they were true renditions of real world events and states of affairs.

If we treat health care as a commodity, then we are prone to "sell it" like any other commodity—that is, by creating a demand among those who can pay. Getting the competitive edge via advertising is standard commercial practice. The first move in this direction came in 1982 when the Federal Trade Commission decided that the then-standing AMA ethical prohibition against advertising constituted a restraint of trade (Federal Trade Commission 1982). The Commission treated medicine as a business and not a profession. In effect, the Commission ordered the AMA to set its ethical code aside in the interests of commerce. The implications of such an action for the ethical integrity of the profession have not been sufficiently appreciated.

Since the FTC order, the ethos of the advertising world, with its all-too-characteristic seductive promises and often-misleading inducements has dominated the promotion of health care in the media. In the name of competition, everything has become a "P.R." problem and an exercise in spin control. The claim that advertising provides information upon which consumers (patients) can base their choice of doctors or health plans is no less spurious than it is in the advertisement of cosmetics. Reliable, clear, unambiguous data on coverage and quality are hard to see through the camouflage and persiflage of marketing.

Does Commodification Work?

Some might agree that treating health care as a commodity does, indeed, carry the ethical risks I have detailed above. However, they might insist that, commodity or not, health care is part of the economy, and it is best distributed in a free market. They can point effectively to the dismal failure of government-controlled markets in socialist economies of recent unhappy memory. They might argue that the benefits of a free market might outweigh the dangers. Three of these putative benefits are (1) cost savings which competition would effect, (2) the subscriber or "consumer's" freedom to spend his or her money for health care as he or she wishes, and (3) the satisfaction the patient would enjoy as providers competed for his or her business. Let us examine these presumed benefits in the light of the realities as they are unfolding in managed care, which does, indeed, make health care a commodity and seeks to improve its distribution and price while retaining its quality via the workings of the market.

It is a fact that rationing and limitations on physician decisions have kept costs from escalating. But there are already clear evidences of a reverse trend (Smith 1997; Anders 1996). Premiums are rising in many states and promise to do so elsewhere. Profits are dropping. Initial savings through mergers, reductions of personnel or acquisitions, and tightened controls on physician decisions are one-time savings. Mergers may be as much signs of weakness as strength. Treating medical and health care as a commodity subject to market forces must face certain inescapable clinical realities.

For one thing, subscribers cannot all be, and remain, young and healthy forever. As subscribers age, they need and demand more services. As time goes by, initial promises to contain costs or to return a profit become more difficult to keep. Subscribers either must be dropped, selected out at the outset, or corners must be cut and quality endangered. When profits drop, investors in for-profit plans will sell and move to better opportunities; non-profit organizations will face bankruptcy, and for-profit plans will tighten approval requirements for care or for inclusion in the plan. Every plan will scramble to enroll young, healthy people who have little need for care. The poor, the under-insured, and the genuinely sick will be pariahs to be avoided or dis-enrolled in some way.

The promise of freedom of choice is even more illusory (Enthoven 1980; Hertzlinger 1997). For the largest majority of those insured, their employers (who are the purchasers of the plans) make the first choice—selection of a plan with which to contract for services. This is done primarily on the basis of cost, not of quality. Indeed, neither the employer nor the employee is in a good position to judge outcomes and quality of care except in the grossest terms. The fragility of these choices is manifest in the employer's constant shifting from plan to plan for the "best" buy, which often translates into the cheapest buy. The employee has no choice but to go with the plan or go it alone and buy his or her own insurance.

Once in a plan, freedom is, again, limited—this time in choice of doctor. Yes, there is choice, as long as it is from the panel of approved physicians and a list of approved services. The same limitation on freedom prevails when it comes to choice of hospital, or specialist, or an MRI or lab facility. The advertisements proclaim "choice," but all have fine print that limit those choices.

Even more uncertain is the choice of how best to spend one's money in health care—whether to buy a plan with a high or low deductible, whether to go naked and use one's money for other things, and which of the complex and confusing array of "products" and "packages" best suits one's health needs at one time of life or another. This illusory freedom flies in the face of realities like the difficulty, even for educated people—even health professionals—of comprehending what the convoluted obscurantist language of the contract covers or the impossibility of predicting how much coverage one will, in fact, need, particularly to meet the uncertainty of an unexpected catastrophic illness. Should one buy limited coverage? Should one opt for a high or a low deductible? How are changing needs to be accommodated—like being married, divorced, having children, retiring, choosing a medical savings account, or unexpectedly picking up the care of elderly parents? What do hospitals, physicians, and society do when those who make bad choices appear for care?

Libertarians might regale in this richness of choices. Yet, even they would have to admit that bad choices can be made by the most educated people. The libertarian could reply that this is the price of freedom: "Better than someone else making the choice! After all, some people do not value health care above other goods. They may wish to run the risk in order to be able to spend their earnings on more immediate needs or pleasures." This is carrying *caveat emptor* to the extreme without resolving the question of what physicians do when the patient who made a poor choice presents himself or herself with a medical emergency or a serious illness.

In a market-driven ethos, theoretically at least, physicians would be justified in refusing care. They could argue that patients are responsible for their own health, that they must live with their choices, and that to provide care under those circumstances is to distribute other people's wealth without their consent. This is a stark but unavoidable conclusion of a strictly libertarian view of property rights, health care, and social governance. Whether this conclusion is consistent with the most minimal rudiments of professional ethics or with a good or just society is highly debatable.

Many managed care plans measure their success in terms of consumer satisfaction. But the relationship between satisfaction and quality is a tenuous one. Consumer satisfaction is not the whole of health care. The genuine difficulties of measuring quality outcomes are vastly under-rated by the satisfaction criterion. The young, those who have not needed the system, or those who make low demands might very well be satisfied with lower premiums and some of the advertising slogans. This is much less the case with the chronically ill, the aged, and those who make demands on the system. Data are appearing that show these patients have poorer outcomes in managed care systems than in fee-for-service systems (Ware et al. 1996). Others go through the "revolving door," leaving their capitated plan for Medicare and Medicaid coverage when they really become ill.

If Not a Commodity, What Is Health Care?

If, as I have argued, health care is not a commodity, if the consequences of treating it as such are morally unpalatable, and if it is a special kind of human activity derived from a universal need of all humans when they become ill, how should it be treated in a just society? Here we enter the complex, much-debated field of distributive justice, in general and in health care, and the very practical issues of health care reform and policy. These large subjects are well beyond the scope of this essay. But, by arguing against the commodity notion and the market ethic, I incur a certain obligation to point to the direction in which a morally tenable answer might lie.

Buchanan (1987) has summarized the major theories of justice associated with the distribution of health care. He has done so with care and with a fair appraisal of the strengths and weaknesses of each. In serial order, Buchanan examines the libertarian theories of Nozick (1974) and

Engelhardt (1996), the contractarian views of Rawls (1971) and Daniels (1985), the egalitarianism of Veatch (1986) and Menzel (1983). These theories all depend on whether or not there is a right of the sick to health care, created by the unfortunate circumstance of illness. The limitation of rights and rights language in public life are receiving more attention (Glendon 1991; Bellah et al. 1991). Rights language focuses too often on the negative rights of freedom from coercion and not enough on obligation and duties. Given the vulnerable and dependent state of sick persons, it is not intrusion on rights they fear, but abandonment to their fates by their fellow humans. As a result, there is a growing interest in communitarian and common good conceptions of justice.

Buchanan includes a non-rights-based approach which contends, instead, that there is a duty in beneficence to aid the needy and those in distress. In this view, health care is a "collective good." Government enforcement is necessary to ensure that this collective good is provided even to those who may not have a discernable "right" to it. In this approach, beneficence is given at least equal weight with justice, and the collective good at least as much weight as the individual good (Buchanan 1987, p. 558).

Another challenge to commodification is to regard medical and health care in a societal context as a public work, that is, as an ". . . organized medical response to illness in a social context and to the practice of caring in a community" (Jennings and Hanson 1995, p. 8). This notion needs further fleshing out. While it intimates a connection with the idea of a common or civic good, it remains somewhat vague. Importantly, it does return our attention to the fundamental questions about the social ethics of health care.

I believe that the moves to a *prima facie* obligation of beneficence on behalf of the sick (Buchanan 1987) or the practice of caring in a community (Jennings and Hanson 1995) are in the right direction. For a morally defensible policy of health care distribution, however, the obligation to provide health care needs firmer grounding in a philosophy of medicine and of society. In a theory built on *prima facie* principles, social beneficence could be overridden for good reason by other principles like autonomy or a competing theory of justice like Engelhardt's or Nozick's. A firmer justification can be found in the origins of a moral claim in the phenomena of illness and healing and in the notion of health care as common good. Together these realities would establish health care as a moral obligation a *good* society owes to all its members.

This is because health, or at least freedom from acute or chronic pain, disability, or disease, is a condition of human flourishing. Human beings cannot attain their fullest potential without some significant measure of health. A good society is one in which each citizen is enabled to flourish, grow, and develop as a human being. A society becomes good if it provides those goods which are most closely linked to being human. Health care is surely one of the first of these goods. It is, to be sure, not the only human good (Aristotle, *Nicomachean Ethics*, 1178b30–34). But other goods, like happiness, wealth, friends, career, etc., are compromised or even impossible without health.

In addition to the claim that arises out of the obligation of a good society to enhance the flourishing of its members, there is the non-proprietary, non-commodity character of medical knowledge alluded to in sections I and II above. The nature of medical knowledge and the way in which it is acquired and transmitted to health professionals make it a collective good on which the members of a society have a substantive claim. Human beings across national boundaries also contribute to the body of knowledge required in health care today. With varying degrees of strength, all humans are linked in a world community which shares in the fruits of medical research.

Health care is both an individual and a social good. A good and well-functioning human society requires healthy members, and healthy members require a good and well-functioning society. This reciprocity of dependence between individual and societal good implies a reciprocity of obligations as well. Aquinas puts the relationship between the individual and common good in this way:

> He who pursues the common good thereby pursues his own good for two reasons. First, because the proper good of the individual cannot exist without the common good of the family or state or realm. . . . Second, since a person is a part of a household or state, he ought to esteem that good for him which provides for the benefit of the community. (Aquinas, *ST* 2a2ae, q. 10, 2)

Any linkage of a social obligation to provide health care as a human good must engage the question of reciprocal responsibility of citizens to care for their own health. In a common good conception, the self-abuser, the person who refuses to buy insurance he or she can afford, or who refuses to take a genuine part in community life, imposes burdens on his fellow humans. Such persons weaken any claim they might have had to societal resources (Boyle 1977). Plato warned about hypochondriac or aged members of society whom he believed should not receive care (Heyd 1995).

This is a harsh judgment which a compassionate society could not impose strictly. It implies refusal to treat in the emergency room the self-abuser whose bleeding from esophageal varices are the result of alcoholic cirrhosis of the liver. Such retributive justice could not be consistent with the primary ethical obligation of physicians as healers. Perhaps a practical compromise is to discriminate against products like alcohol, tobacco, high-risk sports, etc. by taxation or higher premiums but not against persons who do not know how or do not care about their health (Evans 1988). After all, where does one draw the line on irresponsibility? How much exercise, weight-, or stress-reduction is enough to qualify for participation in the societal good? Who has pursued health so sedulously as to be free of lapses for which he is responsible? Where do we draw the bright line?

The role of government here is not forcefully to redistribute wealth in general or to bring about total equality in all things but to assure that collective goods, or the satisfaction of a common claim on such goods, are justly distributed. This approach does not translate into an unlimited claim on all the health care possible. It is not an invitation to "blank check" medicine. Nor does it mean that health care takes priority at all times and in all places over all other societal goods. Nor does it swallow private property rights in central planning. It does mean that there is a moral obligation of a good society to relieve the sufferings of its citizens, to provide what is needed for the fabric of society to hold together, and to see that the collective interest of society's members in health care is assured. This is, in effect, beneficent justice—justice ordered by the obligation to rescue, sustain, and nourish both society and the individual since each suffers if either is neglected or abused. This is a positive obligation that transcends the more negative or legalistic notion of "rights," but it is not an absolute obligation overriding all other obligations.

Treating health care as a common good implies a notion of the solidarity of humanity, i.e., the linkage of humans to each other as social beings. The common good is, however, more than economic good—necessary though this may be in an instrumental sense (Bellah 1991; Glendon 1991). It also implies the development of social and governmental institutions designed to promote justice and the well-being of the whole society in essential things like health, safety, environment, and education.

Nowhere does this conception militate against the protection of individual rights. It stands against the absolutization of the Marxian collective as well as the absolutization of Nozickian property rights. Rather, the morally defensible aim is a mixed economy: one in which private property and private enterprise are protected, but there is enough social control to assure justice, especially in those things that cannot be left to the fortuitous operations of the competitive marketplace (Ryan 1916). These things must always be few and of such nature that a healthy and well-functioning society could not exist without them.

It is especially important to recognize that rejection of a marketplace ethics for the distribution of health care does not make the market an unethical instrument for the distribution of most other goods and services. As Worland has shown, Adam Smith himself recognized that the market was not the preferred device for providing certain public goods like defense, education, or a transportation infrastructure or for setting rates of interest, etc. (Worland 1983, pp. 8–9). Smith had no difficulty reconciling liberty, private property, and government intervention when the rights of a few threatened to endanger the whole. In both *The Wealth of Nations* (1909) and *The Theory of Moral Sentiments* (1817), Smith saw a specific role for moral restraint on self-interest and of government's responsibility to prevent monopoly and to administer justice (Worland 1983, p. 21).

In this view, the role of the government is both to protect personal liberty and attend to those common goods that liberty destroys when it becomes license. How this balance is to be achieved is a constant struggle of democratic societies and institutions. What is crucial in health care is that any policy must take cognizance of the common social good, the shared moral claim on medical knowledge, and the special nature of health care as a human activity.

What is equally crucial is that the physician remain truly a physician, concerned with healing and not money-making (Plato, *Republic* 342c and 342d). In any plan in the future, the physician ought not be the gatekeeper, microallocator, or rationer. Nor should she or he become provider, insurer, or risk-taker simultaneously (O'Reilly 1998; Witten 1997; Wang 1996). The current move to establish the physician-provider organizations in which employers, hospitals, and corporations "buy" health care from groups of doctors are just as dubious morally as other capitated insurance plans. In addition, they deprive patients of their last advocate since the physician is the healer, the risk-taker, and the profit-maker simultaneously (Woolhandler and Himmelstein 1995). The assumption that physicians as administrators are more likely to represent patient interests if they own or administer the system is dubious at best. If earlier studies of higher prices and overutilization of doctor-owned radiology and laboratory facilities are accurate, this assumption is likely to be a dangerous myth.

This is not the place to design a total system of health care, nor to fill in the content of precisely what services constitute a fair share of the common good of health care, nor to speak of the costs, modes of payment, and choices among other societal goods. Obviously, those are the questions most often at issue in policy debates. But, in the end, those are second-order questions. They can be answered properly only in light of the first-order questions: What is health care? What kind of good is it? What moral claim do members of a society have on this good? What are society's obligations, and what are the obligations of the health professional with reference to that good?

Understanding health care to be a commodity takes one down one arm of a bifurcating pathway to the ethic of the marketplace and instrumental resolution of injustices. Taking health care as a human good takes us down a divergent pathway to the resolution of injustice through a moral ordering of societal and individual priorities.

One thing is certain: if health care is a commodity, it is for sale, and the physician is, indeed, a money-maker; if it is a human good, it cannot be for sale and the physician is a healer. Plato's question admits of only one ethically defensible answer.

> Can we deny, then, said I, that neither does any physician, insofar as he is a physician, seek to enjoin the advantage of the physician but that of the patient? (Plato, *Republic* 342c)

References

Anders, G. 1996. *Health Against Wealth: HMOs and the Breakdown of the Medical Trust.* New York: Houghton Mifflin.

Anderson, E. S. 1990. "Is Women's Labor a Commodity?" *Philosophy and Public Affairs* 19: 71–92.

Anderson, E. S. 1996. "The Ethical Limitation of the Market." *Economics and Ethics* 6: 179–205.

Aquinas, St. Thomas. 1974. *Summa Theologiae,* T. Gilby (trans.). New York and London: Blackfriars and McGraw-Hill.

Aristotle. 1984. *Nicomachean Ethics.* In *The Complete Works of Aristotle Volume II,* trans. and ed. J. Barnes. Princeton, NJ: Princeton University Press.

Bellah, R. et al. 1991. *The Good Society. New York:* Alfred A. Knopf.

Blair, M. M. 1995. *Ownership and Control: Rethinking Corporate Governance for the 21st Century.* Washington, DC: Brookings Institute.

Blecher, M. B. 1998. "Size Does Matter." *Hospitals and Health Networks* June 20, 1998: 29–36.

Bowie, N. E. and Duska, R. F. 1990. *Business Ethics, 2nd ed.* Englewood Cliffs, NJ: Prentice Hall.

Boyle, J. 1977. "The Concept of Health and the Right to Health Care." *Social Thought* Summer: 5–17.

Brecher, R. 1991. "Buying Human Kidneys: Autonomy, Commodity, and Power." *Journal of Medical Ethics* 17: 99.

Brink, S. 1996. "How Your HMO Can Hurt You." *U.S. News and World Report* 120: 62–64.

Buchanan, A. E. 1987. "Justice and Charity." *Ethics* 97: 558–575.

Busch, L. and Tanaka, K. 1996. "Rites of Passage: Constructing Quality in a Commodity Subsector." *Science, Technology, and Human Values* 21: 3–27.

Daniels, N. 1985. *Just Health Care.* Cambridge: Cambridge University Press.

Dionne, E. J. 1998. "The Big Idea." *Washington Post,* August 9, 1998: C1–C2.

Elola, J. 1996. "Health Care System Reforms in Western European Countries: The Relevance of Health Care Organization." *International Journal of Health Services* 26: 239–251.

Emanuel, E. J. 1995. "Medical Ethics in an Era of Managed Care: The Need for Institutional Structures instead of Principles in Individual Cases." *Journal of Clinical Ethics* 6(4): 335–338.

Engelhardt, H. T. 1996. *The Foundations of Bioethics,* 2nd ed. New York: Oxford University Press.

Enthoven, A. C. 1980. *Health Plan: The Only Practical Solution to the Soaring Cost of Medical Care.* Reading, MA: Addison-Wesley.

Evan, W. M. and Freeman, R. E. 1988. "A Stakeholder Theory of the Modern Corporation: Kantian Capitalism." In *Ethical Theory and Business* 3rd ed., ed.

T. L. Beauchamp and N. E. Bowie, pp. 97–106. Englewood Cliffs, NJ: Prentice Hall.

Evans, R. G. 1988. "We'll Take Care of It for You: Health Care in the Canadian Community." *Daedalus* 117: 155–189.

Federal Trade Commission. 1982. "In the Matter of the American Medical Association. Docket 9064, May 19, 1982." *Journal of the American Medical Association* 248: 981–982.

Flocke, S. A. et al. 1997. "The Impact of Insurance Type and Forced Discontinuity on the Delivery of Primary Care." *Journal of Family Practice* 45: 129–135.

Friedman, M. 1967. *Capitalism and Freedom. Chicago:* University of Chicago Press.

Friedman, M. 1970. "The Social Responsibility of Business Is to Increase Its Profits." *New York Times Magazine,* September 13, 1970: 33.

Gadamer, H. G. 1996. *The Enigma of Health: The Art of Healing in a Scientific Age. Stanford, CA:* Stanford University Press.

Glendon, M. A. 1991. *Rights Talk: The Impoverishment of Political Discourse. New York:* Free Press.

Greenberg, H. M. 1998. "Is American Medicine on the Right Track?" *Journal of the American Medical Association* 279: 426–428.

Greenberg, W. M. et al. 1989. "The Hospitalizable Patient as Commodity: Selling in a Bear Market." *Hospital and Community Psychiatry* 40(2): 184–185.

Hertzlinger, R. 1997. *Market-Driven Health Care.* Reading, MA: Addison-Wesley.

Heyd, D. 1995. "The Medicalization of Health: Plato's Warning." *Revue Internationale de Philosophie* 193(3): 375–393.

Iglehart, J. K. 1994a. "Health Care Reform and Graduate Medical Education: Part I." *New England Journal of Medicine* 330: 1167–1171.

Iglehart, J. K. 1994b. "Health Care Reform and Graduate Medical Education: Part II." *New England Journal of Medicine* 332: 407–411.

Immershein, A. W. and Lestes, C. 1996. "From Health Services to Medical Markets: The Commodity Transformation of Medical Production and the Non-Profit Sector." *International Journal of Health Services* 26: 221–237.

Jennings, B. and Hanson, M. J. 1995. "Commodity of Public Work? Two Perspectives in Health Care." *Bioethics Forum* Fall: 3–11.

Kassirer, J. 1997. "Managed Care's Tarnished Image." *New England Journal of Medicine* 337: 338–339.

Kuttner, R. 1998. "Must Good HMOs Go Bad?—Second of Two Parts: The Search for Checks and Balances." *New England Journal of Medicine* 338: 1635–1639.

Larson, E. 1996. "The Soul of an HMO." *Time Magazine* 147: 45–52.

McArthur, J. and Moore, F. D. 1997. "The Two Cultures and the Health Care Revolution: Commerce and Professionalism in Medical Care." *Journal of the American Medical Association* 277: 985–1005.

Menzel, P. T. 1983. *Medical Costs, Moral Choices.* New Haven, CT: Yale University Press.

Nozick, R. 1974. *Anarchy, State, and Utopia*. New York: Basic Books.

O'Reilly, B. 1998. "Taking on the HMOs." *Fortune* 137: 96–100.

Outka, G. 1976. "Social Justice and Equal Access to Health Care." In *Social Justice and Equal Access to Health Care*, ed. R. Veatch and R. Branson, pp. 79–126. Cambridge: Ballinger Publishing.

Patient Access and Responsibility Act. 1997. H.R.1415.

Pear, R. 1998. "Government Lags in Steps to Widen Health Coverage." *New York Times (interactive edition)*, August 9, National Desk Section.

Pellegrino, E. D. 1994. "Words *Can* Hurt You: Some Reflections on the Metaphors of Managed Care (First Annual Nicholas J. Pisacano Lecture)." *Journal of the American Board of Family Practice* 6/7: 505–510.

Pellegrino, E. D. 1995. "Medical Education." In *Encyclopedia of Bioethics*, rev. ed., vol. 3, ed. W. T. Reich, pp. 1435–1439. New York: Simon and Schuster/Macmillan.

Pellegrino, E. D. 1997. "Managed Care at the Bedside: How Do we Look in the Moral Mirror?" *Kennedy Institute of Ethics Journal* 7: 321–330.

Pellegrino, E. D. 2000. *The Lived World of Doctor and Patient*. New Haven, CT: Yale University Press.

Pellegrino, E. D. and Thomasma, D. C. 1988. *For the Patient's Good: The Restoration of Beneficence in Health Care*. New York: Oxford University Press.

Piderit, J. J. 1993. *The Ethical Foundations of Economics*. Washington, DC: Georgetown University Press.

Plato. 1982. *Republic*, P. Shorey (trans.). In *The Collected Dialogues of Plato*, ed. E. Hamilton and H. Cairns. Princeton, NJ: Princeton University Press.

President's Commission for the Study of Ethical Problems in Medicine and Behavioral Research. 1983. *Securing Access to Health Care*, vol. 1. Washington, DC: Department of Health, Education and Welfare.

Rawls, J. 1971. *A Theory of Justice*. Cambridge, MA: Harvard University Press

Ray, M. A. 1987. "Health Care and Human Caring in Nursing: Why the Moral Conflict Must Be Resolved." *Family and Community Health* 10: 35–43.

Reynolds, D. 1995. "Not Commodity and Not Public Work." *Bioethics Forum* Winter: 38–39.

Rodwin, M. A. 1995. "Strains in the Fiduciary Metaphor: Divided Physician Loyalties and Obligations in a Changing Health Care System." *American Journal of Law and Medicine* 21: 241–257.

Rodwin, M. A. 1996. "Consumer Protection and Managed Care: Issues, Reform Proposals, and Trade-Offs." *Houston Law Review* 32: 1319–1381.

Roulidis, Z. C. and Schulman, K. A. 1994. "Physician Communication in Managed Care Organizations: Opinions of Primary Care Physicians." *Journal of Family Practice* 39: 446–451.

Ryan, J. A. 1916. *Distributive Justice*. New York: Macmillan.

Sade, R. M. 1971. "Medical Care as a Right: A Refutation." *New England Journal of Medicine* 285: 1288–1292.

Sen, A. 1987. *On Ethics and Economics*. Oxford: Basil Blackwell.

Shortell, S. M. et al. 1996. *Remaking Health Care in America: Building Organized Delivery Systems*. San Francisco: Jossey-Bass.

Smith, A. 1817. *The Theory of Moral Sentiments*. Philadelphia: Anthony Finley.

Smith, A. 1909. *An Inquiry into the Nature and Causes of the Wealth of Nations*, ed. C. J. Bullock. New York: P. F. Collier.

Smith, M. B. 1997. "Trends in Health Care Coverage and Their Implications for Policy." *New England Journal of Medicine* 337: 1000–1003.

Starr, P. 1982. *The Social Transformation of American Medicine*. New York: Basic Books.

Titmuss, R. 1997. *The Gift Relationship: From Human Blood to Social Policy*. London: London School of Economics.

Veatch, R. M. 1986. *The Foundations of Justice*. New York: Oxford University Press.

Wang, C. 1996. "Unions and Equity HMOs: Two Sources of Physician Power in a World of Managed Care." *Family Practice Management* February 1996: 21–27.

Ware, J. E. et al. 1996. "Differences in 4-Year Health Outcomes for Elderly and Poor Chronically Ill Patients in HMO and Fee-for-Service Systems: Results from Medical Outcomes Study." *Journal of the American Medical Association* 216: 1039–1047.

Witten, D. 1997. "Regulation Downstream and Direct Risk Contracting: The Quest for Consumer Protection and a Level Playing Field." *American Journal of Law and Medicine* 23: 449–486.

Woolhandler, S. and Himmelstein, D. 1995. "Extreme Risk—The New Corporate Proposition for Physicians." *New England Journal of Medicine* 333: 1706–1707.

Woolhandler, S. and Himmelstein, D. 1997. "Costs of Care at For-Profit and Other Hospitals in the United States." *New England Journal of Medicine* 336: 769–774.

Worland, S. T. 1983. "Adam Smith, Economic Justice, and the Founding Father." In *New Directions in Economic Justice*, ed. R. Skurski, pp. 1–32. Notre Dame, IN: University of Notre Dame Press.

Zoloth-Dorfman, L. and Rubin, S. 1995. "The Patient as Commodity and the Question of Ethics." *Journal of Clinical Ethics* 6(4): 339–357.

Medicine Today

Its Identity, Its Role, and the Role of Physicians

Models of Medicine

Medicine as a Body of Knowledge

The commonest approach to a definition of medicine is to identify it with some body of knowledge useful in the treatment of illness. The dominant example of this genre is the so-called biomedical model, well articulated by Donald Seldin. Seldin defines medicine as biology applied to the cure and prevention of disease and the postponement of death. He specifically excludes social concerns, psychosocial elements, and bioethics as beyond the boundaries of the physician's knowledge base, though he does not deny their importance in society. Seldin summarizes his view this way: "Medicine is a discipline which subserves a narrow but vital arena. It cannot bring happiness, prescribe the good life, or legislate morality. But it can bring to bear an increasingly powerful conceptual and technical framework for the mitigation of that type of human suffering rooted in biomedical derangements."[1]

Seldin articulates clearly the dominant view of today's practitioners, teachers, and students. It has the virtue of limiting medicine to what it can do well, excluding what it does inadequately, and defining disease in terms of etiologies that are measurable and quantifiable. So attractive is the biomedical model that some investigations urge that it be the paradigm for psychopathology as well as somatic disease.[2]

The limitations of this model are several. For one thing, it is flagrantly reductionistic, limiting medicine to biology, chemistry, and physics. It suffers, therefore, from the logical and epistemological deficiencies of all reductionism.[3] It commits the error of circuitous reasoning—what we need for the proof is itself in need of proof by the settlement of the question we are asking. We cannot prove medicine is only biology unless we know first what medicine is—and that is the question.

The result is that the aims of medicine are determined by a preselected body of knowledge instead of medicine determining what knowledge it needs to achieve its ends. The error of reductionism is that it cannot logically exclude alternative reductions of medicine to applied sociology, psychology, or anthropology. Since these are admittedly elements of illness, why not assign them to the physicians and relegate the biological aspects to the biologists?

Even if we were to accept Seldin's reduction he does not tell us who is to provide the other kinds of knowledge needed to treat patients. How can those other dimensions be related to medicine? Who adjudicates the conflicts? Who decides what *should* be done for the patient? Since man is more than a biological being and his illness is more than biology, who manages the relationships between those different bodies of knowledge needed to heal? Seldin does not deny that human illness may rise in personal, familial, or social contexts or that it cannot be treated by biological means alone. What makes the patient "whole" again—since this is what healing means?

The most serious empirical limitation of the biomedical model is its one-dimensionality, its abnegation of the complexity of the experience of illness and therefore of the complexity of healing those who are ill. François Jacob, the molecular biologist, shows how limited this one-dimensionality can become: "The one-dimensional sequence of bases in the genes determines in some way the production of the two-dimensional cell layers that fold in a precise way to produce the three-dimensional tissues and organs that give the organism its shape, its properties, and, as Seymour Benzer puts it, its four-dimensional behavior."[4]

Since disease and illness involve all four dimensions it is hard to see how biology *qua* biology can be satisfactory as an explanatory principle, to say nothing of a therapeutic one. George Engel responds to the defects in the biomedical model by proposing one that includes biology as well as sociology and psychology and, he says, "will include the patient and his attributes as a person."[5] He (the doctor) must weigh the relative contributions of social and psychological as well as biological factors implicated in the patient's dysphoria and dysfunction as well as his decision to accept patienthood and with it the responsibility to cooperate in his own care. "It is the doctor's, not the patient's, responsibility to establish the nature of the problem and decide whether it is best handled in a medical framework. Hence the physician's basic professional knowledge must span the social, psychological and biological for his decisions on behalf of the patient involve all three."[6]

Engel goes further and offers general systems theory as an explanatory model rather than biology. In this way, he proposes to resolve the controversies between reductionists and holists. Systems theory, he says rather expansively, should be the "... blueprint for research, a framework for teaching and a design for action in the real world of health care."[7] Having expanded the model of medicine, he then confines it in a new mold— not of biology but of applied systems theory. The logical difficulties differ in degree but not in kind from Seldin's.

Engel's model has the virtue of including more of the realities of human illness, and vesting in the physician the task of fusing them in treating patients. It remedies some of the grosser deficiencies of the biomedical model but it still defines medicine in terms of a knowledge base, albeit a broader one. Indeed, so broad is this definition that it errs in the other direction, leaving out very little. It would not take much analysis to stretch the biopsychosocial model to embrace almost as much as the much-criticized WHO definition of health as complete physical, social, and emotional well-being.

Significantly, Engel does leave out one dimension—that is the spiritual, unless he includes it under the social and psychological. This is a dimension that the proponents of "holistic" medicine feel is also a part of medicine and healing.[8] Since religion, or at least some stance with reference to the transcendental, is part of the fabric of human existence, what justifies its exclusion?

Engel's theory, along with Seldin's and the others that define medicine in terms of a knowledge base, always ends up begging the question: What is medicine? Is it only the disconnected sum total of the kinds of knowledge it uses? If so, why is one combination of disciplines more pertinent than any other? The question can only be answered by recourse to something more fundamental in the nature of medicine itself, something which shapes what knowledge is needed and for what purpose. Engel, for a brief moment, touches this question when he refers to what patients are seeking in their encounter with the physician.[9] He quickly leaves it, however, to expatiate on the value of general systems theory as an organizing principle.

Systems theory may well provide a useful explanatory model for the interacting hierarchies of form and function that characterize human health and illness. But to make it, as Engel does, the "blueprint," "design," "framework" of the whole of medicine is to trade on one kind of reductionism—the biological—for another. Granting the utility of such a step, it can become a shackle on medicine. The explanatory utility of a paradigm does not qualify it as a theory of medicine. It has always been perilous to transpose the method and language of one discipline beyond its operational boundaries. We need only mention the misleading and even deleterious effects of the appropriation of such concepts as Darwinian evolution, entropy, relativity, Freudian or Jungian metapsychology, or Wilsonian sociobiology by social, political, and administrative theorists to illustrate this point.[10]

Neither Seldin's restrictionist nor Engel's expansionist theories are adequate as organizing principles. We are still left with the question: What is the nature of medicine, what knowledge does it need, what does it do?

Medicine Defined in Terms of Its End

An alternative approach to viewing medicine as a body of knowledge is to define it in terms of its end, its purpose, the terminus toward which medicine is directed as a human activity. The end then becomes the determining principle that defines what kind of knowledge medicine needs.

Leon Kass is one of the few theorists of medicine who analyzes the nature of medicine this way—a genuinely philosophical way. He declares the healthy human being the only "reasonable" goal of medicine. He rejects such goals as happiness, social adjustment, behavior modification, or the simple prolongation of life. "Health" is the end of medicine and not ". . . pleasure, happiness, civil peace and order, virtue, wisdom, and truth."[11]

Kass admits that he cannot define health precisely but he offers "wholeness" and "well-functioning" as approximations. Health is, he says, a "finite and natural norm," the ". . . well working of the organism as a whole, an activity of the human body in accordance with its specific excellence."[12] It is not only a somatic norm but a psychic one as well. Indeed, "our whole way of life" influences our health.[13]

On Kass's view, attainment of the end of health is the doctor's only business. His role should be limited to the use of only the technology and knowledge that advance therapeutic purposes. It is the physician, not the consumer or the government, that must define health care and the standards of practice. He questions expenditures for costly procedures like dialysis and doubts the validity of such concepts as the right to health and the benefit of national health insurance. Health, while it is a good end in itself, is not the only ingredient of a good life. Those other ingredients are not the domain of medicine.

Having tried to contract the domain of medicine, Kass then opens it up again. He says health is everybody's business—not only the physician's. Medicine itself must become "whole" again by attending to health maintenance as well as cure of illness. He urges more research in "healthiness," disease prevention, and health maintenance and that these become the determinants of health policy.

Kass's analysis has the virtue of defining medicine philosophically in terms of the purpose for which it is ordained or acts. Physicians and patients do in fact seek health through the acts of medicine. That is why health has been recognized as the end of medicine since Hippocrates. The weakness of this theory lies in the indefiniteness of the definition of health. While Kass limits the physician to the attainment of health for his patient, his notion of health has such wavering boundaries that it could include even those things Kass specifically excludes. How, for example, can we place social adjustment or behavior modification outside medicine? Can emotional or psychological illness be ameliorated without some attention to social adjustment? Can prevention which requires a change in lifestyle to be achieved without some modification of established behavior patterns? The doctor is enjoined to seek "wholeness" and well function of psyche and soma. These ends require the same breadth of concern and knowledge that Engel includes in his theory.

Defining medicine by its end is more sound philosophically than defining it as a knowledge base. But unless the end itself can be delineated, the boundaries balloon again when we try to realize that end in actual practice. Seldin's view at least has the virtue of specificity in its end—those illnesses susceptible to biological cure or amelioration. Furthermore, health is an abstract notion, an ideal toward which the doctor is supposed to work. As an ideal it is never fully attained. What is the doctor's function when health is not even relatively restorable, when the illness can only be ameliorated symptomatically or contained? What is the end of medicine when even these limited goals are not attainable? Surely one of the "ends" of medicine is to help the patient to cope with chronic illness or disability, or even to live the last days of life as comfortably and humanely as circumstances will allow.

Kass recognizes that responsibility for health is not solely medicine's. Everyone has some part in promoting his own health and society's. If this is so, we face the recurrent question: When is the pursuit of health the physician's duty and when not? Kass's theory never answers this question satisfactorily. It warns against using technology for "non-medical ends," but this depends on defining "medical"—something Kass does not do. As with Seldin and Engel, the central question remains.

Defining Medicine in the Patient-Physician Encounter

To obviate some of the difficulties of the knowledge and end-determined theories of medicine, one can approach the question more phenomenologically. Mark Siegler, for example, focuses his theory on the nature of the physician-patient relationship—on ". . . how clinical medicine works in the realities of daily practice."[14] He criticizes most theories because they are "context-free" and deductive, to which he opposes his own concept which is "context-dependent" and inductive.

Siegler's major thesis is that ". . . a problem becomes one for clinical medicine only when the patient and doctor agree that it is one."[15] Siegler sees the definition of medicine as the result of a negotiated agreement between individual patients and physicians. He sees the negotiation in four stages: (1) The decision by the patient that he is ill; (2) the physician's application of the clinical method to answer the patient's question of whether he is sick or has a serious disease; (3) the doctor-patient "accommodation" in which each decides whether or not to enter the relationship with the other; and (4) the doctor-patient "relationship" in which an exchange of trust occurs and a stable and prolonged relationship is established.[16]

Except for the second stage, Siegler feels that theories of health and disease have relatively little influence on the definition of clinical medicine. Its nature is defined principally by the resolution of individual doctor-patient accommodations. In that accommodation Siegler clearly leaves the final determination to the physician. He says that "every patient presentation generates a claim to be heard by physicians."[17] But it is the physician who determines whether he will manage *this* problem in *this* patient.

Siegler's formulation has the signal advantage of seeking a definition of medicine in the phenomena of clinical medicine itself—indeed, in what is most characteristic of medicine, the encounter between physician and patient. His description of the four clinical "moments" is sound so far as it goes. I too have used the term "clinical moment" in defining what is unique about medicine—but in a rather different sense from Siegler's.[18]

Unfortunately, Siegler does not really define clinical medicine. What he does is to describe the *process* whereby physician and patient agree to enter the clinical relationship, but not the essence of the relationship itself. The process of negotiation decides whether or not physician and patient will accept each other for what each claims to be—one claims to be sick, one claims to be able to heal. This would make medicine anything the physician and patient want it to be. Even if this were defensible in individual clinical encounters, it could not serve as a basis for public policy.

Siegler's four stages are propaedeutic to some end or purpose. It is what occurs after the decision is made that constitutes the clinical moment that sets medicine off from other activities. Doctor and patient may reject each other, but presumably at some point each engages in some other therapeutic relationship—and what happens once the engagement occurs is what defines clinical medicine. The process of negotiation cannot exhaust what we mean by clinical medicine, hence it cannot *define* clinical medicine. This is not to deny the utility of Siegler's description of the preludes to clinical medicine, but the prelude is not that which is essential to medicine as a human activity. Let us assume that the physician denies the patient's "claim" to be ill. If the patient accepts this decision he has been relieved, reassured, and educated. He has been healed, cured, or helped. Something more than a mere negotiation has occurred. If the patient does not accept the denial of his claim to be ill, the reason he consulted the doctor remains unattended. He will seek another physician who does agree to go beyond the negotiation. In either case some end beyond negotiation of a claim about illness must be served.

The potential latitude of a definition by negotiation makes it difficult to translate into public policy, education, or ethics. The narrowest and the broadest interpretations would be equally tenable. On which of these bases do we establish the physician's ethical obligations, the education he should receive, or the extent of what society should support as medical care?

Siegler's insistence on a definition based in the reality of clinical medicine itself is superior to the knowledge or end-oriented definitions. It does not go far enough, however, into the central phenomenon of the physician-patient encounter. Since it leaves the ultimate definition to the physician who evaluates a patient's claim to be ill, the physician's philosophical conception of medicine is far more influential than Siegler allows.

Siegler shares with Seldin, Kass, and Engel the conviction that it is the physician's specific duty to define what is health, a view Whitbeck and others would contest. Whitbeck defines health as ". . . the psychophysiological capacity to act or respond appropriately in a variety of situations."[19] She argues that medical expertise is not relevant to many health decisions and concludes that some of these decisions are best made by the person whose health is at stake. One might raise the same question about the definition of illness, which is, after all, a subjective experience which the physician penetrates only partially and incompletely.

Fabrega takes the external definition even further, showing how social, personal, and cultural norms determine health, disease, and illness.[20] Since medicine is part of the socio-cultural and ethnic fabric of societies it is related to the dominant characteristics of society. This view has merits for homogeneous cultures with univalent value systems. For multivalent systems like ours, the question remains: What is medicine? If it is defined externally, which of the many possible value systems should predominate?

Every society and era does indeed provide some system of succor for its members who, because of illness or trauma, cannot function in their accustomed social roles. The social and cultural definitions of health and illness may vary, but the need for healing is a constant. It is in that constant fact that we should seek our organizing principle—the universal fact that humans become ill, and in that state seek and need help, healing, and cure. However the cultural milieu may differ, this fact is common to all medical systems. Thus the immediate and practical end of medicine is an action taken in behalf of one who is ill, who has decided that his unease is significant enough to warrant a decision to seek medical help. Health is a more remote end. It is attainable only if the special human relationship of healing is a successful one. It is that relationship which provides the architectonics of medicine as medicine, and not health, which may not even be attainable for many who seek help and healing.

The Goals and Ends of Medicine

The *essentialist* approach is grounded in the nature of medicine, in what sets it apart from other activities as an enterprise of a special kind, and defines it as something in the real world independent of the construction society might put upon that reality. This approach is based in a real definition, a grasp of some extramental reality from which we abstract that which makes a thing what it is and separates it from all those other characteristics it possesses: its so-called accidents, or that which is not crucial to what a thing is.

Before defining the content of this essentialist approach, it is important to take note of the strong objections leveled against any essentialist position today.

First, many contemporary thinkers accept Wittgenstein's rejection of real definitions as imaginary or impossible. For Wittgenstein any congruence between the real world and the language we use to describe it is merely a matter of grammatical articulation. As he puts it, "Essence is expressed as grammar."[21] "Grammar tells what kind of object anything is."[22] On this view, Aristotle's definition of a thing by its essence and all of Socrates' "What is . . ." questions are illusory. They cannot get at real world essences.[23]

Second, if real definitions are not possible, we cannot define ends or goals intrinsic to medicine. We can only define goals by deciding the uses to which we want to put medicine. By defining the goals we choose, we can define what medicine is. On this instrumentalist view, the ends of medicine can only be a project for social construction, generated by what we want to achieve socially, politically, economically, and legally. Theoretically we could "construct" medicine in such a way as to divert it totally, or in part, from its dedication to the care of the sick, or we could add to it any function we might wish, like gatekeeping or assisting in state-ordered executions, or involuntary or nonvoluntary euthanasia.

A third objection is that an essentialist definition puts arbitrary limits on the goals of medicine. Goals, it is argued, could be independent of traditional goals of healing, curing, caring, and helping individual patients. On a socially constructed model, the limits of medicine can be expanded or contracted by societal fiat. Thus, the majority opinions of both the Second and the Ninth Circuit Court include physician assistance in suicide as part of the practice of medicine[24] This inclusion is a sociolegal construction of practice. If the opinions are upheld by the Supreme Court, assisted suicide may be offered to patients as the "standard" of practice. Or a patient or a society could stretch the limits of medicine to include provision of whatever treatment a society might want, even if it is scientifically futile or even harmful to individual patients.

A final objection, which any attempt to derive essences must confront, is the problem of separating what to include in the "essence" from what to leave out. On the view I shall present, this determination is not arbitrary; that is, what is essential is derivable from the phenomena of medicine itself, from the concrete realities of the physician-patient relationship, or from what healing, helping, caring, and curing entail, a point I will develop in more detail later in this essay.

Here is not the place to engage in an epistemological and metaphysical rebuttal of the objections against essentialism. It suffices for my present purposes simply to compare and contrast the logical consequences of essentialism and social construction since the question is which one should have primacy in determining the ends and goals of medicine.

Social Construction: Goals before Ends

An influential approach today is the definition of reality and morals through social construction. The foundation of this approach so far as goal setting goes is that there is little likelihood of agreement on such things as essences, definitions, or ethical norms. In consequence, there can be no universalizable ends of purposes.[25] Rather, these must be defined by each community in terms of its own values and perceptions of reality.[26] On this view, reality itself, knowledge, and nature are social constructs. Medicine becomes primarily a social endeavor since its concepts of disease, illness, healing, and health are all socially defined. Social construction comes in many forms as varied as the social reality of Schutz's everyday world and Marxian praxis.[27] Social constructions have in common an emphasis on subjectivity, intersubjectivity, process, dialogue, and consensus as the sources of social realities like morality, medicine, and social good.

In any case, the term "social construction" as used in the Hasting Center Goals of Medicine project report[28] is not taken in this strictly formal philosophical sense. One therefore need not engage its full epistemic or ontological implications. Rather, "social constructionist" is used in the project report to apply to a process definition of the goals of medicine, arrived at by social dialogue, consensus formation, political process, or negotiation. It is in this latter, more general sense, that I will take the term when comparing it with the essentialist viewpoint.

This is not the place to discuss the various forms of social construction. But there are certain conceptual difficulties common to social construction in general. I will confine myself to the difficulty they present to defining the goals of medicine.

First of all, to accept social constructionism is to accept that there is ultimately nothing permanent or universalizable about medicine. If so, its goals can be defined only in an ephemeral manner. They will change with each new construction and have no permanence. The whole project of goal setting is perilous as a result. If we are continually redefining medicine and its goals, how far beyond the present social moment can we look in confronting the issues the project report so well identifies?

The second difficulty with constructed models is that they conflate the meanings of ends, goals, and purposes and use these terms interchangeably. In the social construction models, goals can stand for whatever political, economic, physician, citizen, or other groups determine them to be. On this view, the ends are simply the uses to which medical knowledge or physicians can be put. It is in this sense that many use the term "goals" when they speak of reshaping the goals of medicine.

Ends are not the same as goals. Ends in the classical sense of *telos* are tied to the nature of medicine, to its essence. Ends serve to define medicine. Without certain ends, the activity in question does not qualify as medicine. The ends of medicine distinguish it from other arts and sciences that have different ends. To convert the ends of medicine to the purposes of economics, politics, or professional prerogative transforms medicine into economics, politics, or professional preference.

Medical science, for example, can be used to advance the ends of medicine, but medical science is not *per se* medicine. It becomes medicine only when it is used to advance the ends of medicine, that is, only in the clinical encounter, with the needs of a particular patient. Medical knowledge *per se* has uses other than cure, care, help, or healing of the sick. It can be used to cure animals, or manipulate their genes, synthesize new organic molecules, attain economic goals or political advantage, and so on. Only when medical knowledge is focused on the healing of *this* patient, here and now, or on promoting the health of society as a whole is it medicine *per se*.

Goals and purposes, unlike ends, are not formally tied to the essence of medicine. They may conform to the ends of medicine, but they may not. The goals and purposes to which we put medical knowledge or activity may even destroy medicine or frustrate its proper ends. The list of possible distortions of the healing purposes of medicine is a long one: torturing political prisoners, genocide, "cleansing" society of the unfit or handicapped, participating in state-ordered executions, making political converts, punishing political dissidents, or managing medical care for nonmedical purposes such as profit or political power. Goals and purposes are therefore unrestrained by the specific ends intrinsic to what medicine is. They are subject to many social interpretations, some quite inimical to the ends of medicine.

Socially constructed goals—as long as they have social sanction—open medicine to possible subversion by economics, politics, social ideology, or government, and this openness is an ever-present threat to the integrity of medicine as a practice. The ends internal to medicine are the compass points by which goals and purposes can be measured. Ends provide the mooring for medical ethics. The enormous extent of medicine's technical power is vulnerable to the pathological use a disordered society may wish to make of it unless it is restrained by the ends proper to medicine.

Finally, which community of values shall determine the goals of medicine? We all belong to many communities—family, neighborhood, school, church, profession, political party, and social group—and the values of these overlapping communities may conflict with each other. Which shall have primacy when this occurs? How do we decide to choose one community's values over another? Is there such a thing as a good society and good medicine? If so, then we are back at a dilemma: either we strive for an essentialist definition of the good society and good medicine, or we submit to constant revision of the ends of both medicine and society.

An Essentialist Construction: Ends over Goals

On the essentialist view, the ends of medicine are defined internally out of the nature of medicine itself. They grow out of the phenomenology of medicine, that is, out of that which is more fundamental than medicine itself—the universal human experience of illness. It is the universality of this experience, its existence beyond time, place, history, or culture—and the need of sick persons for care, cure, help, and healing—that gives medicine its essential character. These ends make medicine what it is. On this view, the ends of medicine are the same for Hippocrates among the Ancient Greeks, Maimonides in the Middle Ages, Sydenham in the eighteenth century, Osler in the nineteenth century, and for the nameless physicians who will take care of those who are ill on the first spaceship to penetrate intergalactic space.

Several things are notable about this way of defining the ends of medicine. First, it depends on a real, not a nominal, definition of medicine, one which describes something in the real world, not just a language game or simply the way we use the word "medicine." Second, the ends of medicine are built into the reality of medicine as a special kind of human activity. Third, the limits of medicine are also built into its ends. When those ends are no longer achievable—when treatment is not effective or beneficial, or when cure cannot be achieved—care and helping become primary ends.

These are the ends of medicine, and they are as old as medicine itself. They define medicine. They are its essence. From the beginning they had to be defined to answer those who denied that medicine existed as a separate endeavor or that it qualified as an art. For example, the Hippocratic authors had to make clear that medicine was distinct from both religion and philosophy, that it was "invented" to care for the sick and had its own practitioners to achieve this end. "Let us consider also whether the acknowledged art of medicine, that was discovered for the treatment of the sick, and has both a name and artists has the same object as the other art and what its origin was. In my opinion, nobody would have even sought for medicine if the same ways of life had suited both the sick and those in health."[29]

Elsewhere the Hippocratic author(s) provide a more specific definition of the ends of medicine, noting its limitations as well. "First I will define what I conceive medicine to be. In general terms, it is to do away with the suffering of the sick, to lessen the violence of their diseases, and to refuse to treat those who are overmastered by their diseases, realizing that in such cases medicine is powerless."[30]

Later on, in the same treatise, the Hippocratic author places limits on what the patient may expect from medicine and insists that it ought not be used when it is futile, that is, when its ends cannot be attained. "Whenever, therefore, a man suffers from an ill which is too strong for the means at the disposal of medicine, he surely must not even expect that it can be overcome by medicine."[31]

But even if a case is not medically curable, the patient is not abandoned. Other ends than cure are recognized as ends for medicine. "Why forsooth trouble one's mind about cases which have become incurable? This is far from the right attitude. The investigation of these matters too belongs to the same science; it is impossible to separate them from one another. In incurable cases we must contrive ways to prevent their becoming incurable [. . .] while one must study incurable cases so as to avoid doing harm by useless efforts."[32]

In later centuries the ends of medicine were spelled out a little differently but in fidelity to the Hippocratic definition with emphasis on the phenomena of healing and helping. Here is one example. "It is the duty of the doctor in the first place to cure us; in the second to be kind to us; in the third to be true to us; in the fourth to keep our secrets; in the fifth to warn us and best of all to forewarn us; in the sixth to be grateful to us; and in the last to keep his time and his temper."[33]

Objection may be made at this point that the ancient texts do not speak of prevention specifically as one of the ends of medicine. This is true, but it does not mean that prevention was not recognized or respected as an end of medicine. Indeed, in the Hippocratic era, the culture of health was closely tied to the whole idea of education.[34] Gymnastics, diet, and hygiene were critical for the Hippocratic physicians and intrinsic to the education of citizens of the Greek state. Prevention was thus the concern not only of medicine but of a good life of body and mind.

Clearly we have in these ancient sources intrinsic definitions of the ends that set medicine apart as a certain kind of human activity. At the same time, we are introduced to the limits of medicine—to the now much-discussed notion of futility—to those times when medicine ought not be used since its ends are no longer attainable. But even then, care and help were recognized as ends intrinsic to the art of medicine.

I would expand the derivation of the ends of medicine by an extension of these concise definitions of the Hippocratic writers. Like them, we must assert the obvious: medicine exists because humans become sick. It is an activity conceived to attain the overall end of coping with the individual and social experience of disordered health. Its end is to heal, help, care and cure, to prevent illness, and cultivate health. Medicine itself is a true art because it pursues its ends with knowledge and understanding for the good of its object—the sick person or social group—and in a practical way.[35]

In its everyday clinical practice, the ends of medicine are technically right and morally good decisions and actions made by, and with, the person who is ill. Both the technical and moral good are essential to the craft of medicine if it is to achieve its ends of healing, helping, caring, and curing.[36] It may achieve those ends by a variety of means, but those means are always constrained by the ends.

On this view, physicians do not determine the ends of medicine; it is their task to realize these ends in a specific clinical encounter with a particular patient. Physicians are charged with ascertaining, together with the patient, the content of the end of healing. Note, the content of healing is not a social construction of the end, but it accepts healing as an end. It is healing which is specific to this patient, not healing as an end. For this healing, technical knowledge is essential, but not sufficient. That knowledge must also be applied within the context of the patient's notion of health and well-being. Thus, medicine could not be defined solely as knowledge-based, but as knowledge, based and directed to a specific end—knowledge directed by an architectonic principle—healing or helping a sick person become whole again.

This forum is not the place to expand on the details of the nature of the healing relationship. Thomasma and I have done so in extenso elsewhere. Here I wish only to note that the ends of medicine are related to the reasons humans established medicine—that is, as a response to a universal and common experience of illness.

It is this healing end of medicine in the context of patient vulnerability that determines not only the technical practice of clinical medicine but also the ethic of medicine. The physician offers to help, professes to have the needed craft and to use that craft in the interests of the person confronting the experience of illness. The ends of medicine thus define the moral obligations, the virtues, duties, and principles that constitute medical ethics. This role is their justification, not the fact that doctors have constructed ethical codes or that society has mandated legal regulation of the profession. Clinical medicine, preventive medicine, nursing, public health, and social and community medicine each have ends arising out of specific health needs. These too are derivable from the phenomena with which they deal. By analogy with our analysis of the ends of clinical medicine, each health profession is shaped by a specific set of ends that set it apart and give it a needed role in the larger spectrum of "health care."

This line of reasoning does not assume that defining the ends of medicine as intrinsic to medicine necessitates that physicians are the arbiters of those ends. In the essentialist view, physicians themselves are bound by the ends internal to medicine as a specific kind of human activity. They can make, have made, are making, and will make errors in defining those ends. If the ends of medicine are derived from a critical examination of the nature of medicine, I argue, these errors can only be identified and corrected by reference to the inherent ends of medical action which are in turn derived from the phenomenon of healing.

But if physicians have no epistemological sovereignty in defining the ends of medicine, neither do economists, politicians, policymakers, or ordinary citizens. What all of us must do is determine how to use medical knowledge and skill to bring the goals and purposes we assign to medicine into conformity with its intrinsic ends. It is the *telos* or goal of the medical craft that provides the ethical restraint in the way medicine is used. No social mechanism, regal fiat, legislative, or professional decree should be immune to the test of congruence with the ends internal to medicine as a special kind of human activity.

Whenever medicine is used for any purpose or goal—however defined—that distorts, frustrates, or impairs its capacity to achieve its proper ends, it loses its integrity as a craft and its moral status as a human activity. This consequence is true whether the distortion is generated by physicians, economics, politics, or exigency of any kind.

We have socially crucial reasons for maintaining the internally defined ends of medicine. Without ends, there is no source of criticism, no counter to the most malevolent uses of the power of medical knowledge and skill by individuals, societies, or governments. To the extent that they are genuinely faithful to the ends of medicine, physicians must set limits on what they will do in the name of medicine, no matter what the social construction of medicine may demand of them. They must know when to say "no." This refusal is what the Nazi and Soviet physicians failed to muster. It is their infamy—not to have resisted a malevolent social construction of medicine.

Economics, politics, cultural and social values, and mores are important. But they are not sovereign. They are subject to restraint, criticism, and even refusal when they seriously impair the ends of medicine. Once we accept a socially constructed external definition of those ends, we eradicate these restraints at the peril of the sick and of society tself.

Notes

1. D. Seldin, "The Boundaries of Medicine. Presidential Address," *Transactions of the Association of American Physicians* 94(1981): 75–86.

2. S. Kety, "From Rationalization to Reason." *American Journal of Psychiatry* 131(1974): 957–963.

3. R. Nozick, *Philosophical Explanations* (Cambridge, MA: Harvard University Press, Cambridge, 1981).

4. F. Jacob, *The Possible and the Actual* (Seattle and London: University of Washington Press, 1982), p. 44.

5. G. Engel, "The Clinical Application of the Biopsychosocial Model," *American Journal of Psychiatry* 137(1980): 535–544.

6. G. Engel, "The Need for a New Medical Model: A Challenge for Biomedicine," *Science* 196(1977): 129–136.

7. Ibid.

8. D. Allen et al., *Whole-Person Medicine* (Downers Grove, IL: Inter-Varsity Press, 1980). See also "The Good" in *The Encyclopedia of Philosophy,* ed. P. Edwards (New York: Free Press, 1967), 3:367–370.

9. G. Engel, "The Clinical Application of the Biopsychosocial Model."

10. E. D. Pellegrino, "Biology and Public Administration: Some Touchstones Scrutinized," in *Critic Cornerstones of Public Administration,* ed. Philip Schorr (Boston: Oelgeschlager, Gunn, and Hain, 1985).

11. L. Kass, "Regarding the End of Medicine and the Pursuit of Health," *The Public Interest* 40(1975): 11–42.

12. Ibid.

13. Ibid.

14. E. D. Pellegrino and D. C. Thomasma, *A Philosophical Basis of Medical Practice: Toward a Philosophy and Ethic of the Healing Professions* (New York: Oxford University Press, 1981).

15. M. Siegler, "The Doctor-Patient Encounter and Its Relationship to Health and Disease," in *Concepts of Health and Disease: Interdisciplinary Perspectives,* ed. A. Caplan et al. (Reading, MA: Addison-Wesley, 1981), pp. 627–644

16. Ibid.

17. Ibid.

18. E. D. Pellegrino, "Philosophy and Medicine: Problematic and Potential," *Journal of Medicine and Philosophy* 1(1976): 5–31.

19. C. Whitbeck, "A Theory of Health," in *Concepts of Health and Disease,* ed. A. Caplan et al., pp. 611–626.

20. H. Fabrega, "Concepts of Disease: Logical Features and Social Implications," *Perspectives in Biology and Medicine* 1(1973): 538–617.

21. L. Wittgenstein, *Philosophical Investigations,* 3rd ed., G. E. M. Anscombe, trans. (New York: Macmillan, 1968), p. 16.

22. Ibid.

23. Ibid., p. 6.

24. *Quill v. Vacco,* 80FBd 716 (2nd Cir. 1996); *Compassion in Dying v. State of Washington* 49FBd 790 (9th Cir. 1996).

25. H. T. Engelhardt, Jr., *The Foundations of Bioethics,* 2nd ed. (New York: Oxford University Press, 1996), pp. 189–238.

26. P. L. Berger and T. Luckmann, *The Social Construction of Reality: A Treatise in the Sociology of Knowledge* (Garden City, NY: Doubleday, 1966).

27. N. Lobkowia, *Theory and Practice: History of a Concept from Aristotle to Marx* (Notre Dame, IN: University of Notre Dame Press 1967); A. Schutz, *Collected Papers,* ed. M. Natanson, vol. 1, *The Problem of Social Reality,* 2nd ed. (The Hague: Martinus Nijhoff, 1967).

28. The Hastings Center, *The Goals of Medicine: Setting New Priorities.* Briarcliff Manor, NY: The Hastings Center, 1996.

29. Hippocrates, "Ancient Medicine," in *Hippocrates,* trans. W. H. S. Jones (Cambridge, MA: Harvard University Press, 1923), 1:21.

30. Hippocrates, "The Art," in *Hippocrates,* trans. W. H. S. Jones (Cambridge, MA: Harvard University Press, 1923), 2:193.

31. Ibid., p. 205.

32. Hippocrates, "On Joints," in *Hippocrates,* trans. W. H. S. Jones (Cambridge, MA: Harvard University Press, 1923) 3:339.

33. J. Brown, *Horae Subsecivae* (London: A. and C. Black, 1907), p. 407.

34. W. Jaeger, *Paideia: The Ideals of Greek Culture,* trans. G. Highet, vol. 3, *The Conflict of Cultural Ideas in the Age of Plato* (New York: Oxford University Press, 1944), pp. 3–45.

35. See W. Jaeger, *Commentary on Plato's Gorgias,"* 465a, 464a, in *Paideia: The Ideals of Greek Culture,* trans. G. Highet, vol. 2, *In Search of the Divine Centre* (New York: Oxford University Press, 1944).

36. E. D. Pellegrino and D. C. Thomasma, *For the Patient's Good: The Restoration of Beneficence in Health Care* (New York: Oxford University Press, 1988).

From Medical Ethics to a Moral Philosophy of the Professions

When I joined the Kennedy Institute of Ethics in 1978, I was no stranger to medical ethics. I had been reading and studying the subject since 1940, my junior year in college. My major field of study was chemistry. However, pre–World War II Catholic colleges required four years of philosophy and four of theology regardless of what undergraduate major field one chose to study. I was fortunate in that these subjects were just as fascinating to me as chemistry. As a result, both fields provided the launching pad for my later scholarly research in the laboratory and in philosophy.

I was first introduced to medical ethics by my college professors, who lent me books and papers in medical ethics taken from the 400-year-old Roman Catholic tradition of medical morality. I was thus sensitized to the indispensability of medical ethics to the practice of medicine and to my personal integrity as a Roman Catholic physician. I read and discussed the issues then current without the slightest doubt about their relevance to my future medical practice. At that time, Aldous Huxley's *Brave New World,* published in 1932, had already provided arresting insights into the complex ethical and social issues that could result from progress in human and animal biology. Debates about genetics, artificial placentas, biotechnology, and technocracy were already under way in class and in conversations outside class. Earlier "sci-fi" novels by Jules Verne and H. G. Wells foresaw the technological possibilities of time and space travel. George Orwell's *1984,* published later in 1949, gave a graphic and chilling picture of a technocratic society. The "brave new world" was already a visible ethical morass, and the need for ethical constraints on the advance of technology was appreciated.

These imaginative literary prognostications were not evident in medical practice when I entered medical school. In 1941, specific treatments that effectively changed the natural history of disease were scant in number. The list was a small one: arsenic for syphilis, liver extract for "pernicious anemia," quinine for malaria, insulin for diabetes, digitalis for heart failure, and a few others. Medicine's dramatic and unprecedented power to alter the human condition was still a promissory note.

To be sure, the sulfonamides had made their appearance a few years earlier. Penicillin came to us in my final year in school as a dirty-colored powder in a vial to be used experimentally to treat pneumonia and subacute bacterial endocarditis. This was the beginning of the era prematurely dubbed the "conquest of infectious disease." The basic science and the pharmacological and genetic intricacies of today's medicine were scarcely imagined. Medical ethics in consequence was largely confined to professional ethics, taught, if at all, as a set of precepts to be followed, not a subject for critical ethical appraisal.

In my own case, I do not recall medical ethics being mentioned, except in small informal discussions among students and residents. Catholic students did worry about certain dilemmas associated with obstetrical practice. For the most part it was assumed that we would discover what was right on our own. Among both Catholics and non-Catholics abortion and euthanasia were almost universally condemned, as were the "corporate practice" of medicine and for-profit doctor-owned hospitals.

Some passing references to the traditions of medical ethics were made in discussions in a medical history club. But since my class was on an accelerated schedule, finishing the whole curriculum in three years because of World War II, there was really no time for reflective thinking. My own reading continued, however, through my medical school residency years.

I myself began to teach medical ethics at the bedside to residents and medical students in 1960 when I became chairman of the department of medicine at the University of Kentucky. I first began then to write and publish on a variety of topics in medical ethics and the humanities in medicine (McElhinney and Pellegrino 2001, pp. 291–317). I approached these topics then, as I do now, from an Aristotelian-Thomist realist stance and with a scholastic taste for distinctions and definitions.

In the mid-1960s, it became clear that most of medical ethics was really medical morality—a set of assertions and moral precepts without a formal groundwork of ethical justification or argumentation. While many of these moral precepts might be valid, without a justifiable ethical foundation they could easily be challenged, denied, or compromised. This is indeed what happened when medical morals were subjected to critical philosophical inquiry in the early 1970s.

Professional philosophers began to take medical ethics seriously and to look for principled arguments for the resolution of professional and clinical ethical dilemmas. This was a departure, since until that time philosophers had largely ignored medical ethics. Even physician-philosophers like John Locke, Karl Jaspers, or William James failed to do a systemic analysis of the ethics of their original professions. To be sure, Plato, Aristotle, and the Stoics used medicine to illustrate their philosophical arguments. But none produced a treatise on medical ethics itself (Jaspers 1963).

When serious study of medical ethics was initiated, it consisted largely in the application of existing philosophical or theological systems to medicine. These systems were "applied" or, better, superimposed on medicine and its practice. None derived an ethic of medicine beginning with medicine or looking at the nature of medicine itself as a special kind of human activity.

At the same time, historical and sociological critics disassembled the Hippocratic ethic and ethos. The ancient idea of a universal set of duties binding all physicians as physicians across time and national boundaries was seriously eroded. Demands for a "new" ethic more suitable to the times and mores multiplied and continue to this day. The whole enterprise of medical and professional ethics was headed to definition by social convention and consensus, a pathway I believed then and believe now to be deleterious to patients and to society.

Contravening these trends, I thought then, and I think now, that the ethics of medicine should be based in the nature of the medical relationship, that is, in a philosophy *of* medicine. My thesis then was, and remains, that the obligations specific to physicians arise from the special features of the personal relationship between the person who is ill and the person the ill person seeks for help. The resulting relationship has certain features that give it a special character that generates special mutual moral duties.

This does not mean that medical ethics is isolated from general ethics or that the principles, rules, and duties of medical ethics as a discipline are self-justifying. It does, I believe, mean that the determination of which principles, duties, and virtues are most pertinent is linked to the nature of the human relationships that are central to the clinical encounter. The exploration of the existential, experiential, and phenomenological aspects of being ill, professing to heal, and healing seemed the most likely starting point for a philosophy of medicine and the first step to the ethics of medicine.

This approach fitted well with my own years of expertise as a clinician and with my earlier training in the realism of existential Thomism and some of its extensions in phenomenological realism (Von Hildebrand 1973; Seifert 1984). I had been introduced to the possibilities of the phenomenological method through my friendship and conversations with Professor Erwin Straus. I did not accept the transcendental dimensions of Husserl's philosophy, but Straus helped me to see in his critique of the Cartesianism of modern psychology that the primacy of the world of the senses could be recovered (Straus 1963).

Indeed, my contact with Professor Straus led me to my first effort to link philosophy and medicine (Pellegrino 1966, pp. 272–284). This was my first effort at a philosophy of medicine in its broadest terms. It revealed my conviction that a philosophical anthropology was an existential element in any moral philosophy for medicine. It was also behind my interest in developing a journal linking philosophy and medicine. These ideas were further developed by others and by me in the early issues of the *Journal of Medicine and Philosophy,* which was first published in 1976.

In 1976 I published my own first attempt to ground an ethic of medicine in a specific philosophy of medicine, that is, in a philosophy of the interpersonal relationship between physician and patient in the "clinical encounter"—that moment when a decision and action must be taken which will be for the good of the patient, both technically and morally (Pellegrino 1976, pp. 35–56). In that paper I argued that three phenomena of the clinical encounter should serve as the starting point of a definition of what makes medicine what it is. This paper later served as the starting point for *A Philosophical Basis of Medical Practice* (Pellegrino and Thomasma 1981), and in fact an extended version of it forms the first chapter of that work.

These three phenomena were (1) the existential fact of illness or disease, (2) the act of promise or profession by the physician who offers to help the patient caught in the predicament of illness, and (3) the act of medicine—making the technically right and the morally good decision that best serves the needs of the sick person as grasped by that person and her physician. The close relationship of these three universal phenomena—being ill, promising to heal, and healing itself—provided a foundation in the real world for the obligations of the physician and patient to each other.

I argued that illness wounded our humanity, challenged our self-image, limited our freedom in special ways, and made us vulnerable ontologically and existentially. A physician who offered to help a human in this altered existential state incurred obligations to act in such a way that the purpose of the encounter—healing, helping, caring, curing—could be achieved. The primacy of the good of the patient was the *locus ethicus* of the relationship. This primacy could only be preserved if physicians are competent, discern the complex nature of the patient's good, are compassionate, practice some degree of suppression of self-interest, and protect the inherent dignity of the patient as a human person.

On this view, the immediate telos of the clinical relationship is the good of the patient or, in more clinical terms, a right and good healing and helping act. If this telos or end is to be achieved, certain character traits are entailed—fidelity, trust, benevolence, truth telling, intellectual honesty, humility, courage, suppression of self-interest—at a minimum. These character traits are entailed not because they are admirable; they are admirable because they are essential to achieving the ends and purposes of medicine. These ends derive from the realities of the clinical encounter and not from societal convention, construction, negotiated agreement, or contract.

Many of these duties and virtues were expressed or implied in the Hippocratic Oath and the deontological books of the corpus. But they do not derive their moral authority because they are in the oath. The oath

simply reflects the moral content of the patient-physician personal healing and helping relationship (Pellegrino 2001, pp. 70–87). My hope has
been that my analysis of the source of the doctor's obligations and virtues
will give moral substance to the oath and explain why it has had such a
long-standing place of influence in medical ethics.

I do not assert that medical ethics is the privileged domain of the doctor, but that it is imposed on the doctor by the very nature of what he purports to do as a physician. Nor do I argue that medicine is the only healing
profession defined by these moral considerations. Indeed, as my subsequent work, alone and with David Thomasma, emphasizes, they are requisite features of the other health professions and of other professions.
Each helping profession confronts vulnerable, dependent, and anxious
human beings and possesses and professes the special knowledge and skill
needed by those persons.

I also hold that these realities of the clinical encounter reflect universal human needs experienced by human beings in whatever era, cultural
milieu, or ethnic category they exist. They are in fact human experiences
modified by culture and history but not in any essential way. These were
the realities that faced the Hippocratic physicians, the Shaman, medicine
man, or curandero, as well as the technologically trained physician of
today and tomorrow. As long as humans are mortal, become ill, and are
altered existentially by illness and disease, they will need help, healing,
caring, and curing. The relationship may be mediated and modulated by
culture, technology, or spiritual belief, but its fundamental human grounding will not disappear.

Thomasma and I developed these themes in a series of books. In the
first, *A Philosophical Basis of Medical Practice,* we developed our most fundamental statement of the philosophical basis of medical practice, which
we grounded in a philosophy of the body and mind phenomenologically
considered (Pellegrino and Thomasma 1981). In a series of books that followed, we explored different dimensions of the vision laid out in *A Philosophical Basis of Medical Practice.* We focused on the complex nature of
the patient's good as the telos of the clinical encounter (Pellegrino and
Thomasma 1988). This led us to a study of the virtues required of the physician if the telos of the relationship—the good of the patient—was to be
attained (Pellegrino and Thomasma 1993). To this we added an analysis of

the spiritual virtues entailed by the fact that some physicians also claimed to be Christian (Pellegrino and Thomasma 1996). Our last book went further into the spiritual and religious dimensions of healing and helping (Pellegrino and Thomasma 1997).

As I was preparing this chapter, my friend and coauthor David Thomasma died suddenly and unexpectedly. At the time of his death we were close to the completion of a second edition of our *Philosophical Basis*. I hope I shall be able to complete the task in a way David would have approved. I will sorely miss my collaborator with whom I have worked and from whom I have profited immensely for a quarter of a century.

I cannot do justice to David Thomasma in this essay. So close was our collaboration that it is difficult for me to know who was responsible for any idea, theme, or argument. I can honestly say that in all the time we worked together we never had a falling out of any kind. This I attribute to David's equitable temper, charity, and sense of humor. I will miss his creative mind, his knowledge of the literature, his skill in dissecting my bad ideas, and his generosity with my failings.

As we argued at the beginning of *A Philosophical Basis of Medical Practice,* we took ourselves to be elucidating a philosophy *of* medicine, which we distinguished from philosophy *and* medicine and philosophy *in* medicine. In *A Philosophical Basis of Medical Practice* and in our other individual and independent writings, we have emphasized different aspects of the philosophy of medicine, but on the basic perceptions we were in agreement. Some of our critics have taken us to task for concentrating too much on individual patients, neglecting preventive and social medicine, and for overuse of the "medical model."

We never intended to exclude such considerations. Our aim was to proceed stepwise to develop a paradigm, a philosophy of medicine that could be applied analogically to social medicine, preventive medicine, and to the healing relationships characteristic of the other health professions as well. In the coming second edition of *A Philosophical Basis for Medical Practice,* we address these issues as well as the criticism that we commit the naturalist fallacy.

We have already addressed some of these perceived omissions in separate papers authored collaboratively or individually. As we expanded our notion of a philosophy of medicine, it became clear that we were really developing an existentially grounded philosophy of healing and helping of humans in a state of vulnerability. It has become increasingly apparent too that our philosophy of medicine was also based in a particular notion of the idea of man, that is, a philosophical anthropology and a metaphysical notion of human and social good. Thus we entered the more foundational realm of moral philosophy beyond simply medicine or health care ethics.

We have expanded our consideration beyond medical ethics going progressively from a philosophy of medicine to a philosophy of healing to a philosophy of the health professions. This approach also suggested a way to define a philosophical basis and moral philosophy for other "helping" professions, e.g., law, ministry, teaching. These professions deal, as medicine does, with vulnerable persons: persons in need of justice, learning, or spiritual healing. Law, teaching, and ministry, like medicine, are based in certain empirical phenomena inherent in specific interhuman relationships that entail a moral relationship between the vulnerable and those who serve them.

Let me close with an attempt to relate my own work to the current state of bioethics.[1] Recently, I have continued to explore the basis of a moral philosophy of the health professions and of the professions of law, ministry, and teaching (Pellegrino 2002a, pp. 556–579). Neither this essay nor any of the others is meant to impose what is pejoratively called the "medical model" on other professions. Rather it suggests that there is a phenomenological and real-world similarity in the human existential realities of persons rendered vulnerable by illness, or by a need for justice, spiritual consolation, or knowledge. These phenomena by their nature entail duties, obligations, and virtues of physicians, lawyers, teachers, and ministers. They help to develop a more extended and more credible moral philosophy for the professions more generally than the current sociological interpretations that now prevail.

Let me point out in response to some of my critics that what we have done thus far is not a *compleat* philosophy and ethic of even medicine or health care. We need a fuller explication of the societal dimensions of medicine and its relationships with other professions and society and with preventative medicine. These questions can be approached by a realist examination of the phenomena of the personal and community relationships specific to each of these ways medicine can be manifested. Some of this will be adumbrated in the coming revision of *A Philosophical Basis for Medical Practice*, other parts in a planned work on the social ethics of medicine.

There are a number of interactions and dissonances between the philosophy of medicine and health care that I have espoused from the publication of *A Philosophical Basis of Medical Practice* through to the present and what I take to be the dominant themes of contemporary bioethics.

First, my view runs contrary to the postmodern insistence on the fallacy of all foundations or overarching ideas in philosophy. It also is "premodern" in its belief in the capacity of reason, albeit limited, to arrive at objective moral truth. The current infatuation with praxis—with what works—is no solid source for either the normative or the morally true.

I do not think a comprehensive moral philosophy, whether in medicine or more generally, is possible without an account of religious and theological sources of moral authority. In the end, faith and reason compliment each other. The ground between them is not an intellectual or conceptual no-man's-land. There are signs of some lessening in the conflict between them, at least among those ethicists who are not willing entirely to foreclose reflection on these two dimensions of the human spirit. Postmodernists who have sought consolation in moral skepticism have no other place to go. Theologians who scorn reason are similarly constrained. As a result, both are beginning to realize that the boundary between them is not impermeable.

The same can be said of the necessity for a philosophical anthropology. Medicine being simultaneously the scientific and humanistic study of man cannot escape being based in an explicit or implicit philosophy of human nature. Even the denial of such a thing as the "nature" of man, and even those who see only his biological nature, are by these assertions holding a philosophical anthropology.

The genome project, the prospects of human cloning, and the fabrication of human-animal or human-machine hybrids force the question of what it is to be human upon us. When all is said and done the Psalmist's question "What is man?" cannot be evaded (Psalm 8). Clearly the articulation of a philosophy of man and a philosophy of medicine are essential elements in a normative moral philosophy. In this inquiry the philosophy of medicine—of man being ill, suffering, and being healed—fills a place in the complex mosaic of what it means to be human. My realism and search for objective foundations contravenes the current bioethical trend toward social convention, social construction, and dialogue as means of arriving at transient moral truths. These are valid as methods of political democracy but dangerous. Society is not *per se* the final arbiter of moral truth. There are sadly too many pathological societies past and present to entrust the canons of morality entirely to politics or social convention. Ethics is not a matter of polls or plebiscites.

My methodological approach is that of Aristotelian-Thomist natural law ethics. While still unpopular with some ethicists, it is enjoying something of a resurgence, but it is distinctly countercultural at the moment, gaining more attention as the poverty of ethical subjectivism becomes more manifest (Lisska 1996).

I do not claim to arrive at perfection in the grasp of moral truths. This can only be done asymptotically, given the limitations of human intellect. But a realist approach is far less likely to miss the truth than some of the current more fashionable methods of philosophizing, which begin with the content of the mind rather than the world "out there."

These divergences notwithstanding, there are areas of fruitful interaction with existing models of ethics to which our approach can offer some insights.

For one thing, our system is consistent with principlism. To be sure, the notion of common morality is an insufficient foundation for a philosophy or ethic of medicine. The four principles, however, fit well with the kinds of obligations we would justify on the basis of the phenomena of medicine. Autonomy derives from a philosophical anthropology grounded in the inherent and essential dignity of every human being. Justice likewise would be the fulfillment of the moral claim of every human to fair and equal treatment. We would add the Aristotelian notion of *epikeia* to adjust justice to the particularities of a particular human being's life, thus addressing the difficulties of balancing principles when they are in conflict (Pellegrino 2002b).

We see hermeneutics and literature, now so popular not as independent theories of ethics, but as important adjuvants to enable decision makers to comprehend their own and their fellow human experiences of the complexities and particular concrete details of the moral life. Narratives and hermeneutics are not normative *per se* but enhance our comprehension of the normative by their evocation of the concrete and detailed moral encounters that characterize every human life.

Feminism and caring we see also as important modulating influences on moral philosophy, raising sensitivities to long-neglected dimensions. But their normative claims, like all others, must pass philosophical muster. The same can be said of casuistry, dialogue, and dialectic. These are essential aspects of moral discourse and crucial to the resolution of conflicts, since the first step must always be understanding the sources of conflict. But again, they are not normative in themselves but helpful methodological aids to a realistically grounded moral philosophy.

We do not accept the powerful current conviction that, given the impossibility of moral consensus, we must abandon the search for the right and the good and instead be satisfied with what we can agree upon. This is simply another way to drive ethics as a discipline away from moral discourse and into "value" exchange and compromise. Values are personal attributions of worth or interest attached to things, ideas, or people. Being personal, they are important and need to be taken account of in ethical discourse. But they are not by that fact norms, principles, duties, or obligations. It is a tribute to modern sensibilities that they occur in ethical discourse, but their limitations are also important to recognize.

Finally, I think that a philosophy of medicine and an ethic of the professions is crucial to the current move to reverse the trend toward deprofessionalization. Admirable as the effort may be, the recent "principles" and rules promulgated by the American Board of Internal Medicine, the American Society for Internal Medicine, and the European Federation of Internists are insufficient (Pellegrino 2001, pp. 70–87; ABIM 2002, pp. 243–246). Like the ancient Hippocratic oath, the current proposal is a set of moral and nonmoral assertions without an explicit moral foundation or justification. A deeper probing of what a profession is, what that entails morally, and what duties it requires is needed. This is true of the parallel efforts now extant in law, ministry, and teaching to "recapture" the idea of professional commitment. Without a reconstruction of the moral foundations of the idea of a profession, these efforts cannot be fully successful. They cannot succeed without clarity of their deeper moral underpinnings.

To be sure, reaffirmation of professionalism in the best sense is a necessary step in reprofessionalization. But the illness is now too deeply seated to be healed without a moral conception of what a profession entails and what makes it different from other occupations. We need much more careful consideration of what makes the professions sufficiently different to warrant designation of a special domain called "professional ethics."

The answer will not be found in constructing a "new" ethic for each profession. Such an exercise usually ends in manipulating long-standing moral precepts, converting duties and virtues into "values" and reformulating them in terms more palatable to modern tastes for "choice," private interpretations, and an atomized morality. When professional ethics becomes only what we can agree on or what we ourselves dictate, it becomes merely self-justifying. This is just as perilous as the older tendency to justify morality on the fact that the profession has defined it in a certain way. Professional codes must ground their authority and binding power in moral reality, not in professional privilege or preference.

We need to return to serious reflection on the nature of the good, the telos of professional activity, and the way both are related to the realities of human beings in predicaments of particular need. No enterprise could be more important in a world in which professional expertise plays so influential a role in the lives of all of us. Sooner or later, no matter what our own expertise may be, we all find ourselves in need of the help of some other professional. As soon as we step outside the narrow perimeter of our own expertise we are vulnerable to the ethical standards and character of those whom we consult.

Professional ethics, its groundings, the sources of its moral authority, and the way they are justified are of concern to all of us. It is not the whole of bioethics to be sure. But it is through professionals that bioethics becomes a benefit or a danger for every human being in a technological society. A philosophy of the profession that grounds the ethics of the professions is therefore more than an idle academic exercise.

The pathway of my scholarly interests has led me from medical ethics as a moral system based in an affirmation of certain moral precepts, to a search for the philosophical foundations of those precepts in a philosophy of medicine derived from the realities of medical practice, to a moral philosophy of healing. Such a moral philosophy has certain foundations common to all healing and helping professions. A better understanding of the moral foundations is essential to any definition of what constitutes a profession and distinguishes it from mere professionalism.

Notes

I have understood the task assigned to me as a contributor to this volume to be a description of how my own thinking about the philosophy and ethics of medicine developed during the two decades of my association with the Kennedy Institute of Ethics. This has occasioned an inordinate concentration on my own writing. I trust this does no injustice to my colleagues.

1. For a more considered statement of my concerns about the future of bioethics, I refer you to a recent paper published in the *Journal of Medicine and Philosophy* (Pellegrino 2000, pp. 655–675). For a look at the direction my work is taking from the philosophy of medicine as a basis of medical ethics, to a philosophy and moral philosophy of the health professions and the professions of law, ministry, and teaching, see my paper published in 2002 in the *Journal of Medicine and Philosophy* (Pellegrino 2002a, pp. 556–579).

References

ABIM Foundation, ACP-ASIM Foundation, and European Federation of Internal Medicine. 2002. "Medical Professionalism in the New Millennium: A Physician Charter." *Annals of Internal Medicine* 136 (3): 243–246.

Jaspers, Karl. 1963. *Philosophy and the World, Selected Essays.* Washington, DC: Regnery.

Lisska, Anthony J. 1996. *Aquinas's Theory of Natural Law: An Analytic Reconstruction.* New York: Oxford University Press.

McElhinney, Thomas K., and Edmund D. Pellegrino. 2001. "The Institute on Human Values in Medicine: Its Role and Influence in the Conception and Evolution of Bioethics." *Theoretical Medicine* 22: 291–317.

Pellegrino, E. D. 1966. "Medicine, Philosophy, and Man's Infirmity in Conditio Humana." In *Edwin Straus on His Seventy-fifth Birthday,* ed. Walter von Baeyer and Richard M. Griffith. New York: Springer.

———. 1976. "Philosophy of Medicine, Problematic and Potential." *Journal of Medicine and Philosophy* 1: 5–31.

———. 2000. "Bioethics at Century's Turn: Can the Normative Be Retrieved?" *Journal of Medicine and Philosophy* 25: 655–675.

———. 2001. "Professional Codes." In *Methods in Medical Ethics,* ed. Jeremy Sugarman and Daniel Sulmasy. Washington, DC: Georgetown University Press.

———. 2002a. "The Internal Morality of Clinical Medicine: A Paradigm for the Ethics of the Helping and Healing Professions." *Journal of Medicine and Philosophy* 26: 556–579.

———. 2002b. "Rationing Health Care: Inherent Conflicts within the Concept of Justice." In *The Ethics of Managed Care: Professional Integrity and Patient Rights,* ed. William Bondeson and H. T. Engelhardt, Jr. Dordrecht: Kluwer.

Pellegrino, E. D., and D. C. Thomasma. 1981. *A Philosophical Basis of Medical Practice: Toward a Philosophy and Ethic of the Healing Professions.* Oxford: Oxford University Press.

———. 1988. *For the Patient's Good: The Restoration of Beneficence in Health Care.* Oxford: Oxford University Press.

———. 1993. *The Virtues in Medical Practice.* Oxford: Oxford University Press.

———. 1996. *The Christian Virtues in Medical Practice.* Washington, DC: Georgetown University Press.

———. 1997. *Helping and Healing: Religious Commitment in Health Care.* Washington, DC: Georgetown University Press.

Seifert, Josef. 1984. "Essence and Infinity: A Dialogue with Existential Thomism." *The New Scholasticism* 58: 84–98.

Straus, Erwin. 1963. *The Primary World of Senses: A Vindication of Sensory Experience,* trans. by Jacob Needleman. New York: The Free Press of Glencoe.

Von Hildebrand, Dietrich. 1973. *What Is Philosophy?* London and New York: W. Kohlhammer.

11

PHYSICIAN-PATIENT RELATIONSHIP

The Healing Relationship

Moral Choice, the Good of the Patient, and the Patient's Good

Introduction

Acting for the good of the patient is the most ancient and universally acknowledged principle of medical ethics. It grounds ethical theories and shapes the way their principles are applied in particular cases. It is the ultimate court of appeal for the morality of medical acts. While it may, on rare occasions be set aside for the common good, this is done with trepidation and in only the most urgent circumstances.

Yet what precisely we may mean by the patient's "good" or the "good of the patient" is subject to the most different interpretations. These divergent interpretations engender some of the most vexing ethical dilemmas, and their solution is impossible without clear understandings of the central terms. But so beguiling is the idea of doing good for the patient that we rarely examine closely what good, and whose good, we are serving.

In a morally diverse society, opposing views of ultimate and immediate good may be held by the parties in clinical decisions involving moral choice. Each participant is a moral agent and as such is bound to uphold, and be accountable for, his, or her, own conception of what is right and good. Making morally defensible decisions in the face of substantive differences in conceptions of patient good has become, therefore, one of the urgent procedural problems in medical ethics.

The problem is, of course, a subset of the problems attendant on the lack of moral consensus in our society. This, in turn, is the consequence of our philosophical and theological disagreement on what constitutes "The Good," and the good life. A theory of good grounds every theory of morals, general and medical. Since we are not likely to agree on our philosophical or theological definitions we are compelled to clarify the various senses in which we may use our terms and establish a morally defensible procedure for dealing with conflicts when they arise.

This essay is an attempt to meet these two requirements—an analysis of the components of patient good and a procedure for handling differences in a morally defensible way. It proposes that the concept of patient good is a compound one, that at least four senses of patient good can be discerned, that they are related to each other, but distinct, that the physician (and other health professionals) are obliged to respect each level of patient good, and that a hierarchy exists among them that determines how conflicts should be resolved. Moreover, each component can be related to the several notions of the good in Aristotle's *Ethics*.

The author's analysis of patient good, together with related essays on the philosophy of the healing relationship and the virtuous physician, constitute an effort to complement and supplement the prevalent emphasis on rights and duty-based ethical systems [23].

Because of their urgency, and their momentous nature, decisions not to resuscitate—so called "No-Code Orders"—will be used to illustrate how different notions of patient good may conflict and why a clarification of the meanings of patient good is necessary. This is so even with the benefit of the recent, admirably cogent analysis of life-sustaining treatments by the President's Commission [6]. That report clearly recognizes the centrality of patient self-determination as well as patient benefit in the decisions to refuse cardiopulmonary resuscitation and other life-sustaining measures. Even with such well-reasoned guidelines, the question of what is the good of the competent and the incompetent patient remains at the heart of each decision.

The Patient's "Good": Its Fourfold Meanings

The good of the patient is a particular kind of good, that which pertains to a human person in a particular existential circumstance—being ill, and needing the help of others to be restored, or to cope with the assault of illness. In a general way the good the patient seeks is restoration of health—a return to his or her definition of what constitutes a worthwhile way of life—one that permits the pursuit of personal goals with a minimum of pain, discomfort, or disability. This is the end the patient seeks in the medical encounter, and the physician promises to serve by his act of "profession"—his promise to help with the special knowledge at his disposal. The physician thus becomes an instrument for the attainment of the good the patient seeks.

Inherent in the nature of the physician's offer to help is a tacit promise to use his knowledge and skill to advance the patient's good [10, 22]. This may be interpreted differently by the patient, the physician or the family. Unless the patient is incompetent, however, the physician is obligated to act for the good conceived by the patient and to support his goals. In the event those goals are morally unpalatable to the physician, he is free to withdraw from the case under the usual conditions.

If he accepts the case, and as long as he maintains his relationship with the patient, the physician is obligated to promote four components of the patient's good: (1) *Ultimate good*—that which constitutes the patient's ultimate standard for his life's choices, that which has the highest meaning for him; (2) *Biomedical or techno-medical good,* that which results from the correct application of medical knowledge and skill; (3) *The patient's perception of his own good* at the particular time and circumstance of the clinical decision and how he prefers to advance his own life plan; (4) *The good of the patient as a human person,* capable of reasoned choices. Where the patient may have confused or conflicting notions of his own good, full congruence may not be possible. Nonetheless, I will argue that the physician is bound to advance each of these four senses of good to the extent possible.

Good, the Good, and the Patient's Concept of Ultimate Good

At the outset, and throughout this discussion, we must remain clear about the distinction between the good as perceived by the participants in clinical decisions and the ontological nature of good. This essay cannot presume to deal adequately with the prickly question of the objectivity or non-objectivity of the good. The point of this essay is not whether particular interpretations of patient good are metaphysically sound. Rather its focus is on the fact that widely divergent interpretations do occur, that in spite of that fact, physicians, patients and families must make decisions together, and that the conflicts, when they occur, must be dealt with in a morally defensible way.

But even if all the participants in a clinical decision were to agree on each of the four levels in their interpretations of patient good, that would not make the decision ontologically good. One could conceive of agreement on interpretations that would be intrinsically evil—e.g., falsification of disability or cause of death to gain compensation or insurance benefits; withholding public information of a diagnosis of plague or cholera or of a patient's homicidal intent; the practice of killing defective infants or adults.

The aim of the essay is to encourage a clearer identification of each component of patient good, to clarify the use of this universal notion, to understand the conflicts that can result from its varying interpretations by the participants in clinical decisions involving moral choice, and to examine how to resolve these conflicts in some orderly, and morally reliable way.

The good of the patient is a particular good and like all particular goods it is related to, and shaped by, the conception we hold of the notion of good and "The Good." This is the first component to be examined in mapping the content of the good of the patient. What we think of the nature of good and "The Good" ultimately shapes all the other components.

The history of philosophical debate about the nature of "the" good is too long and unsettled to be repeated here [26, 5, 19, 11]. The perennial question remains—what is the nature of "the" good? Is it properly understood as one thing or many? Does it rest on some factual aspect of the nature of man or the world? Is it primarily a psychological, intuitive or self-evident concept? Is it even susceptible of rational justification? Is the ultimate good the contemplation of truth, living in accordance with God's will, developing one's potential, wealth, honor, pleasure, power, the good of the species, or some combination of these things that adds up to "happiness"? We need not resolve these questions to appreciate that how we answer conditions the subsidiary notions contained in the ideas of the patient's good.

The concept we hold of the ultimate good is the reference standard for all decisions including clinical decisions. It serves to justify and define the nature and aim of moral choices. In clinical decisions, some take the ultimate standard to be whatever the patient desires, others what the physician judges to be good, for still others conformity with philosophical, theological, or socially determined principles like the will or law of God, or freedom, self-determination, social utility, quality of life, or the good of the species. The list is long, and the competing concepts are often incompatible.

Equally incompatible are the opposing theories of those who hold that the good is whatever humans desire, or have an interest in, and those who hold the good to inhere in certain things and actions whether humans desire them or not [6]. Without trying to resolve these theoretical questions, it is sufficient to realize that in any particular moral choice some final concept of the good, some "good of last resort," underlies the other components of patient good. That final concept is the most pervasive, the least negotiable and often the least explicit presupposition when conflicts arise in making clinical decisions with moral overtones.

Biomedical or Techno-Medical Good: What Medicine Can Achieve Technically

Biomedical or techno-medical good encompasses the effects of medical interventions on the natural history of the disease being treated. It is the good that can be achieved by the application of expert technical medical knowledge—cure, containment of disease, prevention, amelioration of symptoms, or prolongation of life. It is directly related to the physician's technical competence; it is the first step in fulfillment of the moral obligations of his or her promise to help. Biomedical good is the *instrumental* good the patient seeks from the physician. It is also a good internal to medicine—part of its claim to be a special kind of human activity. It is the good that results from the physician's craftsmanship—his capacity to make the technically correct decision and to carry it out safely, competently, and with minimal discomfort to the patient. Biomedical or techno-medical good is usually subsumed under the phrase "medically indicated."

⌈There always is an unfortunate tendency for physicians to equate bio-medical or techno-medical good with the whole of the patient's good. Techno-medical good does not exhaust the good the physician is obliged to do. It is an essential. but not a sufficient component of good medicine. Two ethical errors may result from the conflation of techno-medical good with the good of the patient. ⌉

The first error is to make the patient a victim of the medical impera-tive to insist that if a procedure offers any physiological or therapeutic benefit then it must be done. On this view, ethical medicine is limited to technically right interventions. Ethical quandaries are thus ignored since the only good acknowledged is medical good in its narrowest sense, and this is ascertained by scientific means and not by ethical discourse or analysis.

The second error is to confuse the physician's judgment of the toler-ability of the quality of life that would ensue from a treatment with the medical indications for that treatment. On this view, if treatment of a de-fective infant results in a life without "meaningful relationships," then it is not medically indicated and should not be done. This is an unjustifiable extension of medical judgment beyond its legitimate limits. Whether a life is worth living is a value decision only the patient who must live that life can decide. Moreover, it is not a matter determinable by the capabilities of medicine *qua* medicine, in the first place.

It is the obligation of the physician to ascertain, by the most careful method, the kind of life that might ensue from a particular treatment in a particular patient. These are matters of scientific judgment proper to medicine. They are essential in helping the patient to decide if the life that ensues from treatment is worthwhile. It is he who must judge, with the physician's help, the kind of life he wishes to lead and the risks or discom-fort he is willing to bear to attain the benefits medical treatment might offer.

On this view, I would argue that medical good but not medicine should be interpreted narrowly—as that which can be ascertained scien-tifically and technically to be possible in altering the natural history of *this* disease in *this* person. I recognize that certain value judgments are in-volved but these should be kept to a minimum and limited to scientific competence, sound clinical reasoning and valid probabilistic statements about diagnosis, prognosis and therapeutics. I must repeat here that while techno-medical good should be defined narrowly, this is *not* the whole of the physician's responsibility or of medicine as a practice.

Let us examine this concept of biomedical good more specifically in the context of cardiopulmonary resuscitation (CPR). CPR was introduced in 1962 to reinitiate the heartbeat in patients about to die suddenly due to electrical dysfunction of the heart, in the presence of a mechanically intact heart muscle. A variety of dysrhythmias—ventricular, fibrillation, asystole or bradycardia—may lead to ineffective output of the heart with cessation of blood flow to the brain. Within a few minutes cerebral damage becomes irreversible and death ensues.

The ideal and unequivocal clinical indication, the highest techno-medical good that CPR can achieve, is in cases of sudden death resulting from acute cessation of flow through a coronary artery in an otherwise normal heart. Resuscitation offers the probability of a complete recovery and subsequent use of effective medical and surgical procedures for the underlying disorder. This is true also in drowning, electroshock, or when someone is struck by lightning. In these situations, the medical good is unequivocal.

Sudden cessation of cardiopulmonary function may also occur under other clinical circumstances in which the final medical outcome may be less clearly predictable. Cardiopulmonary arrest, for example, can accompany any severe acute illness from a variety of causes—medical and surgical shock, overwhelming infection, diseases of the brain and meninges, diabetic ketoacidosis, poisonings, or renal failure. In these situations the heart muscle may or may not be intact, but if the patient can be resuscitated, treatment can be instituted for the underlying disorder. CPR is medically indicated, though the eventual good is problematic and cannot usually be foreseen at the time CPR is instituted. The techno-medical "good" here is to gain time to diagnose and treat the underlying disease.

The most controversial use of CPR is in the patient who is known to be dying—one whose underlying disease has progressed to the point of no return, and in whom further treatment offers little or no prospect of success. Here cardiac and pulmonary arrest, and the accompanying cardiac dysrhythmias, are simply part of an inevitable process of dying. From a strictly biomedical point of view, in these situations CPR only temporarily interrupts the inevitable last stages of dying. If CPR is successful, a series of other measures will usually be required to keep the patient alive—intubation, mechanically assisted respiration or circulation, drugs to support circulation, infusions, dialysis, etc. These measures offer a very limited medical good—to sustain life (usually for other than medical reasons)—until some decision is made to permit the process of dying to resume its inexorable course.

In cardiopulmonary arrest outside the hospital, it is rarely possible to determine accurately whether the patient will be medically assisted by CPR. CPR could achieve some techno-medical good since it gains time for the patient to be transported to the hospital where more deliberative and definitive diagnosis and prognosis are possible. Generally speaking, CPR under these circumstances would also coincide with patient good as we shall describe it shortly unless the patient had previously been diagnosed as terminally ill on good clinical grounds or has executed a valid living will. Whenever prognosis and diagnosis are uncertain, CPR can serve some medical good by allowing time for a better assessment of what medical interventions can offer but also what the patient's desires might be with respect to a no-code order.

The Patient's Best Interests: The Patient's Concept of His Own Good

A biomedically or techno-medically good treatment is not automatically a good from the patient's point of view. It must be examined in the context of the patient's life situation and his or her value system. To be good in the fuller sense, the choice must square with what the patient thinks worthwhile given the circumstances and alternatives his illness forces upon him. The patient must weigh the probable medical benefits of a treatment or a no-code order against some ultimate good (e.g., his religious beliefs). When he is competent, only the patient can decide ultimately whether the quality of the life that remains is "worthwhile," consistent with his belief system or with some plan he may have for his life. The range of satisfactions left to the sick and disabled is narrowed. But what is left may still be savored by the patient in ways the healthy person cannot comprehend.

When the patient is competent it is he who can best ascertain what is in his best interests. When he is not, then his surrogates must ascertain as closely as possible what he would have chosen as in his best interests were he able to make the choice himself. Our concern must be for the person who is to live the life illness imposes, not what we think of the quality of that life.

The court in the Shirley Dinnerstein case [14] asserted the legal import of the distinction between the medical decision—based on diagnosis and prognosis—and the personal decision—based on the surrogate choice by the family of what was in their mother's best interests [31]. The medical good of a no-code order was deemed within the doctor's province; the patient's interests were placed in the hands of the family. Both were relevant for a legal decision not to resuscitate.

The patient's "interests" then, are the aims, plans, and preferences peculiar to him and chosen by him at a particular time. Any object of desire may become an object of interest for this patient at a particular time. The "good" in this sense can be anything which is an object of interest for this patient.

Patient interest defined in this way is necessarily subjective and relative, since it is rooted in *the patient's view* of what is in his own best interests at this time, and in this circumstance. We cannot know what that is until we ask the patient. This view does not deny the possibility that some objects of interest will be bad or injurious—it requires only that they have been freely chosen by this patient. It is no revelation that we may know the good, but do not infallibly choose it. Because someone has chosen something as good does not make it good intrinsically, or instrumentally. To accept the patient's definition of his own best interests does not necessitate that the doctor agree nor is he bound morally to promote those interests. What the physician must do is to give the most serious weight to the patient's judgment of his own interest in making decisions. Indeed, that judgment must be accorded primacy, since it arises from the operation of an even more fundamental good—the human capacity to choose.

Can something outside of incompetence override that decision?

The Good of the Patient as a Person

The fourth sense of patient good is that which is most proper to being a human person. It is a somewhat different category from the other three senses of good which I have defined. Each of these may be individually determined for, or by, a particular person in a particular circumstance and weighted differently in different persons and circumstances. The fourth good is the operation of the capacity to use reason to *make* choices and to communicate those choices through speech. One cherished and distinctive feature of human existence is this capacity to establish a life plan and to select from a variety of goods those things that are preferred for reasons that are unique and personal. Humans may not reason wisely, prudently or correctly, but the freedom to do so is a good without which it is impossible for the mentally competent person to live a good life.

Those humans who by virtue of pathological or physiological abnormalities of brain function cannot make choices—the comatose or psychotic—or those who have never been competent—infants—are still humans. Their choices must perforce be represented by others but they must be represented nonetheless. Even though their capacities to make reasoned choices cannot be expressed because of brain dysfunction, they are still beings whose nature it is to be rational. We are compelled to respect their good in this manner to the extent possible by the alternative means of surrogate or proxy decision.

Choice requires freedom, and freedom implies that some choices may be wrong or evil. Liberty and the power to choose are therefore intrinsically bound to each other. Louis Lavelle puts it well:

> For liberty is nothing if it is not the power of choosing . . . Thus the perfect unity of the self lies in the possibility it has of choosing. But it can only choose between alternatives and the self's unity is the living unity of the act which postulates and resolves this alternative . . . We can see therefore that by a kind of paradox our liberty can determine itself only by distinguishing between good and evil in the world. ([16], p. 18)

If we are not to violate the humanity of the patient in medical decisions, so long as the patient is competent, we must allow him to make his own choices. We cannot override those choices even if they run counter to what we think is good for the patient. To manipulate the patient's consent, to deceive or misinform him, even to do what we think is good, is to violate his good as a human being. Only the patient can free us of the obligation to abide by his choices by giving us a mandate to make decisions for him if he feels emotionally or intellectually overwhelmed by the complexity of the choices. But even in the act of yielding up his prerogative, the patient exercises his freedom because he can choose not to exercise his capacity if he wishes. The physician can never presume to usurp that prerogative. The freedom to choose, and to be responsible for the outcome of those choices, is the ground upon which any reasonable notion of autonomy is built.

The good of the patient as a human is therefore a more general good than the others. It is the basis for our respect for the personal interpretations particular patients in particular circumstances may place on technomedical good, their immediate interests and their ultimate good. While the ultimate good is the highest good, it too must freely be chosen by the individual. Without freedom to choose and reject there would be little merit in subscribing to some ultimate good, no matter how lofty.

In every human decision, and especially in clinical decisions, these four senses of the good are intermingled. The configuration of choices we make at each of these levels and the way we relate one to the other in large part defines us as persons. Each level must be understood and respected. When they are in conflict with each other, or are interpreted differently by the parties making medical decisions, some hierarchical order must be established among them. Without such an order decision making is paralyzed or, worse still, results in the capitulation to or superimposition of one person's choices on another.

To acknowledge that these four levels of good can differ among interacting humans is not to accede to the idea that all choices are equally valid logically, epistemologically or metaphysically. No capitulation is being made here to moral relativism or emotivism. There are morally good and bad choices at each level, and those distinctions must not be abandoned. They must be recognized, and morally sound procedures established, so that each element of patient good is adequately promoted in the face of potential conflicts among the interacting parties. The ethics of the procedure must be distinguished carefully from the ethical substance of the decisions.   *procedure vs substance*

No-Code Orders and the Components of Patient Good

No-code orders illustrate some of the conflicts and confusions that may occur in clinical decisions among persons all of whom would argue that they are pursuing the good of the patient, or avoiding harm, or respecting patient autonomy [1, 2, 7, 9, 12, 15, 17, 18, 25, 27].

The most difficult situation occurs when CPR is not medically indicated because the patient's underlying disorder is incurable or the patient is in a terminal state. CPR will then only interrupt the last stages of dying; that is, no techno-medical good can be achieved in the sense that the natural history of the illness cannot be reversed.

Under these circumstances, the patient, physician, or family might still wish to use CPR because of some "interest" of the patient. For example, the patient or physician might be an Orthodox Jew who feels that the doctor's dedication must always be to preserve life at all costs—as long as something can be done it must be done. Many Christians hold this view also. On this view, life will end only when God wishes it to end. God would not have given man the knowledge of CPR if it were not to be used to preserve life. Any relaxation of efforts to sustain life would be interpreted as nothing short of assisted suicide, perhaps even homicide.

On a more secular level, CPR might be chosen, even when its benefits are dubious, to take advantage of the remote possibility of diagnostic or prognostic error. Even with the best of human knowledge prognosis can be a risky exercise in probabilities. Any clinician with extensive experience can recall patients he consigned to inevitable death who confounded him by surviving. Also, there is always the remote possibility that if the patient is kept alive some new treatment for the underlying disease might be discovered. Or, some bold therapeutic idea might occur to clinicians or consultants that might overturn the hopeless prognosis. Obviously such cases are vastly in the minority. Still, for some patients whose values dispose them to a last ditch stand, CPR might be chosen even though its utility may be virtually nonexistent.

Another example is the case in which patient, physician and family agree with the prognosis and the medical futility of CPR yet find that the patient perceives a few additional hours, days, or weeks of life to be in his interests. The patient, before he dies, may wish to see a child or grandchild born, a son graduate, a long absent relative, or friend. Or, he may wish to finish some work, or attend to some final arrangement regarding his estate, or fulfill some obligation.

CPR may also be in the family's or physician's interest (but not in the patient's); it may assuage their guilt, real or imagined, for the way they may have treated the patient during his life. If "everything" is done, they might feel some part of their past guilt to have been expiated. In this way also the physician might assure himself that he is not "responsible" for the death. Sometimes medical attendants are reluctant to let a patient die when they have invested months of work and personal involvement in his care. In these situations the patient's good is in conflict with the needs and interests of his family or medical attendants. Under the guise of serving the "good" of the patient, they may violate the patient's perception of his own good and his freedom to make his own choice as a human being.

There are also cases where the physician does not wish to use CPR even when it might be medically indicated, because he believes he would thereby "condemn" the patient to a life not worth living. To avoid "doing harm" the physician might withhold CPR, for example, in an elderly man who had a stroke or suffered an acute coronary episode. Or, the physician might decide that preserving the life of a malformed infant or a retarded, aged, or otherwise disabled patient might impose too large a burden on society, or family, or on the patient himself. The doctor might see his role as an agent of social and economic good as well as the patient's "good." In such cases he might refuse to satisfy the particular request for CPR, or perform it ineffectively to mollify the staff, or family, or to avoid legal liabilities. Even less commendably, the physician might allow his own estimate of a patient's moral or social worth to influence his decision to withhold CPR from patients he considers social "misfits"—sociopaths, chronic alcoholics, vagrants, criminals, or drug addicts. In these instances the good of the patient is usurped by the physician's concept of good.

Social Good

We have concentrated on the meanings of the patient's good because this is the *raison dêtre* of all clinical medicine. But as the cumulative effects of individual medical decisions alter the world's demography, and high technology consumes an ever larger percentage of its resources, the other good things a society seeks come more and more into conflict with the good of individual patients. Already, the economic and social costs of prolonging the lives of many aged and disabled patients are intruding themselves into clinical decisions. Medicine's more vocal critics often take it to task for over-emphasizing the good of the individual patient and neglecting the good of society. As a result, the principles of social and distributive justice are increasingly invoked in clinical decisions.

With respect to CPR, some questions of justice can be legitimately raised: Is the patient really free to choose CPR simply to achieve something he deems in his best interest, i.e., arranging his affairs, seeing a grandchild graduate from medical school? Are not the costs he incurs a burden on others? Recall that cardiopulmonary arrest outside the hospital is generally considered an automatic indication for CPR since neither rational decisions nor proper diagnosis and prognosis are possible under such urgent conditions. Is this policy tenable if the probability of eventual survival or return of socially active life is small and the costs to society high? Is the surrogate of a severely impaired infant or neonate free to choose CPR if that infant's future life is to require the use of extensive resources and expenditures which the patient cannot afford and the whole of society must bear? What if these expenditures are likely to continue long after the proxy is able to help in defraying them?

These questions bring the patient's interests and even his agency squarely into conflict with the good of others. Some advocate a form of social paternalism to protect society against the economic and social consequences of CPR in seriously ill patients. The possibility of a public policy in the U.S. that would deny CPR to certain categories of patients is not beyond contemplation.

As a result, physicians are being pressured to assume the role of monitors of the social and economic good of society. When patient good and social good are thus intermingled they may well come into conflict. How consistent is a concern for social good with the traditional ethical commitment of physicians to do everything to advance the interests and medical good of their patients?

The foregoing questions illustrate the complexity of the concept of the good of the patient. They underscore the need not only for more explicit analysis of the points of conflict but also for their resolution. That resolution in its turn requires establishment of some hierarchical order among the various notions of *good* if decisions are to be made on any principled basis.

hierarchy of "good" necessary for procedural fairness

Making Moral Choices — The Hierarchical Order of Patient Good

Making clinical decisions with moral implications necessitates some ranking of the four senses of patient good because they can come into conflict. I would now like to examine more closely the hierarchical relationship which should obtain among these several levels of patient good when they are in conflict. Conflicts between good things can only be resolved according to some rational organizing principle.

Some of us clearly organize our lives around one good that is the highest good in our lives, traditionally the *summum bonum.* For those who reject that idea, I would refer simply to the "good of last resort"—that good to which we tend to return whenever we are forced to make choices between competing goods, the one good we tend to place above others. For the religious person the highest good is accommodation to the will or law of the Creator. For the non-religious person it may be seeking the greatest pleasure, the least harm, the greatest utility, enlightened self-interest, the good of the least advantaged person in a society, the absolute autonomy of patients to choose or the survival of the species. Without arguing at this point about what that ultimate good should be, we need only accept that there is *de facto* such a good for all who attempt to make rational choices. Even pluralistic intuitionists must base their intuitions on a final good, in this sense.

Clearly, the ultimate good, or the good of last resort, will take precedence over the other forms of patient good. Strong paternalism with respect to a patient's choice of ultimate good is morally offensive. The ultimate good is the starting point of a person's moral reasoning, his first act of intellectual faith so to speak. If he or she is competent, it must be respected over medical good, and the physician's, society's, the family's, or the law's construal of ultimate good. The patient may abandon or subjugate his conception of ultimate good to his more immediate personal interests, but others may not do so.

There has never been, nor is there likely ever to be, universal agreement on the ultimate good. Societies that wish to be homogeneous in their choice of ultimate good usually do so by some form of coercion. In democratic societies it is a civic right of competent persons to choose their own belief systems. To pursue a moral life we are under compulsion to act with fidelity to some ultimate source or concept of good though our choices of that source or concept may vary widely.

When conflicts occur in decisions involving human life—as for example with no-code orders, discontinuing life support measures, artificial insemination, abortion, etc. they often involve disagreements about the ultimate good and are therefore reconcilable with great difficulty if at all. Under such circumstances the patient-physician relationship should be respectfully and courteously discontinued since neither physician nor patient can morally compromise his belief system—particularly when the issue involves ultimate good.

The good next in order of priority is the good of the patient as a human person, his freedom to make his own decisions. To place even medical good or the quality of life ahead of freedom to choose is to rob the patient of his humanity. The physician instead has the obligation to enhance the patient's competence in every way—treating pathophysiological disturbances of brain function, freely providing accurate information needed to make choices, and refraining from coercion or deception even to overcome resistance to needed treatments.

The once-competent patient who at the time of decision is comatose, psychotic or otherwise unable to reason and choose does not lose his claim as a human being to have his interests respected. We turn therefore to surrogates, who can act on behalf of those interests. Presumably the surrogate knows the patient better than the physician or is closer to his cultural or ethical value system. His choices are more likely to approximate what the patient would have wanted were he able to express his choice. If the surrogate or proxy is competent and is clearly acting in the interests of the patient, his or her choices take precedence over the physician's. In the difficult situation in which there is doubt about the capability or good intention of the surrogate, then the physician must attend to the good of the patient. This may require resort to the courts if the physician thinks the surrogate's decision is not in the patient's interests. Under these circumstances, at least the patient's legal rights can be protected, and the intentions of both the surrogate and the physician examined a little more objectively, recognizing always that a legal decision may not be necessarily a morally correct one.

In the case of the never-competent—infants and the retarded—we have no way of knowing what the patient would have chosen, nor do the surrogates, even when they are the parents. Here there is no way to determine what is or would be the patient's perception of his own good or of his ultimate good. Neither will the patient ever be free to choose. Under these circumstances three of the four components of patient good, as we have been discussing them, cannot be ascertained. Biomedical or techno-medical good therefore assumes a dominant role. It is probably a safer guide than presumptions about what an infant would consider in his interest as his life evolves in the presence of a severe handicap. I would, under these circumstances, tend to Paul Ramsey's position, i.e., if some clinical benefit, easing of pain, discomfort, or physiological improvement can be obtained for the patient, then treatment probably should be undertaken ([25], pp. 189–227). Obviously we cannot know at the time of decision whether in the long run the patient will thank us or not. But at least, the decision will be taken on the basis of what can be known, and not on what can only be presumed with the greatest uncertainty about another person's future preferences.

With the never-competent patient, it is still the good of the patient that ordinarily remains our concern—not that of the parents, or guardians, or society in general. The possibilities for disagreement on what is "best" in such cases are evident from the wide range of arguments in the current literature. For some, spiritual good may accrue to the family and society from the care of a deformed, defective or disabled infant. For a utilitarian the social costs of a life of total dependency may be totally unjustifiable. Obviously the case of the never-competent will occasion the greatest difficulty in applying any hierarchical order to patient good. Yet some attempt must be made, otherwise decisions will be unpredictable, intuitive and fortuitous.

The choice of competent surrogates is limited if it violates the conscience of the medical attendant or contravenes any of the senses of patient good we have outlined. The physician or nurse must remain faithful to his or her conscience. His or her humanity is as precious as that of the patient. Coercion by court order, law, or other means of the physician's decision is as indefensible as coercion of the patient's decision.

All the moral obligations that derive from this schema of patient good are obviously not spelled out here. All health professionals, health care

*For Pellegrino, physician's conscience must not be coerced

institutions, ministers, families and friends—all who participate in decisions that affect those who are ill—must take into account the many dimensions of "patient good." In the best decisions, the four senses I have outlined should be closely congruent with each other. When they are not, the differences should be spelled out as clearly as possible and negotiated with honesty and sensitivity. This is an instance in which the quality of the personal relationships and the character traits of the interacting parties will often be more important than rules or procedures.

The hierarchical order I have suggested has implications for the way the common principles of medical ethics are applied in particular instances. This is pertinent for each of the several varieties of paternalism ([8], pp. 16–22). The physician who is a strong paternalist, for example, might place techno-medical good above other senses of patient good. For him the patient's perceptions of his own immediate or ultimate good and his freedom, as a person, to make his own choices are not primary concerns. For some strong paternalists techno-medical good justifies withholding or manipulating information or breaking promises. Even the use of deceit or force might be rationalized to assure compliance with what is medically indicated.

Conversely, the libertarian typically places personal autonomy at the head of the list of what is good for the patient. A Rawlsian contractarian would opt for the good of the least advantaged member of society, though a Hobbesian would not. For the utilitarian social good would seem most defensible. Some sociobiologists deem the preservation of the gene pool the highest good. Some economists might choose just distribution of scarce resources and others the unimpeded operation of the free market.

The way the principles of beneficence, non-maleficence, justice, truth telling and promise keeping are applied is linked to the interpretation we put on the good of the patient. The hierarchical order we choose for arranging the four senses of patient good will differ with the ethical theory we espouse because every theory is grounded in some concept of the good. That order may vary even with different fields of medicine. For example, in preventive medicine, and public health as contrasted with curative medicine, certain strictures must be placed on the patient's expression of his own interests and even his freedom to refuse certain interventions like immunization [2].

Patient Good and Aristotle's Notion of Good

These problems are further exemplified when the question of patient good is set in the context of contemporary views of the good and contrasted with Aristotle's classical account.[1] In a recent study Henry Veatch, in part following Leo Strauss, contrasts the teleology of the modern view—of contractarians and consequentialists—with that of Aristotle [29]. The "moderns" interpret morality in terms of rights, particularly the right to define good for oneself limited only by the rights of others to do likewise. Rights then precede duty and morality enters when the pursuit of one's own ends and interests conflicts with the same pursuit by others. On the "modern" view we cannot know what is good for the patient without knowing his desires. The patient's choice is a good simply because he desires it. To do good for the patient we should do the good he desires. This concept of good is most consistent with a libertarian or permissive, anti-paternalist stance that permits the patient to choose a course even when it may seem wrong to a reasonable observer so long as the consequences are not harmful to others.

On the classical-medieval view, the good is objective and intrinsic to things that are good. These things ought to be done because they perfect our humanity and are most fitting for humans as humans. Good therefore is to be determined without reference to whether the patient wants it. Indeed he *ought* to want it and has a duty to want it. Duty precedes rights. Indeed rights exist because we must be unimpeded to do the good we ought to do. Patients ought not to be free to choose an evil course of action. For their good, their wishes can be overriden.

Veatch's interpretation of Aristotelian teleology may slide somewhat too easily over the controversies about precisely what Aristotle meant by the good. Nicholas White, for example, holds that Aristotle used good in the *Ethics* in at least three senses: (1) that which is good in itself and desired for itself and for which all other things are sought, (2) that which is good for a human being, or (3) that which is the aim or desire of an individual [30]. White attempts valiantly to reconcile these views in terms of *the good*, but his efforts are not entirely convincing. It seems far more likely that Aristotle too had to confront the fact that humans do in fact see the good in at least these three ways and that they are probably not completely reconcilable with each other.

W. F. R. Hardie, on the other hand, suggests that Aristotle's doctrine of the good may be taken in two ways: the first he calls "inclusive," i.e., encompassing a wide variety of aims consistent with the kind of life one wants to live [14]. Man is distinguished from other creatures as the responsible planner of his own life. His choices therefore are apt to be quite individual and peculiar to each person's plan of life. Hardie's second idea is of good as the dominant end. Here good is the overall plan that most fully makes a man a man, i.e., the attainment of theoretical knowledge. Hardie says, "Aristotle's doctrine of the final good is a doctrine about what is proper to a man. The power to reflect on his own abilities and desires and to conceive and choose for himself a satisfactory way of life" ([13], p. 321). This is reminiscent of Ralph Barton Perry's general theory of value which distinguishes man from animal by his ability to plan ahead in accord with his interests [24].

Let us return, briefly, to the three senses of "good" in Aristotle listed by White: (1) good *simpliciter,* that is, ultimate good for which all other things are chosen; (2) good for someone, i.e., a particular person; and (3) good for a human being. I would like to suggest a correspondence between these three senses of "good" and the four senses of *patient good* I have offered.

Aristotle's good *simpliciter* is, of course, *the good* or ultimate good. It is always in the background in clinical decisions. Even those who deny the usefulness of such a concept nonetheless tend to have a "good of last resort," so to speak, on which they found their sense of what is morally defensible.

It is the second and third senses of good, as used by Aristotle, i.e., the good of a particular person and the good of a human being, that correspond more closely with the several senses of patient good I have discussed.

The "patient's interests," his idea of what is good for him and fits his life plan, corresponds rather well with Aristotle's notion of the good as something at which people aim, the good of particular persons. Medical good is then the instrumental good that enables the patient to achieve his aims given the exigencies of illness.

"Freedom to choose" corresponds to Aristotle's third sense of the good as what is proper to a human being—someone endowed with reason—". . . for man therefore the life according to reason is best and pleasantest since reason more than anything else is man" ([4], 1178a 6–8). This passage has been interpreted as pointing to the life of contemplation, but as Hardie argues, it also points to the good of choosing, planning one's own life, and defining one's selfhood. Without freedom to choose it is impossible to use one's reason in an effective way.

Preeminent realist that he was, Aristotle's struggle with the conception of the good probably reflects his sensitivity to the actual difficulties of any simple definition of such a compound term. The realities of clinical decisions and the trifold notion of patient good argue somewhat against those who attempt to conflate Aristotle's three conceptions into one.

Medical good, the goal of medical interest, namely the health of the body, was for Aristotle a subsidiary good. It was a necessary condition and a means for the pursuit of the good life and the ultimate good but not itself ultimate [21]. Thus in the *Rhetoric* he says, "The excellence of the body is health; that is a condition which allows us while keeping free from disease to have use of our bodies" ([3], 1361b3). But he did not think health should override other human concerns, ". . . for many people are healthy as we are told Herodotus was, and these no one can congratulate on their health for they have to abstain from everything or nearly everything that men do" ([3], 1361b4). Aristotle's assignment of health in the hierarchy of good is not very far from the position we have given medical good in our analysis.

Recapitulation

Everyone who participates in a clinical decision justifies his or her actions as being in behalf of the patient's good. I have tried in this essay to clarify that all-inclusive notion by analyzing it into four components, identifying conflicts among these components as interpreted by the patient, the physician, the family and society, and suggesting how these conflicts might be resolved in making clinical decisions. I have confined myself to the patient's good as perceived by the patient and have avoided the more profound issues of the good of the patient metaphysically. I have used the example of decisions not to resuscitate as a paradigm case for the issues involving the patient's good, though the analysis is applicable to most clinical decisions involving moral choice. Finally I have suggested that a proper analysis of the patient's good will make for an ethically sounder physician-patient relationship and a clearer interpretation of the usual principles of medical ethics.[2]

Notes

1. See [4], especially Book I; Book X, Chapters 2, 7–8; and Book XII, Chapters 6–7, 9–10.

2. The author owes special thanks to the editors, Loretta Kopelman and John Moskop, for their careful editing and helpful suggestions which are incorporated into the text.

References

1. G. J. Annas, "CPR: The Beat Goes On." *Hastings Center Report* 12(4) (August 1982): 24–25.
2. G. J. Annas, "CPR: When the Beat Should Stop." *Hastings Center Report* 12(5) (October 1991): 30–31.
3. Aristotle, *Rhetoric.*
4. Aristotle, *Nichomachean Ethics.*
5. R. B. Brandt, *A Theory of the Good and the Right* (Oxford: Clarendon Press, 1979).
6. D. W. Brock, "Paternalism and Promoting the Good." In *Paternalism,* ed. R. Sartorius, pp. 237–260 (Minneapolis: University of Minnesota Press, 1983).
7. R. A. Carson and M. Siegler, "Does 'Doing Everything' Include CPR?" Case Study, *Hastings Center Report* 12(5) (October 1982): 27–29.
8. James F. Childress. *Who Should Decide? Paternalism in Health Care* (New York: Oxford University Press, 1982).
9. Clinical Care Committee of the Massachusetts General Hospital, "Optimum Care for Hopelessly Ill Patients." *New England Journal of Medicine* 295(7) (1976): 362–369.

10. E. L. Erde, "The Place of the Good in the Science and Art of Medicine." *Man and Medicine* 3(2) (1978): 89–100.

11. W. K. Frankena, *Ethics* (Englewood Cliffs, NJ: Prentice Hall, 1963).

12. B. Gruzalski, "When to Keep Patients Alive Against Their Will." In *Value Conflicts in Health Care Delivery,* ed. B. Gruzalski and C. E. Nelson, pp. 171–191 (Cambridge, MA: Ballinger, 1982).

13. W. F. R. Hardie, "The Final Good in Aristotle's Ethics." In *Aristotle: A Collection of Critical Essays,* ed. J. M. E. Moravcsik, pp. 296–322 (Garden City, NY: Anchor, 1967).

14. *In re Dinnerstein,* 380 N.E. 2d 134 (Mass. App. 1978).

15. D. L. Jackson and S. Youngner, "Patient Autonomy and Death with Dignity." *New England Journal of Medicine* 301(8) (1973): 404–408.

16. L. Lavelle, *The Problem of Evil in Contemporary European Ethics,* ed. J. J. Kochelmans (Garden City, NY: Anchor Books, 1972).

17. R. J. Levine, "Do Not Resuscitate Decisions and Their Implications." In *Dilemmas of Dying: Policies and Procedures for Decisions Not to Treat,* ed. C. Wong and J. P. Swazey, pp. 23–41 (Boston: Hall Medical, 1981).

18. S. H. Miles, R. Cranford and A. L. Schultz, "The Do-Not-Resuscitate Order in a Teaching Hospital." *Annals of Internal Medicine* 96(5) (1982): 660–664.

19. R. G. Olson, "The Good." In *The Encyclopedia of Philosophy,* vol. 3, ed. P. Edwards, pp. 367–370 (New York: Macmillan., 1982).

20. J. Owens, "Aristotelian Ethics and Medicine." In *Philosophical Medical Ethics: Its Nature and Significance,* ed. S. F. Spicker and H. T. Engelhardt, Jr., pp. 127–142 (Dordrecht, Holland: D. Reidel, 1977).

21. E. D. Pellegrino, "Autonomy and Coercion in Disease Prevention and Health Promotion." *Theoretical Medicine* 5(1) (1983): 83–91.

22. E. D. Pellegrino, "Towards a Reconstruction of Medical Morality: The Primacy of the Act of Profession and the Fact of Illness." *Journal of Medicine and Philosophy* 4(1) (1979): 32–56.

23. E. D. Pellegrino, "The Virtuous Physician and the Ethics of Medicine." In *Virtue and Medicine,* ed. E. Shelp (Dordrecht, Holland: D. Reidel, 1985).

24. R. B. Perry, *General Theory of Value* (New York: Longmans, Green, 1926).

25. P. Ramsey, *Ethics at the Edges of Life,* pp. 189–227 (New Haven, CT: Yale University Press, 1978).

26. W. D. Ross, *The Right and the Good* (London: Oxford University Press, 1930).

27. S. S. Spencer, "Code or No Code: A Nonlegal Opinion." *New England Journal of Medicine* 300(3) (1979): 138–140.

28. U.S. President's Commission for the Study of Ethical Problems in Medicine and Biomedical and Behavioral Research, *Deciding to Forego Life-Sustaining Treatment* (Washington, DC, 1983).

29. H. B. Veatch, "Telos and Teleology in Aristotelian Ethics." In *Studies in Aristotle,* ed. D. O'Meara, pp. 279–296 (Washington, DC: Catholic University of America Press, 1981).
30. N. P. White, "Goodness and Human Aims in Aristotle's Ethics." In *Studies in Aristotle,* ed. D. O'Meara, pp. 225–246 (Washington, DC: Catholic University of America Press, 1981).
31. C. B. Wong and J. P. Swazey, *Dilemmas of Dying: Policies and Procedures for Decisions Not to Treat* (Boston: Hall Medical, 1981).

The Four Principles and
the Doctor-Patient Relationship

1994

The Need for a Better Linkage

Introduction

1978

A little more than a decade ago, Beauchamp and Childress published the first edition of what has since become the most influential guide to biomedical ethics (1). They adapted W. D. Ross's notion of *prima facie* principles to the emerging field of medical ethics (2). Today, non-maleficence, beneficence, autonomy, and justice have become the reference *tetrad par excellence* which doctors and ethicists use to resolve ethical dilemmas and define the right conduct of doctors and patients.

As experience in the use of the four-principle framework has widened, shortcomings in its application to the clinical realities of the doctor-patient relationship have begun to appear. As a result, some moral philosophers today have called for the abandonment of "principlism" (3) or its replacement by alternative theories based in virtue, feminist psychology, casuistry, or experience (4, 5).

In this chapter I shall argue that the four principles should not be abandoned. Rather, they need to be redefined and grounded in the reality of the doctor-patient relationship. This grounding can provide a standard against which the fundamental conceptual problem of conflict among *prima facie* principles can be resolved. This approach is also more congenial than "principlism" to enrichment by moral insights from a variety of non-principle-based ethical perspectives.

The first part of this chapter describes how the emergence of autonomy as a dominant principle has altered our construal of the doctor-patient relationship. The second part details the conflicts that can occur among the four *prima facie* principles when they are applied in clinical ethical decision-making. The third part offers a teleological foundation for the four principles as obligations of the good doctor. The last section re-examines the way philosophy itself is used as a tool in critical reflections on medicine.

Autonomy and Models of the Doctor-Patient Relationship

Nothing in medical ethics has changed so dramatically and drastically in the last quarter-century as the standards of ethical conduct governing the relationship between doctors and patients. In that time the center of gravity of clinical decision-making has shifted almost completely from the doctor to the patient. The traditional benign and respected image of the doctor as both moral and technical authority has been replaced by the doctor as protector, facilitator, and advocate for the self-determination of the patient. Now, every facet of care, from the choice among preferred treatments to requests not to be resuscitated, and even for active euthanasia and assisted suicide, are construed as moral and civil rights with which doctors in good conscience are expected to comply.

This metamorphosis has been most evident and most advanced in the United States. But the sociopolitical and cultural forces that have nurtured such a drastic change are effecting similar transformations in almost every country of the world. Among these forces are the actualization of participatory democracy, the increasing moral pluralism and moral heterogeneity of modem society, expansions in public education by the media, the weakening of religion as an ultimate source of morality, a general mistrust of the exercise of authority in all spheres of life, and, of course, the unprecedented expansion of medical power through technology.

Not the least of the forces effecting change was the entry of the professional philosopher into the study of medical ethics. Curiously, philosophers historically paid little formal attention to the ethics of medicine. To be sure, there were "philosophical" reflections by doctors on the nature of medicine and medical ethics, but this was philosophy only in the loosest sense. Until the mid-sixties, professional philosophers paid little formal attention to medical ethics.

This changed when medical ethics first came under serious philosophical scrutiny. Surely the most influential thrust in this direction was Beauchamp and Childress's *Principles of Biomedical Ethics,* first published in 1978, in which the four-principle approach around which this whole book is organized was first introduced (1). This book added the reinforcement of formal analysis to the more inchoate stirrings of social change which had already weakened the pediments of the traditional Hippocratic model of the doctor-patient relationship. In its place a variety of autonomy-based models have gained pre-eminence.

Given the confluence of forces we mentioned above as characteristic of modern democratic, secular, morally heterogeneous societies, the principle of autonomy has had understandable worldwide appeal within and outside medicine. Autonomy, self-governance, and the right to privacy have become symbols of resistance to the misuse of authority by professionals, institutions, and governments. Respect for autonomy seeks to balance the enormous power of expert knowledge which figures so prominently in private and public decisions in industrialized and technologically oriented societies. Autonomy calls for protection of the moral and personal values of each individual and, thus, of the integrity of the person.

Autonomy has had a particular appeal in medical relationships. It counters the historical dominance of benign authoritarianism or paternalism in the traditional ethics of medicine. It assures that patients may choose among treatment alternatives and accept or reject any of them and, thus, retain control over some of the most intimate and personal decisions in their lives. Respect for autonomy also protects patients against submergence of their moral values and beliefs. In morally diverse societies where doctors and patients may come from markedly different cultural, ethnic, and religious origins, observance of this facet of autonomy is especially and justifiably cherished.

The assertion of autonomy in medical ethics has been salubrious on the whole. It has become a powerful and increasingly effective deterrent to abuses of doctor power. It has served particularly well in placing the ultimate control of decisions at the beginning and ending of life more fully in control of the patient. It is the driving force behind judicial opinion and legislation which confirm the legal rights of patients to make their own decisions and to make use of advance directives to assure control of decisions if competence to do so is lost in the course of an illness.

The emphasis on autonomy has also fostered the emergence of several models of the doctor-patient relationship sharply divergent from traditional models (6). Two examples are the consumer and the negotiated contract models.

In the consumer model, health care is viewed as a commodity or service, like any other commodity, to be purchased in the marketplace on the consumer's terms, i.e., in terms of his personal assessment of alternative modes of treatment, their cost, benefits and risks. The doctor is a provider whose task it is to provide reliable information, perhaps to advise, but not to interject her own values. The patient's values must predominate, and the doctor's moral obligations are to inform, to perform with competence, and to protect and enhance the patient's capabilities for self-determination.

In the negotiated contract model, doctor and patient discuss their relative values in advance—those related to health and those related to moral values in general. As in the consumer model, the doctor and patient are both autonomous persons entering a contract, but in the negotiated model the details of the contract are more intensively examined before any medical relationship is entered. Moreover, the nature of the relationship is determinable only by the contracting parties. In essence, they alone must determine what conduct is expected so that the ethics of the relationship varies with the ethics of the contracting parties. On this view, the notion of a universally applicable set of ethical principles beyond autonomy is irrelevant: doctor and patient may pursue any course they wish, provided it is mutually agreed upon. That which is agreed upon is no concern of third parties. It might include active euthanasia, assisted suicide or an advance directive that calls for involuntary or non-voluntary euthanasia.

These two examples of autonomy-driven models of the doctor-patient relationship make the relationship largely instrumental and procedural. They are legalistic in spirit, and the ethic they engender is one of minimal personal commitment and trust. Indeed, they are more based in distrust than trust. They are also destructive of the idea of a common medical morality since the participants give medical ethics any meaning they choose. The only ethical failure is failure to abide by a prearranged contract.

While these autonomy-inspired models seem to protect the patient's right of self-determination, on closer inspection they are also, in considerable measure, illusory and even dangerous to both parties. First, one thing they neglect is the fact that doctor and patient are not Lockean free agents equal in bargaining power. The patient is vulnerable since she is the one in need of help, has not the power to heal herself, is in pain, anxious, frightened, perhaps distressed. It is hard to imagine a valid contract in which one of the parties is so dependent upon the other for the information necessary to a choice and upon the competence of the other to carry out the choice once it is made.

Autonomy-based models thus seem oblivious to the incontestable fact of doctor power, a power that arises from several sources. There is the *de facto* power mentioned above, which derives from the fact of illness itself. But there is also the power of the doctor's personality or charisma which operates in subtle ways often inapparent to both doctor and patient but, nonetheless, a powerful force in shaping even the independently minded patient's decisions. Finally, there is the force of social sanction of medicine and its monopoly of medical knowledge which operate regardless of the details of a negotiated contract.

The realities of these forms of ("Aesculapian power") make it amply evident that the desire to limit trust in the doctor which lies behind the autonomy models is often deceptive. There is no way to circumvent the doctor's character or her construal of what autonomy means in actual practice. In fact, to execute a contract is to send a signal of distrust of the doctor and to put her on her guard. As a result she might restrain her inclinations to be beneficent when the clinical situation changes in ways that could not be anticipated. In any case, there is no evidence that a relationship based in mistrust is any more protective of patient autonomy than one based in trust, i.e., in a covenant rather than a contract (7).

The deficiences of autonomy-based models of the doctor-patient relationship do not, of course, vitiate the validity of autonomy as a moral principle. There is no question that the centuries-old neglect of the role of the patient in decisions that affect him is not, and was not, morally defensible, even if it was socially tolerable. Respect for the patient's self-determination and, thus, for the integrity of the person, is a moral requirement in all human relationships and especially in those like medicine in which there is a *de facto* imbalance of power. What the deficiencies of the models that try to optimize autonomy reveal is not that autonomy is to be abandoned, but that absolutization is morally perilous. If autonomy itself is to be safeguarded, its expression must be more closely related with the other major principles of beneficence and justice, as well as with theories of medical ethics which are not principle based.

Conflicts of Autonomy with Beneficence

A second consequence of the autonomy movement is the degree to which patient self-determination is set in polar opposition to beneficence. This emerges very clearly in Beauchamp's book with L. B. McCullough (8). Here, beneficence is erroneously equated with paternalism. The case examples used to illustrate the conceptual content of the text choices are framed almost exclusively as conflicts between beneficence and autonomy. Several misconceptions arise as a result.

First of all, beneficence and paternalism are not synonymous. Paternalism (or maternalism) assumes that the doctor knows better than the patient what is in the patient's best interests or that a mentally competent patient cannot possibly know enough about the choices to be able to make intelligent decisions. Or, less benignly, the doctor may assume that it is her prerogative as the privileged proprietor of medical knowledge and skill to dispense it as she sees fit without the patient's interference.

Paternalism, whether benignly intended or not, cannot be beneficent in any true sense of that word. Beneficence and its corollary, non-maleficence, require acting to advance the patient's interests, or at least not harming them. It is difficult to see how violating the patient's own perception of his welfare can be a beneficent act. Paternalism is obviously in a polar relationship with autonomy, but it is also diametrically opposed to beneficence and non-maleficence as well.

True beneficence, on the other hand, seeks the good of the patient. That good is a compound idea consisting in an ascending hierarchical order starting with (a) what is medically good, i.e., restoration of physio-logical functioning and emotional balance; (b) what is defined as good by the patient in terms of his perception of his own good; (c) what is good for humans as humans and members of the human community; and (d) what is good for humans as spiritual beings (9).

In this hierarchical order, autonomy is a good of humans as humans. Without freedom and the capacity to make choices about our own lives, to be responsible for those choices and to carry out a life plan, we cannot express our humanity fully. To violate or impede a patient's autonomy is a maleficent act. To facilitate, enhance, and restore the capability for self-governance is a beneficent act. Beneficence and respect for persons, which is the moral foundation for autonomy, are, therefore, congruent, and it is a misconception to see them as antithetical as some interpreters of the four principles do. Later in this chapter I will suggest an alternative per-spective on the four principles which may help to resolve potential con-flicts between autonomy and beneficence as well as the potential conflict with justice.

does this not merely resituate the conflict around the concept of competence, or is there some advantage gained thereby?

Conflicts of Autonomy and Justice

If the antinomy between respect for autonomy and beneficence is more apparent than real, this is not the case with autonomy and justice. It can happen that respecting the autonomy of the patient may inflict harm on third parties near to, or distant from, the patient. Here we face a funda-mental dilemma of the idea of *prima facie* principles. When two such principles are in conflict with each other, we must choose between them. To do so, one principle must trump the other. But how do we decide which one?

Justice is the most complex of the four principles, and the only one that is simultaneously a virtue and a principle. As a virtue it is a character trait, a habitual disposition to render to each what is due him. As a prin-ciple it ordains that we act in such fashion that we render to each what is due her, and that we treat like cases alike. There is, thus, an element of jus-tice in each of the other principles since we owe it to humans not to harm them, to respect their autonomy, and to do good when we can. Justice, therefore, has a certain prior status in determining the right and the good.

how is it distinguished from "fairness"?

In this sense it limits the exercise of our own autonomy and our obligation to respect the autonomy of others. Justice thus sets limits on the absolutization of autonomy to which the autonomy-based models of the doctor-patient relationship tend.

Some examples in which respect for the autonomy of one person may impose injustice on another are these: the patient, seropositive for HIV infection, who refuses to disclose the fact to her sexual partners or persists in unprotected sexual intercourse; the airline pilot or railroad engineer who refuses to disclose her substance abuse to her employer; the patient who demands marginally beneficial treatments that use up inordinate amounts of health care resources; the psychiatric patient who intends to harm others (10).

Respecting the patient's autonomy can also compromise the autonomy of the doctor—not his autonomy to treat as he sees fit without reference to the patient's best interests, but his autonomy as a human being with his own values and beliefs. An example of this type is the demands of some patients, on grounds of patient autonomy, that the doctor violate standards of good care to provide treatments that are scientifically dubious. Of like kind are demands that the doctor perform abortion, participate in euthanasia, or withdraw artificial feeding and hydration when these actions would violate his personal conscience.

Instances of this kind are increasing as the pressure to absolutize the individual's autonomy become more insistent. There is a growing sentiment in certain public and private quarters that the doctor is merely the instrument of the patient's will. Some have even argued that the doctor should leave personal morality behind in her professional life. On this view, not to provide what the patient wants, or what institutional policy or financial considerations dictate, is to violate not only the rule of autonomy but also beneficence and, indeed, justice. On this view, the doctor's monopoly of medical knowledge is taken as warrant to justify the patient's claim irrespective of the doctor's values.

Judgments about how best to resolve the conflict between *prima facie* principles, or, perhaps more accurately, individual interpretations of how those principles ought to be applied, are difficult. I have suggested justice has a trumping function. Under what circumstances should it take moral precedence over autonomy? These circumstances would obtain when there is an identifiable harm of serious nature to a third party or parties and all other measures to protect autonomy have been taken. These conditions would be met in the case of the patient with HIV infection or the operators of public conveyances where even the small possibility of grievous harm to others outweighs the claim to autonomy and preservation of confidentiality. The harm to others is more remote and less clearly identifiable in cases where patients demand dubious, marginal, or excessively costly treatments. Here the doctor might more readily balance the psychological benefits to the patient against possible indefinite harm to others.

When the patient or social policy dictates that the doctor submerge her own moral values to accommodate patient demands, even if what is demanded is accepted practice, then the conflict is between the patient's and the doctor's autonomy. Here we must argue that the doctor, no less than the patient, is a moral agent, that her autonomy is as deserving of respect as the patient's, and that justice would require that neither doctor nor patient impose her values on the other. If it is maleficent to violate the autonomy of the patient, it is equally maleficent to violate that of the doctor.

In practical terms this will mean that, institutionally and ethically, mechanisms must be devised to permit doctors as well as patients to withdraw from their relationship. This must be done amicably, respectfully, and only after another doctor has agreed to accept the transfer of responsibility for the care of the patient. The doctor cannot withdraw without first making provisions for transfer to another doctor, because to do so would constitute abandonment, in itself a serious breach of ethical obligation.

Proxy and Surrogate Decisions

The potential conflict between autonomy, justice, and beneficence becomes more acute and more complex when the moral right of autonomy is exercised by a surrogate. This is the case with infants and with adults rendered incapable of self-governance by virtue of severe illness, mental retardation, or severe brain damage. Under these circumstances the moral right to autonomous decisions is transferred to a morally valid surrogate or to an advance directive (living will or (durable power of attorney) for health care). The surrogate or living will are intended to assess what the patient would have wanted were he able to understand and evaluate his clinical state as it is when the decision is actually about to be made.

Here, again, autonomy cannot be absolutized, although doing so would simplify decision-making for doctors and families. The doctor can be caught in a serious conflict of obligations. On the one hand, she is bound to respect the delegated moral authority of the surrogate or advance directive; on the other hand, she is also bound in beneficence and justice to safeguard the welfare of the patient against possible abuse by the surrogate. Doctors must daily resolve these conflicts in obligation. They cannot debate endlessly. They must make a decision. They must sign the order. They are moral accomplices unavoidably.

Many practical problems complicate the doctor's decision to agree with, modify, or refuse to comply with the surrogate decision. Application of the four principles is dependent on many factual questions with moral implications. First, is the surrogate morally empowered to act for the patient? To be so qualified, the surrogate should, in fact, know the patient's values and give some evidence of the same; she must be free of obvious conflicts of interest, such as having a large stake in the patient's will; she must not be in an emotionally pathological relationship with the patient which might lead to unconscious over- or under-treatment.

Even if the surrogate is free of impediments to act on behalf of the patient, there are many other possible sources of difficulty (11). We must know whether the surrogate actually discussed the patient's preferences with her, whether they were understood in the same way by surrogate and patient, and whether the surrogate is transmitting the patient's meanings faithfully. When the time lapse between execution and application of an advance directive is long, the diagnosis/prognosis may have changed substantially. One might then question whether it is a beneficent act to follow the patient's advance statement of preferences. What about psychological discontinuity? Is the patient now before us in a permanent vegetative state the same person who told us her preferences when she was well? When, in the interests of beneficence and justice, may the (projected autonomy) which a surrogate or advance directive represents be overridden? May there be times when a "best interests" or "reasonable person" standard is more in the patient's interests? (12).

My purpose in reciting some of these difficulties is not to suggest that the four principles should be abandoned—as others have suggested. It is rather to point to some important philosophical questions that arise from the experience of applying principles in the moment of truth, i.e., in the actualities of the doctor-patient relationship. These experiences indicate that the four principles cannot stand alone, that they need linkages with other sources of ethical insight, and that they need a closer grounding in the phenomena of the relationship itself.

"Tuning" the Four Principles Philosophically and Clinically

To bring the four-principles approach into closer congruence with some of the realities of clinical decision-making, we need to examine at least three questions: (a) How are conflicts between *prima facie* principles to be resolved? (b) How may other sources of ethical insight be incorporated? (c) What, finally, should the relationship be of formal philosophy to medical ethics?

The Conflict between *Prima Facie* Principles

The framework of *prima facie* principles has unquestionably advanced the quality of ethical decision-making at the bedside. Its utility must not be lost in the current zeal for replacing it with alternative approaches which have their own inherent difficulties. The four principles have put the whole process of moral decision-making on a more orderly, less idiosyncratic, and more explicit basis. They have raised sensitivities to ethical issues among all health workers, patients, and their families. The general moral precepts of the Hippocratic ethics have been "fleshed out" where they have been deficient and provided with philosophical grounding where this has been lacking. Principle-based ethics has also provided a *lingua franca* for communication among doctors and ethicists whose moral presuppositions might otherwise have been incommensurable with one another.

It would be a retrogressive step, indeed, to drop the principles and return to some simplistic conviction of the sufficiency of the Hippocratic Oath to which many doctors subscribe. Equally unsatisfactory would be a too-ready acquiescence to the arguments of the anti-principlists who would substitute important but insufficient bases for medical ethics drawn from virtue, feminist, or experiential systems. These alternatives, valuable as they are, also lead to subjectivism, emotivism, and egoism, the major dangers to which non-principle-based approaches are susceptible.

This is not to deny a central difficulty in the design of the system of *prima facie* principles. If these principles are to be honored, unless there is an overwhelming reason to do so, what constitutes an overwhelming reason? Is the justification for overriding made in terms of some other *prima facie* principle or some special circumstance? If it is another *prima facie* principle, then we face the problem of one principle having greater moral weight than another. There is no formal mechanism or convincing argument that would grant trumping privileges to one principle over another.

Clearly, *prima facie* principles cannot be used to resolve conflicts among *prima facie* principles unless some external ordering mechanism is adduced, as I have done above in my discussion of the autonomy-beneficence polarity. Could the trumping justification then simply be the circumstances? If this were the case, the circumstances would, themselves, take on the moral force of a *prima facie* principle, or they would have to be justified by one of the *prima facie* principles—but which one?

Any and all of these attempts to resolve the conflict between *prima facie* principles must eventually put one *prima facie* principle against another. This leads to the logical errors of begging the question or circular reasoning. If this is so, then some resolution must be sought beyond *prima facie* principles, and this could come about in one of five ways: 1. abandon principlism altogether in favor of some alternative theory like virtue, experience, or feminist psychology; 2. retain principlism, but supplement it by insights from other ethical theories; 3. ground principlism more fully in the phenomena of the doctor-patient relationship; 4. some combination of options 2 and 3; 5. retain the four-principle approach without emendation.

From what I have already shown thus far, it is clear that options 1 and 5 are not adequate in the face of the practical and theoretical complexities described here. Option 4 seems the most promising, and this option will be examined briefly, leaving to another occasion its more extended development.

Principlism has sustained its most radical criticism in the work of Clouser and Gert and others (3, 13). These authors point out what they take to be fundamental conceptual flaws in principlism as they are exemplified specifically in the work of Frankena (14) and Beauchamp and Childress. Clouser and Gert (3) assert that principlism lacks systematic unity and thus creates both practical and theoretical problems.

> Since there is no moral theory that ties "principles" together, there is no unified guide to action which generates clear, coherent, comprehensive, and specific rules for action nor any justification of those rules. (ref. 3, p. 227)

On Clouser and Gert's view these inadequacies lead to relativism, since principles seem to stand free of any grounding and since they may conflict with each other without offering a path to resolution. Similar criticisms can be found in the articles by Brody (15) and Green (13). Criticism of another kind comes from the protagonists of virtue theory, feminist psychology, casuistry, or ethics as narrative, experiential or existential phenomena. Space limitations prohibit serious examination of these alternatives. However, they share certain perceptions that principle-based ethics is too abstract, too removed from the actual moral and psychological realities of actual people making actual choices, and too male oriented in its psychology and reasoning. They also aver that principlism ignores the character, gender, life stories, and cultural identity of moral agents. On this view ethics is more than a technical exercise drawing clear conclusions from clear premises. It is a personal act nuanced in a variety of subtle ways principles do not touch. As Oakeshott puts it, "Moral conduct is art, not nature" (16).

One may agree that there is substance in each of these varied criticisms of principle-based ethics without also agreeing that they do away with principles or are themselves fully adequate replacements. It is too soon to know how, and to what extent, they will modify the four-principle approach. The likelihood is that they will enrich and refine principle-based ethics but not replace it (17, 18). It seems clear that a unifying theory of biomedical ethics will need to link principles with insights from these other sources. This is the most serious conceptual task biomedical ethics faces in the immediate future.

Principles, Philosophy, and the Doctor-Patient Relationship

If principles do remain integral to biomedical ethics, they will have to be more firmly grounded in the phenomena of the doctor-patient relationship. One may approach this linkage in two ways: one is externally, by the application of an already developed philosophical or ethical system to the medical relationship. This is the method used by the four principles, whether those principles are conceived consequentially or deontologically. The second way is to examine the doctor-patient relationship with the method of philosophy (critical reflection) but without the content of a specific philosophy in order to derive from the relationship what is required ethically and what principles best exemplify what is required. This is the approach via the internal morality of medicine. This is essentially a teleological approach in the classical, not the consequentialist, sense—that is, it is oriented to the ends and purposes of the relationship, and it is the degree to which decisions and actions of the moral agents—doctors and patients—approximate these ends that determines whether they are right and good.

Briefly, the ends of medicine are ultimately the restoration or improvement of health, and more proximately, to heal, i.e., to cure illness and disease or, when this is not possible, to care and help the patient to live with residual pain, discomfort, or disability. There are many decisions along the way to these ends, but in each decision there is a fusion of technical and moral elements. If it were merely a matter of technical correctness, of medical good alone, the major moral principle would be competence. But the subjects of medical decisions are humans, and humans in special states of vulnerability—anxious, in pain, dependent upon the doctor's knowledge, skill, and trustworthiness, and responsible management of the power his professional status confers *de facto*. Moreover, the doctor offers to help and, thus, promises the vulnerable patient that she will help attain the ends for which the patient seeks medical help. This implies that the doctor will use her promised competence not for her own ends but for those of the patient and will, in ordinary circumstances, efface her own interests in respect for the patient, i.e., she promises to serve the patient's good. But this good is more than simple medical good; it includes the patient's perception of good, material, emotional or spiritual.

If these ends are to be achieved, the good of the patient provides the architectonic of the relationship. Beneficence becomes a requirement not of a system of philosophy applied to medicine, but of the nature of medical activity. Respect for autonomy is required to achieve the ends of medicine because to violate the patient's values is to violate his person and, therefore, a maleficent act which distorts the healing end of the relationship. Justice is a requisite duty because what we owe the patient is fidelity to the trust we elicited when we offered to help, when we invoked confidence in our willingness to act beneficently. In like fashion the derivative obligations are mandatory if we examine the nature of the relationship. We must keep the promise we made, implicitly or explicitly, to be beneficent, to protect the confidentiality (except as outlined earlier when harm to others is at stake), and to tell the truth, since to violate any of these trusts and obligations is to go counter to the nature of the relationship itself.

On the view I am taking, the four principles are derived from obligations owed by doctors. These obligations, in turn, derive from the promise to provide competent help, which is at the heart of the medical relationship. The primary obligation which unifies the theory of medical ethics is beneficence—beneficence not mistakenly equated with paternalism, but beneficence-in-trust, beneficence which fuses respect for the person of the patient with the obligation not just to prevent or remove harm, but to do good. The primary obligation is not non-maleficence, which is a negative obligation required even by law. Beneficence requires preventing harm, removing harm and doing good even at some cost and risk to oneself. Thus, there is an implicit promise of some degree of self-effacement of the doctor's interests in favor of the patient's interests.

The obligations that arise from the nature of the relationship provide the theoretical grounding lacking in the approach through *prima facie* principles. Rather than principles, we can speak of obligations freely undertaken when we freely offer to help a sick person. Beneficence-in-trust—that is to say, beneficence that encompasses the whole of the patient's well-being and not simply his medical well-being—becomes the ordering

✳ author emphasizes "beneficence-in-trust" to distinguish from a paternalistic form of beneficence principle. This form of beneficence cannot obtain if we violate autonomy, justice, truth-telling, fidelity to trust, or promise-keeping.

Beneficence thus becomes a principle that is also a guide to action. "So act in your relationship with your patients that your actions are directed by the good of the patient, the primary telos of the healing relationship." Beneficence as a principle is grounded in the humanity of the persons interacting in the medical relationship. That relationship is, as Oakeshott says of all ethics, a relationship *inter homines* (16).

This approach has the advantage of deriving its obligations and its principles from real phenomena of the real world of clinical medicine. It reverses the usual way philosophy is used to determine medical ethics. Rather than taking principles already formulated in an ethical theory—consequentialist, utilitarian, or deontological—it begins with the phenomena peculiar to the activity in question and examines them philosophically—i.e., critically, formally, systematically, in terms of the human realities they exemplify. It may indeed happen, as in the present inquiry, that the results are similar to the four-principle approach. But the principles are grounded in a more systematic use of theory; its principles flow from obligations grounded in the special character of the medical relationship. They become more than a checklist of considerations for ethical discourse. They have a moral binding power grounded firmly in clinical realities.

Clearly, the teleological approach suggested here does not, by itself, constitute a complete system of medical ethics. To do so, it would also have to link obligations and its primary principles to virtue ethics and incorporate insights from casuistry, moral psychology, and experiential ethical systems.

The four-principle approach does have its theoretical and practical inadequacies. However, it should not be abandoned, because it still has much to offer. Its shortcomings can be remedied. The one direction for refinement I have suggested is a closer and firmer grounding in the doctor-patient relationship. Another direction, which I do not examine here, is to incorporate insights from experience, moral psychology, casuistry, and virtue theories. In the years ahead, such efforts could produce a more complete theory and practice of medical ethics provided that theory is firmly situated in the central pediment of all biomedical ethics, the doctor-patient relationship.

References

1. Beauchamp, T. L., and J. F. Childress. 1978. *Principles of Biomedical Ethics.* Oxford: Oxford University Press.
2. Ross, W. D. 1939. *The Foundations of Ethics.* Oxford: Clarendon Press.
3. Clouser, K. D., and B. Gert. 1990. "A Critique of Principlism." *Journal of Medicine and Philosophy* 15(2): 219–236.
4. Gilligan, C. 1982. *In a Different Voice: Psychological Theory and Women's Development.* Cambridge, MA: Harvard University Press.
5. Drane, J. F. 1988. *Becoming a Good Doctor: The Place of Virtue and Character in Medical Ethics.* Kansas City, MO: Sheed & Ward.
6. Emanuel, E. J., and L. Emanuel. 1992. "Four Models of the Physician-Patient Relationship." *Journal of the American Medical Association* 267(16): 2221–2226.
7. May, W. F. 1983. *The Physician's Covenant.* Philadelphia, PA: Westminster Press.
8. Beauchamp, T. L., and L. B. McCullough. 1984. *Medical Ethics: The Moral Responsibilities of Physicians.* Englewood Cliffs, NJ: Prentice Hall.
9. Pellegrino, E. D., and D. C. Thomasma. 1988. *For the Patient's Good.* New York: Oxford University Press.
10. Beck, J. C. (Ed.). 1990. *Confidentiality versus the Duty to Protect: Foreseeable Harm in the Practice of Psychiatry.* Washington, DC: American Psychiatric Press.
11. Buchanan, A. E., and D. Brock. 1989. *Deciding for Others: The Ethics of Surrogate Decision-Making.* New York: Cambridge University Press.
12. Robertson, J. A. 1991. "Cruzan and the Constitutional Status of Non-treatment Decisions for Incompetent patients." *Georgia Law Review* 25(5): 1139–1202.
13. Green, R. M. 1990. "Method in Bioethics: A Troubled Assessment." *Journal of Medicine and Philosophy* 15(2): 179–197.
14. Frankena, W. K. 1973. *Ethics.* Englewood Cliffs, NJ: Prentice Hall.
15. Brody, B. A. 1990. "Quality of Scholarship in Bioethics." *Journal of Medicine and Philosophy* 15(2): 161–178.
16. Oakeshott, M. J. 1991. *Rationalism in Politics and Other Essays,* p. 296. Indianapolis: Liberty Press.
17. Carse, A. L. 1991. "The Voice of Care: Implications for Bioethical Education." *Journal of Medicine and Philosophy* 16(1): 5–28.
18. Jonsen, A. R., and S. Toulmin. 1988. *The Abuse of Casuistry: A History of Moral Reasoning.* Los Angeles: University of California Press.

Patient and Physician Autonomy

Conflicting Rights and Obligations in the Physician-Patient Relationship

L— 1994

For centuries, physician beneficence went unchallenged as the first principle of medical ethics. To be sure, some physicians had, at times, violated this principle. But no creditable ethical opposition was mounted until a quarter of a century ago when patient autonomy was asserted as a *prima facie* moral principle of equal or greater weight than beneficence.[1] Progressively since then, patient autonomy has become the dominant principle shaping physician-patient relationships.

Three serious moral conflicts have emerged as a result: first, beneficence and autonomy have been polarized against each other when they should be complementary; second, the physician's moral claim to autonomy has received little attention; and third, the "autonomy" of medical ethics, itself, has come under a serious threat. This essay will examine each of these three consequences resulting from the rise of patient autonomy. It shall do so from the point of view that the physician-patient relationship is a moral equation with rights and obligations on both sides and that it must be balanced so that physicians and patients act beneficently toward each other while respecting each other's autonomy. Effecting this balance is a morally mandatory and exacting exercise. The compass points that might guide this balancing are to be found in a reflection on the concepts of autonomy and beneficence, the way the content of these abstract notions is provided by the clinical encounter, and the way conflicts may be resolved in particular clinical situations.

Out of this reflection, five conclusions will emerge: (1) in concept, autonomy and beneficence are complementary and not contradictory; (2) in theory and in practice, autonomy is a positive as well as a negative principle; (3) the actual content of the concepts of beneficence and autonomy is defined in specific actions and decisions in the light of which conflicts are best understood and resolved; (4) the physician's autonomy as a person and a professional must be factored into the equation; and (5) medical ethics, as an enterprise, must maintain a certain "autonomy" in the face of political and socio-economic pressures.

The Concept of Autonomy

Autonomy in General

Autonomy is one of those widely applauded concepts which, on closer inspection, turns out to be difficult to define with precision.[2] This is not the place to review the range of construals of the term. Rather, I will limit myself to that construal which centers on the etymology of the word itself, which means "self-rule." What is common to most definitions is the notion that an autonomous person is one who, in his thoughts, words, and actions, is able to follow those norms he chooses as his own without external constraints or coercion by others.[3]

The history of the concept is complex, and its roots are political as well as moral. Politically, autonomy came into prominence during the Enlightenment as an assertion of the individual's right to be free from tyrannous government—not of law *per se*, but of unjust law.[4] Morally, autonomy encompasses the right of persons to freedom of conscience and to respect as agents capable of making their own judgments in accord with universal moral principles,[5] or in accord with freely arrived at decisions.[6]

Autonomy gets its status as a moral right of humans from the fact that human beings have the capacity to make rational judgments about their own lives, choices, and interests. Self-governance deserves respect because it is the way human beings actualize their powers of choice, and choice is a distinctly human activity. To obstruct the capacity for autonomy is to assault an essential part of a person's humanity, because the choices we make are so much an expression of our membership in the human community, of who we are or what we want to be as individual members of that community. Human beings are owed respect for their autonomy because they have an inherent dignity. They do not have dignity because they are autonomous. Human beings who lack or have lost the capacity for autonomous actions are nonetheless humans who retain their inherent dignity. Respect for persons comprises more than respect for autonomy.

Autonomy has taken on a distinctive negative connotation. Arising, as it did, as a moral claim against invasion of human rights by tyrannous government, it has come to mean a right of self-determination *against* those who would usurp that right. In medical ethics, it is conceived largely as a moral and legal defense against physician paternalism and against those who would impose their values—social, moral, or otherwise—on others.

But autonomy is also a positive concept. It implies an obligation to foster the human capacity for self-determination, to enhance it, and to remove the obstacles to its full operation. This is especially important in clinical medical ethics where pathophysiological, emotional, and social realities complicate the actualization of patient autonomy. If taken as a strictly negative concept of non-interference, autonomy can be self-defeating for patients and self-serving for physicians. This positive aspect of autonomy will become clearer as I fill in the content of the concept as it operates in the clinical situation.

Patient Autonomy and Physician Beneficence

Twenty-five years ago, the political and moral notion of autonomy was appropriated as one of the *prima facie* principles of medical ethics.[7] There were good reasons for the emergence of patient autonomy at that time. The rights of patients to refuse unwanted treatment had been neglected for entirely too long. In the mid-sixties, these rights could no longer be denied as participatory democracy, better public education, and the civil rights movements became realities. All authority claims came under suspicion. The abuses of professional and bureaucratic power were widely publicized and no longer tolerable. Moreover, the unprecedented powers of medicine made the choice of medical treatments a far more significant matter than it had ever been in the past.

The principle of patient autonomy was seen as the patient's protection against usurpation of his right to participate in decisions that affected his life. This amounted to a denial of the long tradition of medical paternalism (or parentalism), which considered the duty of physicians to decide what was best because the patient lacked medical knowledge and might lose hope if he knew the whole truth about his options or prognosis.

Since paternalists acted in the name of beneficence, beneficence was equated with paternalism and thereby came to be interpreted as a counter-principle to autonomy. Morally valid and invalid forms of beneficence and autonomy were not distinguished from each other. The dilemmas of medical decision-making soon were reduced to weighing the principles of autonomy and beneficence against each other.[8]

Medical paternalism and parentalism, however, are not to be equated with beneficence, conceptually or in practice. Paternalism does not account for the patient's preferences or values that are part and parcel of her good or best interests.[9] Paternalism makes the medical good of the patient the only good and subverts other goods to that good. Paternalism violates the patient's autonomy in the name of the patient's best interests while ignoring or overriding some of the most vital of those interests. This cannot be a beneficent act because the patient's own choices are so much an expression of his or her own life story or personhood. To violate or ignore the patient's choices is, by definition, a maleficent act, an injury to the patient's humanity. Only when the patient's human capacity to act autonomously is impaired (i.e., when the patient is incompetent) may we resort to paternalism as a beneficent act to override objections to treatment.[10]

This is the negative aspect of autonomy. Important as it is, it is a distortion of the idea of autonomy to equate it with total independence from the physician or others in making treatment decisions. The cultural bias against dependence or even the semblance of dependence is strong in American life. However, total independence is unrealistic in any walk of life. Human beings live in community and personal association, especially when they are patients. Patients especially need the input of others if their own choices are to be genuine ones. Physicians are needed to provide information and to discuss this information with patients to enable and empower them to use their autonomy wisely. Patients must compare their values with those of others in the context of some community of belief which they accept in whole or in part. Patients cannot identify with their current choices without reference to some structure of values which they formed in the past and which they reaffirm or reject at the moment of choice. This is part of knowing ourselves, and we know ourselves largely in relation to others.

As Dworkin points out, autonomy implies a "capacity to reflect upon one's motivational structure and make changes in that structure."[11] Without associating with others and drawing on their preferences and values, we lack the opportunity to alter or reaffirm our values because we do not know what alternatives are available and why they might be preferable. To move from the abstract realm of concept to actual decisions, autonomy needs content, and this comes from reflection not only on our own past values but on the values of others at the moment of choice. It is the physician's obligation to enhance, empower, and enrich the patient's capacity to be autonomous. An autonomous choice requires that we fill in, to the extent possible, the action or choice that maximizes realization of the patient's values. Thus, autonomy has a positive as well as a negative aspect. To become a reality, patient autonomy requires cooperation and assistance from the physician. In short, it requires the physician's beneficent attention to make the patient's autonomy an authentic as well as an independent, reality.

Physician Autonomy

In all the current discussions about the moral status of patient autonomy, the autonomy of the physician is often neglected. This philosophy has serious defects. The physician-patient relationship is one of mutual obligation—like any truly ethical relationship. The physician as a human being has the same claim to respect for his or her capacity to make personal choices, to follow his or her conscience about what is good medicine and what is morally acceptable as a person. Personal and professional ethics are not fully separable from each other. Therefore, the patient's moral right of autonomy must be balanced with respect for the physician's autonomy. Autonomy cannot be a unilateral moral right for either patients or physicians.

Physician autonomy may be considered under three headings: (1) autonomy as a person, which gives moral status to the physician's personal moral values and conscience; (2) autonomy as a physician, which gives moral status to the physician's knowledge and obligation to use it wisely and well; and (3) autonomy as a member of a profession, of a moral community with collective obligations to patients and society. I have written elsewhere[12] of the moral obligations and the autonomy of medicine as a moral community and will confine myself here only to the first two construals of the physician's autonomy as an individual.

The autonomy of the physician as a person has its roots in the same ground as the autonomy of any other person (i.e., the physician's capacity as a person for rational judgment and expression of preference with respect to values and choices). The physician, therefore, cannot be expected to lay aside or ignore his deeper personal beliefs, values, or religious commitments. To be sure, patient autonomy requires that the physician not impose his values in his decisions for the patient. But patient autonomy cannot require the physician to sacrifice his personal moral integrity even for what the patient may believe to be a morally good purpose.

Respect for the physician's autonomy also derives from the fact that, under normal circumstances, the physician must write the orders that are carried out by others. The physician cannot avoid the fact that she is the focal point through which harm and benefit of a clinical decision will flow in a majority of cases. The physician therefore is a *de facto* moral accomplice in what happens to her patient. She cannot place responsibility on others for morally indefensible decisions or for cooperation in decisions that violate her conscience. This inescapable fact of the physician-patient relationship places unavoidable obligation on the physician to avoid action she deems harmful to her patient, even if that action is "required" by state regulation, policy, or law.[13]

The physician's autonomy as a physician is also grounded in the possession of expert knowledge needed by sick people and society. The power, itself, conferred *de facto* by the possession of such knowledge, demands that the physician be free to use it according to her best judgment.[14] If the physician is to fulfill the moral requirement to make her knowledge available to those who need it, she must be allowed sufficient discretionary latitude to apply that knowledge as rationally, efficiently, and safely as possible. This is essential if physicians are to fulfill their part of the covenant with society and with individual patients. Physicians enter this covenant from the first day in medical school, when they accept the privileges and the obligations that go with the acquisition of medical knowledge and skill.[15]

Clearly, this third sense of physician autonomy can never be absolute. If the physician is incompetent, acts in his own self-interest, or acts paternalistically in the sense I defined earlier, he misuses his expertise and violates his covenant with both the patient and society. That covenant is based on trust in the doctor's Oath which commits him to use his knowledge primarily in the service of the sick.

The physician's autonomy as a physician is also limited when she mistakes medical expertise and authority for expertise in questions of values. The physician has no standing as an expert in human values and no authority to set the goals or priorities of public policy relative to the allocation or distribution of health care resources. To be sure, the physician's knowledge provides essential factual data on which rational social policy should be based. But the actual choices of values are not the prerogative of physicians or any other "experts"—politicians, economists, or even ethicists. Social value questions are a matter of concern for the whole of society. In this respect, the expert is like any other member of society with no authority over the values of other individual members of that society or over the society as a whole. The arguments of experts may have more cogency but no more authority than those of others.

Autonomy: Its Content in the Clinical Context

Autonomy in general, and physician and patient autonomy in particular, might conceivably be defined in the abstract in some general way congenial to a large number of people. However, when we begin to give it content in the context of illness, the problems with absolutism and abstraction become evident, as do the implications of autonomy as a solely negative moral right.

First of all, no two persons experience illness the same way. No two persons have the same way of expressing their capacity for autonomous choice. Very few patients demand only "the facts." Some will seek a wide variety of opinions before deciding on their own; some will not. Some patients will prefer to exercise their autonomy by giving it up to a surrogate (i.e., someone they trust to make the decision for them, or perhaps even the physician). The majority will want to express their own way of being autonomous by asking not only for facts, but also for the doctor's opinion and the opinions of family and friends.

Thus, the content of the idea of autonomy, when it is actualized, will vary with the patient's prior values and cultural, personal, and social relationships. These, in turn, condition a patient's response to illness. Sickness forces a confrontation with the self and with the need to adapt to *this* illness, here and now. Sickness is a test of our values. For each of us, our response to sickness is unique, and thus the way we express our autonomy is also unique.[16] Patients will vary in the degree of dependence or independence they desire depending on their relationship with the physician, on their relationship to their society or community, and on the degree of trust they impute to others.

Second, no matter what degree and kind of autonomy a patient chooses, the very fact of illness physiologically or psychologically compromises the actual expression of autonomy to some degree. The sick person is dependent on the physician's knowledge and help; otherwise she would not need or seek medical help. In addition, in varying degrees, she is in pain, anxious, fearful, and vulnerable. Brain function may be temporarily or permanently compromised by fever, shock, medication, age, or dementia.

To restore autonomy, physicians must first attend to reversing these physiological and psychological impediments to the optimal exercise of autonomy. In such cases, medical treatment is essential to restore autonomy. This may require temporarily downplaying or overriding the patient's autonomy until normal sensorial states are attained, and then enhancing and empowering it as the capacity for self-determination returns. During this transition, beneficence (i.e., acting in the patient's best interest) modulates the physician's move from "weak" paternalism to enhancement of the patient's full autonomy.

Third, no matter what degree of autonomy a patient may want or in what way he wants to express it, the patient is vulnerable to deception in the information he receives. The patient is dependent on the physician's disclosure of diagnosis, prognosis, treatment options, side effects, effectiveness, outcomes, etc. Which facts the physician chooses, which she emphasizes, and which she represses are often subtly or frankly conditioned by her judgment of what she thinks is in the patient's best interests. As any clinician knows, she can get almost any decision she wants from most patients. Therefore, even the most conscientious physician must exert great care to avoid manipulating the patient's choices, even for good reasons. The fact that physicians can so easily influence the patient's choice makes the full operation of patient autonomy problematic. For that very reason, it is morally incumbent on the physician to protect patient autonomy as scrupulously as possible and to try to help the patient realize its positive content.

This cannot mean, as some erroneously argue, that autonomy in a sick person is a fiction, that to try to enhance it is a sham, and that we should return to the Hippocratic tradition of benign authoritarianism. Such a reversal would be an intolerable suppression of the patient's human right as a rational being to make uncoerced choices. Physicians and others, therefore, have an obligation not to take advantage of the patient's vulnerability. Informed consent is an empty notion or a charade if the information on which it is based is biased in favor of the physician's preferences.

None of this means that physicians cannot advise or persuade patients to do what they think is right. Not to do so is a species of moral abandonment. Patients are entitled to know what physicians think is "best," all things considered. Although the extremes of this spectrum are not difficult to identify, no one can draw precise lines between advice, persuasion, manipulation, and coercion. But the difficulty of drawing a line does not justify a presumption in favor of paternalism. Rather, it increases the physician's obligation in beneficence to protect autonomy by the most scrupulous self-examination of his own motives in obtaining consent.

Much, therefore, still depends on the physician's character and sensitivity and her possession of the virtue of benevolence. The physician's character may turn out to be the last safeguard of the patient's autonomy and well-being. But, ultimately, the physician and patient must decide together what is to be done. Only in this way can patient autonomy become a cooperative and beneficent enterprise, rather than an adversarial one.

All of this applies with special force to surrogate decision-making and to advance directives, which become operative when a competent patient loses the capacity to make his own decisions. Here, the patient's wishes are represented by others or by a written document. The surrogate's wishes have the moral status we usually attribute to a competent patient and should be respected as such. However, family and friends can be in a financial or emotional conflict of interest with the welfare of an incompetent patient. They may even wish, consciously or subconsciously, to relieve themselves of the emotional and physical burdens of caring for a chronically ill person. Their representations of what the patient's autonomous decision would have been were he competent are open to serious question.

When "autonomy" is expressed in a living will or other advance directive, an assessment must be made of whether the decision executed in the past, when a person was competent, represents what the patient would want now, when the patient is no longer competent. Is *this* person, now in a persistent vegetative state, the same person who originally made out that living will? Is autonomy, in its full meaning, so absolute that it binds us to decisions the benefits and the import of which the patient could not possibly have anticipated, and which, in the actual context of a particular decision, may not be in his present interests?

In these circumstances, the patient is in need of a beneficent agent—one who can be trusted to protect him or her from the autonomous decisions of others, even those who might be legally, but not morally, valid surrogates. This agent may have to be the physician, nurse, or other health professional who acts under the principle of beneficence. Regardless of whether the surrogate is a family member, friend, or the health professional, when the patient's autonomy has been transferred to others, it must be held in trust. If that trust is violated, the surrogate loses her moral status as well as her "autonomy" to make choices for the patient.

Not enough attention has been given to the limitations placed on the "Western" notion of autonomy when applied to the care of patients from different cultural backgrounds. Even in the "West," as Surbone points out in the case of Italian culture, patients may not expect or want to make decisions, preferring to leave them to families or the physician.[17] Is it a beneficent or maleficent act to insist on or offer autonomous decision-making in these circumstances? Is it morally wrong, or rather a legitimate compromise, to work within the patient's cultural confines? Are we compelled by the fundamental nature of the principle of "respect for persons" to impose our view of autonomy, or may we compromise it in the name of cultural integrity?

These nuances in the full expression of patient autonomy in clinical decisions underscore the fact that autonomy cannot function in actuality without beneficence. Beneficence, properly exercised, is the guarantor of autonomy, rather than its enemy. Enhancing autonomy, enabling and empowering the patient to make her own choices, and helping the patient to understand the choices before her in terms of her own past values are all acts of beneficence. These acts enhance the positive content of autonomy and are crucial to any comprehensive notion of the patient's welfare. On this view, the health professional holds the patient's autonomy in trust. While it must be protected, it cannot be divorced from beneficence. It requires the physician's involvement, not her disengagement. In short, if the positive content of the concept of autonomy is to be realized, it will require beneficent action on the part of the health professional.

I must emphasize this point because the current pressure to assure patient independence is eliciting two morally dangerous responses on the part of health professionals. One response is to emphasize the negative non-interference dimension of autonomy. This negative conception of autonomy reduces the ethics of the physician-patient encounter to procedure rather than substance. On this view, as long as the procedure allows for autonomy, all is well. Autonomy is absolutized in principle and practice. This may lead to the second response, namely, that physicians will accede to whatever the patient or valid surrogate wants. This prompts the physician to transfer all responsibility to patients, family, or friends. This occurs with alarming frequency in the care of infants, the elderly, and demented patients who may be over- or under-treated because their surrogates demand it.

Indeed, one of the most important contributing factors to disagreement between family surrogates and health professionals is the psychological burden family surrogates carry when they must decide whether to discontinue life support measures. Here, the autonomy owed the patient is transferred to the valid surrogate. In such cases, families often feel they are

Pellegrino : principle of beneficience
requires that doctor cannot disengage from the moral
Patient and Physician Autonomy   215   dimension

being asked to sentence a loved one to death or, by their decision, are actually participating in the death of the patient. They need reassurance when the medical situation is one which, in the eyes of the physician, is "hopeless." Physicians cannot simply leave the entire burden to the surrogate or even the patient. They must share that burden.

Thus, detachment is not a beneficent act. Often, when families or patients ask that "everything" be done, they are seeking reassurance that everything that could be *effective* or *beneficial* be done, not that "everything"—irrespective of probabilities of success—be done. They also want to share their responsibility for cessation of life support with the doctor. The focus of ethical concern may well shift, however, from the substantive to the procedural when (irreconcilable conflict) about what constitutes beneficence or the patient's best interests occurs.

Challenges to Physician Autonomy

A seriously neglected facet of the growing dominance of patient autonomy is its impact on the physician's autonomy. The physician-patient relationship, like any ethical relationship, is a reciprocal one. In the justifiable concern for patient autonomy, it is easy to forget that the physician is a moral agent as well as the patient. As such, the physician's autonomy, as well as the patient's, is deserving of respect. When the two are in conflict, the patient's wish does not automatically trump the physician's. The physician's autonomy, like the patient's, has its (negative and positive construals).

It may seem paradoxical to worry about physician autonomy when it is the patient who is vulnerable and the doctor who holds the knowledge and power the patient needs. This fact rightly imposes the heavier moral burden on the physician in the equilibration of the autonomy relationship. He cannot use his claim to autonomy to violate the patient's capacity to make self-governing choices. But the physician is, like the patient, a human being, entitled to respect for his capacity to reason, judge, and make choices that are authentically "his." He cannot impose his values on the patient, just as the patient cannot impose hers on the physician. The physician-patient relationship is a moral equation with reciprocal rights and obligations.

* "authentic" choice

Today, that equation is becoming unbalanced as patient autonomy is elevated to the status of a trumping principle, morally as well as legally. For some, this even implies or includes overriding the physician's values, his discretionary latitude in clinical decisions, and, in some cases, even his rights of conscience. As patient autonomy receives more and more legal sanction, the problem of preserving the physician's moral integrity will grow. This danger is accentuated by the deficiency of "conscience clauses," which could provide statutory protection for physicians who refuse to provide or participate in procedures they find repugnant on moral or religious grounds.[18]

In the United States, these threats to the physician's autonomy and conscience derive from the evolution of autonomy from a negative to a positive right. The rights of patients to make decisions consistent with their own values was first noted as a right to refuse unwanted treatment in 1914.[19] In 1976, it was extended to a right of valid surrogates to refuse life-saving measures over the physician's objections.[20] In 1983, the President's Commission extended autonomy to include the right of participation in "Do Not Resuscitate" orders. This meant that physicians should offer treatments (like resuscitation) that patients might want even if they were not judged medically indicated.[21] As a result, the pristine right of refusal of unwanted treatment is now becoming, for some, a right to demand treatment—even over the doctor's best medical judgment.[22] Elevating patients' demands for specific kinds of care to moral status under the rubric of autonomy poses several challenges to the physician's right to her own moral integrity.

First, there is the challenge to the physician's judgment of what is good medicine (i.e., medicine that is rationally sound in diagnosis, prognosis, and therapeutics). For patients to claim a right to any procedures they wish is to challenge a conscientious physician's integrity as a physician. It depreciates his expertise, reduces his discretionary latitude in decision-making, and makes him a technical instrument of another person's wishes. What is more important is that this can pose a risk to the patient's well-being and subvert the healing purpose for which medicine is intended in the first place. What is demanded may not be indicated, effective, or beneficial. Such demands violate the internal morality of medicine as a practice.[23] They can redound to the patient's harm by undermining the physician's moral obligation to provide sound advice and sound practice and to avoid medically useless or futile treatments.

This threat is especially pressing today in the debate over medical futility and who defines it. Some would do away with the concept entirely because they consider that defining "futility" is not, and cannot be, an objective determination. They argue that the idea of futility is so freighted with both the patient's and physician's values that it should be abandoned entirely.[24] Others would retain the concept only for obvious situations of total brain death, permanent vegetative state, far advanced malignant disease,[25] or when a treatment has failed in the last 100 cases.[26] Still others would institutionalize the criteria for futility in hospital policies that would bind the physician to compliance.[27] Underlying this debate is the challenge to the physician's expertise to determine when a treatment—or all treatment—is useless, ineffective, or not indicated because the healing, caring, or curing ends of medicine can no longer be attained. One of the Hippocratic authors made it an ethical obligation for the physician and the patient[28] to desist from treatment when the limits of medicine's power had been reached.

This limitation on the clinician's discretionary latitude in the use of medical knowledge and skills is especially dangerous when dealing with surrogate decisions for incompetent patients. Do patients or surrogates really know what doing "everything possible" means? Must we respect orders for "no tubes" or "extraordinary measures" when these may well be effective and beneficial and might have been desired if the patient were now competent? Did the previously competent patient really intend to foreswear such measures? Is it ever possible in a living will or medical directive to anticipate what one would wish at the moment of actual decision-making? Must vigorous, ineffective, burdensome, and futile treatment be continued because the living will or surrogate requires it?

These difficulties do not vitiate living wills or surrogate decisions by those with a durable power of attorney for health. They do warrant caution about the content of autonomy and its actualization in particular cases in which there is doubt about what the patient wanted to be done. They alert us to the fact that the physician's discretion can be so restricted by advance directives that the patient's welfare is compromised. Moreover, a mistaken respect for autonomy or the physician's fear of violating autonomy becomes an excuse for moral detachment, which is actually moral abandonment.

The physician is accorded discretionary latitude in clinical decisions because medical knowledge must be applied to individual cases. The care of individual cases is not reduced to a set formula, but rather must be modulated by a host of clinical and personal factors peculiar to each patient. Without discretionary latitude, the physician cannot personalize and individualize care; she cannot fulfill her obligation to use her knowledge for the patient's best interests. Without constraints on discretionary latitude, the physician's decisions can violate the patient's values or produce physical harm. The balance between too narrow and too wide a definition of discretionary space is a delicate, but increasingly important, one to strike.

Another place where physician autonomy is endangered is in the sensitive realm of the physician's religious beliefs. In the future, the secular trend in our society and the drive for autonomy may converge to place constraints on the physician's religious convictions and values. Current legal literature already reflects instances of subtle, and sometimes not so subtle, coercion of the consciences of nurses and physicians who oppose or refuse to participate in abortion, sterilization, the use of abortifacient, or to carry out directives to withdraw feeding tubes.[29] Medical students and residents are under increasing pressure to learn and to participate in abortion training by practice. Applicants to medical schools are now frequently asked about their views on abortion. No solid data are available on whether their answers influence the admission committee's or interviewer's decision to accept or reject them. Nevertheless, the question is asked so often that it seems unlikely to be of only passing interest to interviewers.

Fortunately, the right of conscientious refusal on grounds of personal beliefs is currently protected.[30] However, past statements of official bodies like the American College of Obstetricians and Gynecologists with respect to training in abortion techniques as a condition of residency approval are worrisome, even though superseded at the present time.[31]

Another possible challenge to physician autonomy presents itself in the current debate about voluntary euthanasia and assisted suicide. It seems very likely, in view of the current drift of public and professional opinion, that one or both of these practices will become legal. When this happens, these procedures will also very likely become "benefits" or entitlements in our future health care system. The Clinton Administration is likely to include abortion among "reproductive services" in its proposed Health Security Act. Pressures on physicians are then sure to mount to provide abortions as part of the "benefit package." We are promised that the rights of conscience of those who find abortion morally reprehensible are to be protected. However, in a climate of moral pluralism, self-determination, and consensus ethics, this could change.

I cite these examples not to provoke furious debates about the moral status of the procedures in question, but because whatever one's position may be, the moral problem of the integrity of the physician's autonomy and moral rights of expression of conscience cannot be ignored. If legal or societal sanction for a certain procedure becomes widespread, will this warrant violation of the physician's conscience? Some see these as matters of such societal benefit that the physician's private moral and religious beliefs should be dissociated from his professional life.[32] This will pose an impossible situation for the morally conscientious Orthodox Jew, Roman Catholic, or Muslim in certain fields of medicine.

Another challenge to the physician's moral integrity and autonomy is one encountered by physicians in countries with "managed" health care systems. The political and economic pressures of health care policy and reform already place the physician in a position of moral conflict. The economic and fiscal drive behind such programs can make the physician a moral accomplice in practices he deems injurious to his patient's well-being. No matter what setting he is in—cost containment, rationing, acting as a gatekeeper, an institutional milieu of managed health care or managed competition, a publicly funded clinic adhering to clinical guidelines, etc.—all place the physician in the position of double or triple agency.

The physician's professional commitment to advocacy for her patient may put her at odds with an institution's or society's well-being. Exigency, expediency, and economics, not ethics, drive such systems. Does the "autonomy" of the institution or health policy override the autonomy of either, or both, the patient and physician? How are "good" business, economic, political, and fiscal policy and the moral purpose of medicine to be reconciled? Which takes precedence when conflict is unavoidable? Such questions are sure to become more widespread in the future as the zeal for cost containment and managerial ideologies, rather than the welfare of patients, is enshrined in law and public policy.

Procedural Ethics and Conflict Resolution

The central moral issues in any attempt to balance patient and physician autonomy are substantive. But, when substantive moral issues are unresolvable, procedures for ethically dealing with the conflict are necessary. The autonomy of patients, their surrogates, and physicians all carry moral weight and, on that account, command respect. The ethical goal of any procedure aimed at conflict resolution should be to protect each agent's autonomy to the extent possible. To this end, a variety of procedural moves are morally plausible when a conflict in moral or professional values reaches an impasse.

To begin with, the patient or patient's valid surrogate can discharge the physician and engage one who will take care of the patient on his or her terms. Alternatively, the physician can withdraw, respectfully and without recrimination, on grounds of preservation of his moral integrity. However, these alternatives are possible only if another physician is willing to undertake the care of the patient. To withdraw without transferring care to another competent physician is morally and legally unacceptable and constitutes abandonment. Hence, the question about how the transfer should be made arises.

In both situations, patients or surrogates might claim a right to assistance in selection of another physician specifically congenial to their moral values. In cases that do not involve a fundamental moral principle (e.g., a patient's choice of a "lump" resection and radiation as against radial mastectomy for breast cancer, or the use of non-standard, but not harmful, medical treatment), such cooperation could be ethically appropriate. The issue may be more fundamental, however, when it involves voluntary euthanasia, abortion, physician-assisted suicide, or withdrawal of care from patients in a persistent vegetative state. In such instances, some would argue that the physician who withdraws has an obligation to find another physician to undertake the patient's care under the family's or patient's terms. For others, this would constitute an unacceptable degree of moral complicity by cooperation in an act one considers morally untenable.[33]

The most difficult situation, for which there is no totally satisfactory solution, is when physicians and patients or their surrogates disagree on a serious and fundamental ethical issue, and the possibilities of physician withdrawal, or discharge of the physician by patient or surrogate, are foreclosed by external circumstances. There may be no physician willing to undertake care on the patient's or surrogate's terms. No other physician may be available for reasons of geography or urgency of the clinical situation or lack of the required expertise. Or, the physician may be employed in an institutional setting (i.e., prisons, the military, certain managed care plans, or residency training programs), in which physician choice is limited by virtue of his occupying a specific, socially defined role. In these settings, failure to perform the expected role (i.e., participation in state-ordered executions), could result in significant fiscal penalties, discharge from one's job, and legal or disciplinary action.

When there are irreconcilable differences in moral commitments and the physician cannot extricate herself by reasons of exigency or limitations imposed by patient or society, the physician must still be faithful to her conscience. This may mean acceptance of the attendant penalties for refusal to comply with institutional, legal, or socially defined goals (e.g., refusal to participate in state-ordered executions or in coerced interrogation of war prisoners). Just when and how individual physicians should refuse to comply with social conventions is not a matter of precise formulation. No one can enter the mind and heart of another and untangle the moral psychology of a particular moral choice, but this fact does not vitiate judgment about the ethical probity of the act in question.

Some of the most complex and difficult situations occur when surrogates are acting for infants whose future values cannot be known.[34] In such cases, the conflict will often be between the surrogate's and the physician's estimates of what is "best" for the infant. The vagaries of "quality of life" estimates complicate the issue because of the impossibility of assessing how the infant would make that evaluation when he or she becomes aware it must live with the infirmities the physicians prognosticate.

These infirmities are often complex, may result in a life of prolonged disability and discomfort, and constitute grave emotional, physical, and fiscal burdens for parents and society. In a society propelled by economic constraint, reluctance to sacrifice material goods even for disabled children, and an obsession with physical beauty, it is not uncommon for even conscientious parents to decide to withhold or withdraw life-sustaining treatment in order to spare the infant a "life of suffering" or poor quality. But "quality of life" and "value of life" are not synonymous terms. The modern tendency to use them synonymously is a serious point of discord between secular and religious perspectives on ethical decisions. What is right and good in these circumstances is problematic and may be interpreted in contradictory ways by physicians, nurses, parents, and even governmental regulation.[35] In these circumstances, we may search for procedures which will protect the autonomy of all participants, but the substantive ethical disagreement remains.

When the physician believes the parents' decision would constitute grave harm to the infant, she has several procedural alternatives. One alternative is to withdraw and ask the parents to engage another physician. This would be permissible if the physician did not think that withdrawal would result in grave moral and physical harm to the infant. Where the physician might judge otherwise, whether treatment is withheld or continued, then that is medically futile.[36] At such a time, the physician has an obligation to take whatever measures are available to avert harm, such as appeal to an ethics committee or, if necessary, to the courts.

A proponent of absolute parental autonomy might justifiably ask what moral claim a physician can have to judge, or even question, a parent's surrogacy rights. This point of view assumes that parents have absolute dominion over their children and that their decisions will invariably be benevolent and altruistic; it also ignores the covenantal trust relationship between the physician and the patient. For a variety of reasons—pride, shame, or unwillingness to confront the expense, financial and emotional, of caring for a disabled child—parents may decide to undertreat. On the other hand, they may opt for futile overtreatment out of lack of information, religious conviction, or fear of being in some way responsible for their infant's death.

Furthermore, the autonomy imputed to parents cannot be absolute. Physicians and nurses are obliged by virtue of their commitment to the well-being of their patients to act in the interests of the infant. They must, of course, appreciate that decisions surrounding the care of very sick and potentially disabled infants must involve the family. Indeed, in a real sense, the whole family becomes a "patient," whose collective interests must be safeguarded. The implications of the decision on the future lives of the whole family are, therefore, not to be denied; however, these considerations by themselves do not justify withholding or withdrawing treatment that is effective, beneficial, and not disproportionately burdensome.

When there is obvious and overt conflict between the good seen by parents and the medical good of the infant, the obligation is greater to the most vulnerable person (in this case, the infant). Situations involving such irreconcilable conflicts of obligation are sometimes unavoidable. Still, we are obliged to do as much as possible to respect the physician's obligations as physician as well as the autonomy of surrogates or patients. Sometimes both cannot be respected without unacceptable compromises, on one side or the other.

Before such an impasse is reached, all other methods of conflict resolution should be exhausted. Ethics committees can serve to clarify the issues and perhaps suggest a way in which compromise could effectively be reached in a manner that preserves the moral integrity of all the participants. Appointment of legal guardians and appeals to the courts are far less satisfactory. In any case, all of these devices address only the procedural resolution of the practical conflict. They certainly do not resolve the ethical dilemma of conflicting claims to autonomous decision-making.

The Integrity of Medical Ethics

Some would suggest that the problem is with medical ethics itself, with the insistence on universal rules of moral conduct on which physicians base their moral claim to autonomy as physicians. Why not change medical ethics, itself? Why not leave it to be negotiated between physician and patient? Perhaps medical ethics should be a changing, socially constructed contract varying from society to society, era to era, and patient to patient. Some argue that medicine and its ethics must be whatever is negotiated politically between the profession and government. Other socially and politically constructed forms of ethical justification are currently popular as well. They imply that there is no such thing as a universally binding medical ethic, only an ethic of political expediency or societal convention.

Some of us, however, think this would be disastrous for medicine, the physician, and the patient. The autonomy—that is really to say the moral integrity—of both physicians and patients must somehow be preserved. So, too, must the integrity of the ethics of medicine itself. Medical knowledge is too powerful a tool to become an instrument of governmental or social pressures, or private negotiation, however benign their motives may appear to be. Medicine is also too powerful to go wholly unregulated. There are too many examples of the subversion of the powers of medicine to evil purpose by unjust political regimes to make the ethics of medicine a subject for political negotiation.[37] There are too many examples of the way unregulated medical "entrepreneurs" or morally bankrupt physicians can exploit the vulnerability of the sick.

Medical ethics must maintain a degree of independence if it is to protect the sick person. It must remain subject to public criticism, but not be controlled by social convention. It must also be protected from subversion by the profession itself. This requires a much firmer philosophical grounding for medical ethics than we now possess. The possibility of achieving universal approbation for a commonly held ethic of the profession seems to be receding today in the face of the multicultural, morally pluralistic, and morally relativistic temper of the times. This climate, however, cannot justify abandoning the effort. Nothing less is called for than a reconstruction of the ethics of the relationship between patient and doctor. This will be difficult, indeed, because the "remarkable solidarity" and "singular beneficence," which Osler praised,[38] are rapidly disappearing in the worldwide questioning of the moral values that have traditionally undergirded medical ethics.

I have purposely said little about the principle of justice, which must also be factored into the equation. On the whole, this facet of the physician-patient relationship has been underdeveloped. It is now necessary to establish the conceptual relationships among justice, autonomy, and beneficence, as well as their actualization in the clinical context. Justice has the interesting facet of being both a principle and a virtue. The incorporation of justice into the autonomy-beneficence equation will require a prior clarification of how principles and virtues are conceptually and practically related.

Despite the difficulties, the effort to balance the autonomy equation is not futile. Its importance impels us to the effort to try to find the points of balance. Autonomy and beneficence are two principles so closely tied to the healing ends of medicine that to violate either is to imperil the moral integrity of both patients and physicians. Nevertheless, any comprehensive moral philosophy for the health professions must encompass more than these two principles. Justice must be included and account taken of both virtue and the moral psychological insights of non-principle-based theories.

In any case, one step in the larger effort is to try to achieve a better balance between the two most powerful principles shaping physician-patient relations today. Several precepts need to be built into the current reexamination of the foundations of professional ethics:

1) Patient autonomy is a moral right of patients, and it is a duty of physicians to respect it.

2) Integrity of conscience and professional judgment are moral rights of physicians. Society and patients have an obligation to respect them.

3) Physician autonomy is limited by a competent patient's or valid surrogate's moral right to refuse proffered treatment. The physician is obliged, however, to help the patient arrive at an autonomous decision by enhancing or empowering the patient's capacity to make authentic, self-governing choices.

4) The patient's autonomy is limited when it becomes a demand for treatment the physician honestly believes is not medically indicated, is injurious to the patient, or is morally repugnant.

5) The physician's autonomy is limited on questions of value, e.g., on questions of the goals or purposes to which medical knowledge may be put for particular individuals or societies.

6) Societies and institutions must establish mechanisms, with only minimal recourse to law, for unilateral discontinuance of the relationship when either patient or physician feels personal integrity is being compromised.

7) The first principle of medical ethics is still beneficence. Beneficence is essential if autonomy is to be authentically expressed and actualized.

In sum, beneficence and autonomy must be mutually re-enforcing if the patient's good is to be served, if the physician's ability to serve that good is not to be compromised, and if the physician's moral claim to autonomy and the integrity of the whole enterprise of medical ethics are to be respected.

Notes

1. Tom L. Beauchamp & James F. Childress, *Principles of Biomedical Ethics* 67–119 (3rd ed. 1989).

2. Gerald Dworkin, *The Theory and Practice of Autonomy* 3–6, 12–20 (1988).

3. This is a paraphrase of the essentials of Dworkin's use of the term. *Id.* at 7–12.

4. See John Locke, *Locke's Second Treatise on Civil Government* (Lester DeKoster ed., 1978).

5. See Immanuel Kant, *Grounding for the Metaphysics of Morals* (James W. Ellington trans., 1981).

6. See John Stuart Mill, *On Liberty* (Elizabeth Rapaport ed., 1978).

7. Beauchamp & Childress, *supra* note 1.

8. Tom L. Beauchamp & Lawrence B. McCullough, *Medical Ethics: The Moral Responsibilities of Physicians* 22–51 (1984).

9. See Edmund D. Pellegrino & David C. Thomasma, *For the Patient's Good: The Restoration of Beneficence in Health Care* 23–25 (1988).

10. James F. Childress, *Who Should Decide?: Paternalism in Health Care* 102 (1982).

11. Dworkin, *supra* note 2, at 108.

12. Edmund D. Pellegrino, "The Medical Profession as a Moral Community," 66 *Bull. N.Y. Acad. Med.* 221 (1990).

13. Edmund D. Pellegrino, "Societal Duty and Moral Complicity: The Physician's Dilemma of Divided Loyalty," 16 *Int'l J.L. & Psychiatry* 371 (1993).

14. See David M. Mirvis, "Physicians' Autonomy—The Relation between Public and Professional Expectations," 328 *New Eng. J. Med.* 1346 (1993).

15. Edmund D. Pellegrino, "The Ethics of Medical Education," in *The Encyclopedia of Bioethics* (Warren T. Reich ed., 1995).

16. George J. Agich, "Reassessing Autonomy in Long-Term Care," *Hastings Center Rep.*, Nov.–Dec. 1990, at 12.

17. See Antonella Surbone, "Truth Telling to the Patient," 268 *JAMA* 1661 (1992).

18. See Lynn D. Wardle, "Protecting the Rights of Conscience of Health Care Providers," 14 *J. Legal Med.* 177 (1993).

19. *Schloendorff v. Society of N.Y. Hosps.*, 105 N.E. 92, 93 (N.Y. 1914).

20. In *re Quinlan*, 355 A.2d 647 (N.J. 1976).

21. President's Comm'n for the Study of Ethical Problems in Medicine and Biomedical and Behavioral Research, *Deciding to Forego Life-Sustaining Treatment: A Report on the Ethical, Medical, and Legal Issues in Treatment Decisions* 241 (1983).

22. In *re Wanglie*, No. Px-91-283 (D. Minn. July, 1991).

23. For a further discussion of the morality issues in medicine, see John Ladd, "The Internal Morality of Medicine: An Essential Dimension of the Patient-Physician Relationship," in *The Clinical Encounter: The Moral Fabric of the Patient-Physician Relationship* 209 (Earl E. Shelp ed., 1983).

24. R. D. Truog et al., "The Problem with Futility," 326 *New Eng. J. Med.* 1560 (1992).

25. Stuart J. Youngner, "Who Defines Futility?," 260 *JAMA* 2094 (1988).

26. Nancy S. Jecker & Lawrence J. Schneiderman, "Medical Futility: The Duty Not to Treat," 2 *Cambridge Q. Healthcare Ethics* 151 (1993).

27. Lance K. Stell, "Stopping Treatment on Grounds of Futility: A Role for Institutional Policy," 11 *St. Louis U. Pub. L. Rev.* 481 (1992).

28. Hippocrates, "The Art," in 2 *Hippocrates* 185–217 (W. H. S. Jones trans., 1981).

29. Wardle, *supra* note 18.

30. Executive Board Minutes from the American College of Obstetrics and Gynecology at 12, Item 6.2 (Jan. 1992) (on file with organization).

31. See Barbara L. Lindheim & Maureen A. Cotterill, "Training in Induced Abortion by Obstetrics and Gynecology Residency Programs," 10 *Fam. Plan. Persp.* 24 (1978).

32. This dissociation is one I have encountered already in private conversation with medical students, colleagues, and influential laypeople.

33. Pellegrino, *supra* note 12.

34. See Arthur E. Kopelman, "Dilemmas in the Neonatal Intensive Care Unit," in *Ethics and Mental Retardation* 243 (Loretta Kopelman & John C. Moskop eds., 1984).

35. Child Abuse Amendments of 1984, Pub. L. No. 98-457, 98 Stat. 1749 (1984) (amending 42 U.S.C. 5101 (1974)).

36. See Anne Bannon, "The Case of the Bloomington Baby," *Hum. Life Rev.*, Fall 1982, at 63; Michael McCarthy, "Anencephalic Baby's Right to Life?", 342 *Lancet* 919 (1993); John J. Paris et al., "Physicians' Refusal of Requested Treatment: The Case of Baby L," 322 *New Eng. J. Med.* 1012 (1990).

37. See Edmund D. Pellegrino, "Societal Duty and Moral Complicity: The Physician's Dilemma of Divided Loyalty," 16 *Int'l J. Law. & Psychiatry* 371–391 (1993).

38. William Osler, "Chauvinism in Medicine," in *Aequanimitas: With Other Addresses to Medical Students, Nurses and Practitioners of Medicine* 267 (1943).

III

VIRTUE IN MEDICAL PRACTICE

The Physician as Moral Agent

ELEVEN

Character, Virtue, and Self-Interest in the Ethics of the Professions

Introduction

The professions today are afflicted with a species of moral malaise that may prove fatal to their moral identities and perilous to our whole society. This malaise is manifest in a growing conviction even among conscientious doctors, lawyers, and ministers that it is no longer possible to practice their professions within traditional ethical constraints. For reasons which are explained below, this discussion focuses specifically on the "learned" professions: medicine, law and ministry. More specifically, the belief is taking hold that unless he looks out for his own self-interest, the professional will be crushed by the forces of commercialization, competition, government regulation, malpractice, advertising, public and media hostility and a host of other inimical socio-economic forces.

These forces, it is asserted, are conspiring to transform the learned professions into crafts, businesses, or technologies. They are beyond the control of the professions. The fault lies not with the professions. Unless there is some upheaval in conventional morality, professional ethics as we have known it has no future. Indeed, perhaps given the realities of professional practice, professional ethics has rested on faulty philosophical foundations from its very beginnings. This line of reasoning leads to the conclusion that the self-interest of the professional justifies the compromises in, and even the rejection of, obligations imposed by traditional concepts of professional ethics.

231

In this article, strong exception is taken to this line of reasoning both in its foundations and in its conclusions. I argue to the contrary: 1) that what deficiencies there are in professional morality are, as they have always been, deficiencies in character and virtue; 2) that a firm philosophical foundation exists for altruism and fidelity to trust in the ethics of the professions; 3) that professional ethics must at times be independent of conventional morality; and 4) that the professions are moral communities with enormous moral power which, properly used, can sustain the moral integrity of the practitioner and the professions. Moreover, if they use their moral power well, the professions can become paradigms of disinterested service that can raise the level of conventional morality.

This is an ambitious set of assertions. To speak of character and virtue in today's moral climate is to be suspected of the sanctimoniousness of hypocrisy. We must admit that the concepts of virtue and character are two of the oldest and most slippery in moral philosophy. Also, the proper place of self-interest in virtue ethics has never been satisfactorily settled. Finally, we still lack a coherent moral philosophy of the professions in which to locate the concepts of character, altruism, and self-interest and to define the relationships between them. These difficulties notwithstanding, we cannot avoid engagement with what I take to be the central crisis in the professions—today the confusion about who, and what we are, and what we should be.

The moral malaise to which I refer centers on more subtle issues than those more egregious infractions of professional ethics, which everyone will condemn. There is no need, therefore, to assault you with a Jeremiad of gross immorality like incompetence, fraud, deception, mismanagement of funds, violations of confidentiality, or sexual abuse of clients or patients. The more immediate concern is with those practices which are more at the "moral margin."[1] These practices are often legal, often socially acceptable, and are often tolerated, though with some misgivings. They occupy a moral grey zone where the interests of the professional and the patient or client intersect and where the vulnerability of the latter makes him exploitable by the former. They are ethical "ozone holes" that open up when moral sensitivities are blunted. Like their physical counterparts at the earth's poles, ethical ozone holes can spread and have dire consequences unless repaired.

Each of our professions has its own list of morally questionable practices that its members would justify on the grounds of threatened self-interest. I will list a few from my own profession and leave to you in law and the ministry to fill in your own analogues. For medicine, I would select these examples: refusing to treat patients with HIV infection for fear of contagion; denying service to the poor and those with inadequate or exhausted insurance benefits; turning away complicated cases from the emergency room for fear of malpractice; cooperating with hospital or public policies that require early discharge; economic transfer or the "dumping" of those who cannot pay on other hospitals; the various forms of medical entrepreneurism like investment in health care facilities; for-profit medical ventures of all sorts; marketing to increase demand for dubious or unnecessary treatment or tests; and accepting bonuses for denying needed care or enjoying the many emoluments proffered by pharmaceutical companies.

Other professions can draw up their own lists of morally dubious practices. All such practices will, however, have three features in common. First, they are based on the use of privilege and power for the personal gain of the professional. Second, they reflect a failure to take certain risks required for the well-being of those whom the profession serves. Finally, in the case of both of these features, justification is sought on the grounds of legitimate self-interest. It is my conviction that these practices and the justification sought for them derive from the de-emphasis on character and virtue in the three professions we are examining.

In what follows, I will examine three questions about the current moral malaise of the professions: 1) What are the reasons for the erosion of virtue ethics and the moral legitimation of self-interest in the ethics of the professions? 2) Is there a philosophical basis for restoring virtue ethics to the professions? 3) What are the practical and theoretical implications of such a return of virtue ethics? Before examining these questions, I should define the sense in which I shall use each of the key terms in my title—virtue, character, profession, ethics of the professions, altruism, and self-interest.

The definition of virtue, the virtues, and the virtuous person has occupied philosophers since Plato first raised the question of virtue, its nature, number, and teachability. Despite numerous efforts since then, no one has improved on Aristotle's imperfect but still useful definition. Aristotle identifies moral virtues as states of character, by which he means "the things in virtue of which we stand well or badly with reference to the passions. . . ."[2] Virtue is a particular state of character, one which "both brings into good condition the thing of which it is the excellence and makes the work of that thing be done well."[3] And further, "the virtue of a man also will be the state of character which makes a man good and which makes him do his work well."[4]

Implicit in Aristotle's definition are several crucial ideas. First, virtues are, as they were for Socrates, excellence (areté). They have a functional and teleological character since they make things do their work well (cutting, in the case of a knife, and seeing, in the case of the eye are Aristotle's examples) and by that fact make the thing itself good.

In the case of humans, virtue makes us function well as humans to achieve our ends or purposes. We are thereby made good humans. Defining human excellence is more difficult than defining the excellence of a knife. Aristotle addresses that question in both the *Nichomachean* and the *Eudemian Ethics*. I cannot hope to summarize that discussion here.

What is important, however, is that Aristotle's definition of virtue is linked to two other concepts—the concepts of the nature and the good of man. It is the fragmentation of the unity among these concepts that is largely responsible for the confusion we experience today in arriving at some consensus about the meaning of virtue. Plato, Aristotle, and the Stoics were in general agreement, as was Aquinas (with the additional consideration of man's spiritual nature), on a comprehensive moral philosophy of which virtue was a part. The post-medieval dissolution of this moral philosophy, which we shall shortly examine has left the idea of virtue without roots.

I have no pretensions in this article that would lead me to attempt to define the virtuous person, the one who possesses to an excellent degree the character traits that make for a good person. But I do believe it is possible to define the virtues that make for a good physician, lawyer, or clergyman in terms of the ends to which those professions are dedicated.

The term character may be taken in two ways. In a general sense it summates the kind of person one is, as revealed by the virtues and vices we exhibit in our attitudes and actions. More specifically, a person of character is one who can predictably be trusted to act well in most circumstances, to consider others in his or her decisions, to look at the long-term meanings of immediate impulses, and to order those impulses according to the canons of morality. In Aristotle's sense, a person of character (and here I mean virtuous character) is one who "stands well" with reference to the passions, who does not yield to extremes of self-interest, pleasure, or desires for power.

By "ethics of the professions," I do not mean the norms actually followed by professionals, or the professional codes they espouse, but rather the moral obligations deductible from the kinds of activity in which they are engaged. The ethics of the professions, therefore, consists in a rational and systematic ordering of the principles, rules, duties, and virtues intrinsic to achieving the ends to which a profession is dedicated. This is the "internal morality" of a profession.[5]

By a profession, I mean something more than the usual, sociological definition. A profession is, literally speaking, a declaration of a way of life that is specific, a way of life in which expert knowledge is used not primarily for personal gain but for the benefit of those who need that knowledge. The fuller meaning of this definition will emerge as my line of argument unfolds.

Altruism and self-interest, as I shall use these terms in this article, are opposing moral concepts. Without entering into a detailed history of these two ideas I would make the following distinctions: altruism is that trait which disposes a person to take the interests of others into account in using power, privilege, position, and knowledge. It was first introduced by Auguste Comte (1798–1857). One need not accept, as I assuredly do not, Comte's philosophy of humanity and his positivism to use the term as I do. The key term for the ethics of the professions is altruistic beneficence. This means not only taking the interests of others into account but doing so in such fashion that our intentions and acts give some degree of preference to the intention of others. This is a more elevated notion of beneficence than simple benevolence, wishing others well, and non-maleficence, not doing them harm. It implies some degree of effacement of self-interest. Altruistic beneficence is particularly important for the professions given the special phenomenology of the professional relationship, which I shall define later in this article.

Self-interest, too, has several meanings. There is a legitimate self-interest which pertains to the duties we owe to ourselves—duties which guard health, life, some measure of material well-being, the good of our families, friends, etc. Aristotle made clear the two senses of self-love which may exist in humans.[6] There is also an illegitimate sense of self-interest—at least in the moral philosophy of virtue—and that is selfish self-interest. Here we take into account the interests of others, but we discount them in favor of our own self-interests. This may be legitimate when taking into account that the good of others involves heroic degrees of self-sacrifice to the point of discomfort, financial loss, harm to family, or even death. Whether degrees of altruistic beneficence which require some cost in time, effort, or discomfort are required in ordinary affairs is a debatable question which I shall not engage for want of time.

The major point in my argument, however, is that, given the nature of professional relationships, some degree of effacement of self-interest—which I shall take to mean the same as beneficent altruism—is morally obligatory on health professionals. A virtuous professional, then, is one who can be expected with reasonable certainty to exhibit as one of his traits of character altruistic beneficence construed as effacement of self-interest. The precise limits of such a trait, the way in which it would be defined in a specific instance, is not definable by formula.

Finally, I shall focus only on the three traditional "learned" professions of medicine, law, and ministry. Other occupations like teaching and the military have been called professions in the past and now almost every activity that requires skill and is done for a living is called a profession. Indeed, some of the features I shall describe for the learned three will be possessed by other occupations. But the traditional three are paradigms of professional ethics because the characteristics which define them are clustered in a unique way as to degree, kind and number. To the extent that other professions commit themselves to other than self-interest, they approach the paradigm professions and what I say applies analogically to them.

What Accounts for the Erosion of Virtue and the Rise of Self-Interest?

Let me turn now to the first of my three questions. What accounts for the erosion of virtue ethics? I select four factors: a) the unresolved conceptual tension between virtue and self-interest; b) the conceptual difficulties of virtue ethics itself; c) the modern turn in ethics from the character of the moral agent to the resolution of dilemmas; and d) the shift in economic and political values in the last decade.

The Inherent Tension between Virtue and Self-Interest

The tension between self-interest and virtue was recognized at the beginning of western moral philosophy. Plato has Socrates confront this dilemma in the *Republic* when Thrasymachus asserts that "justice is simply the interest of the stronger."[7] Glaucon for his part contends that man by nature pursues self-interest and is deflected only by law—an idea also advanced by other ethical "relativists" like Thucydides and Gorgias. Callicles goes further and insists that virtue consists in acting selfishly and tyrannically. W. K. C. Guthrie shows how persistent the idea of self-interest and self-love was in the thought of the Sophists.[8]

Aristotle too had difficulties with the reality of self-interest and its reconciliation with his doctrine of moral virtue. He asks if one should love one's self primarily, or one's neighbor.[9] At one point, he tries to show, like so many philosophers thereafter, that acting to benefit others contributes to happiness and therefore is in one's own self-interest.[10] But this is a weak argument because Aristotle also asserts that the truly virtuous person ought to practice altruism for its own sake.[11] In his interesting analysis of this problem in Books VIII and IX of the *Eudemian Ethics,* Engberg-Pedersen concludes that Aristotle's position is that justice is the basis of all the virtues. The virtuous person assigns no more of natural goods to himself than to others. In this way he encompasses altruism, places restraints on inordinate self-interest, and serves legitimate self-interest.[12]

Despite the unresolved difficulties of dealing with the reality of self-interest, the ethics of Aristotle, Plato, and the Stoics placed the emphasis squarely on virtues. Virtue ethics dominated classical and Hellenistic moral philosophy. It came to its highest development in the moral philosophy of Aquinas, who joined the supernatural to the natural virtues. Thus the classical and medieval philosophies of virtue constituted a continuum.

This continuum centered on a conception of the virtuous person as one who exhibited the traits of character essential to human flourishing and to optimal fulfillment of the capabilities inherent in human nature.

For such a person, self-interest was recognized as a responsibility, but it was to be submerged to varying degrees of noble acts in the interests of others. The good life called for a rational balance between personal good and the good of others.[13] But the cardinal virtues—temperance, justice, courage, and prudence—all implied some degree of effacement of self-interest as a mark of the virtuous person. At a minimum the virtuous person was not to take advantage of the vulnerability of others. As examples: Socrates chose death to teach a moral lesson to his fellow Athenians; Plato distinguished the art of making money from the art of healing;[14] Cicero admonished the corn merchant not to raise prices when the crop was small;[15] Hippocrates makes beneficent concern for the welfare of his patients the first principle of medical ethics.[16] Thus while they recognized the reality of self-interest, the ancient and medieval moral philosophers held firmly to virtue as the touchstone of the moral life.

In the post-medieval period two philosophical assaults were launched on virtue ethics, one by Machiavelli and the other by Thomas Hobbes. Both are conceptual descendents of Thrasymachus, Callicles, and the anti-virtue pre-Socratics. Both replaced the optimistic view of human nature with moral pessimism. Both found the traditional concepts of virtue anti-ethical to human nature and self-interest. Machiavelli simply converted the traditional virtues into vices, while Hobbes psychologized them as a form of self-interest. The Machiavellian and Hobbesian strains are the heart of today's moral malaise and cynicism which seeks to give moral legitimacy to the professional's self-interest.

The Machiavellian Strain

Machiavelli (1469–1527) was too well educated in classical humanism to deny totally the value of virtue as an ideal in human conduct. But his observation of the real world in which men lived, in warfare, tyranny, and political upheaval, convinced him that there was no survival value in living virtuously. The good man simply could not thrive in a world in which so many others were not good.[17] And so Machiavelli advised the Prince he would be successful to use whatever means would ensure his survival and the continuance of his power. The classical cardinal virtues of temperance, justice, even at times, fortitude and prudence could be impediments when dealing with those who ignored these constraints on self-interest. In these circumstances the virtues, thus, became vices. Moreover, in the Machiavellian view, virtue itself became an instrumental notion, a power to effect a given end, rather than a behavioral ideal. Indeed for Machiavelli, virtue became *virtù*, "manliness"—an expression of power, rather than a disposition to act well as it was understood in the classical-medieval continuum.

Bernard Mandeville (1670–1773), a physician, went further than Machiavelli in some ways. Not only did he think the virtues were impractical, but he held them to be vices—destructive not only for personal, but social, good. It is through greed, the desire for luxury, pleasure, and power that society prospers and things get done. The satisfaction of acquisitiveness, intemperance, and gluttony makes for jobs, puts money into the economy and provides a livelihood for many.[18] Mandeville's *Fable of the Bees*, whether tongue-in-cheek or not, has been influential in encouraging an anti-virtue bias which has always found supporters and has many today.

Nietzsche's (1844–1900) anti-virtue stance was of a different kind but still in the Machiavellian spirit. For Nietzsche's "ubermensch," the traditional virtues were meaningless. They were simply impediments to the achievement of greatness. The virtues were for lesser mortals. For the superman, virtues like temperance or justice would be vices.[19]

A more modern exponent of a similar moral viewpoint is Ayn Rand. Her ideas, though far less well argued than those of Machiavelli, Mandeville, or Nietzsche, are a current compound of all three. Rand's novels of the successful architect or industrialist extol the "virtues" of individualism, ruthlessness, power, and uninhibited pursuit of wealth and self-interest.[20] Her ideas have had a considerable influence on those who seek moral justification for their acquisitive instincts. In this regard it is interesting to note that the slogan of *Regardie's* magazine is "Money, Power, Greed."

Moral Machiavellianism—whether in its original version or its later varieties in Mandeville, Nietzsche, or Rand—is very much alive today. We see it in the medical entrepreneurs who own hospital or nursing homes, the lawyer/power broker who sells influence or leveraged buyouts, and in the multimillion dollar ministries. Indeed, all who hold that virtue simply does not pay and that it is a fool's enterprise are moral Machiavellians.

The Hobbesian Strain

Machiavelli made the virtues into vices. Thomas Hobbes (1588–1679), on the other hand, tried to maintain some idea of virtue which was reconcilable and yet reconcile it with self-interest. His was a formal philosophical break with the medieval tradition. His aim was to establish ethics on purely naturalistic grounds, free of the theological spirit that characterized the medieval synthesis. He built his moral philosophy on a pessimistic view of human nature that departed sharply from the essentially optimistic classical-medieval view.

Aristotle opens his *Politics* by asserting that man is a social animal. Man, Hobbes said, was unsocial by nature. He enters society only to satisfy his most fundamental urges. His selfishness is primary and is expressed in a desire to preserve his own life, enhance pleasure, avoid pain, and become secure from attack by others. Hobbes does not make the virtues into vices, rather he puts them at the service of self-interest. We pity others because we see the possibility of being in the position of those we pity. We are benevolent in return. "All society," he said, "is for gain or glory."[21] We obey society's rules only because we feel if we do not, others will threaten our security. In Hobbes' view, effacement of self-interest is unnatural, because it makes us the victims of others. Self-interest determines what is good and bad. But self-interest alone will not secure a peaceable society—that must finally be secured by an absolute sovereign or society will be torn apart by competing self-interests.

Hobbes' view on self-interest was coupled with a scorn for the idea of the good which had been vital to classical and medieval philosophy. If the good is reducible to what we like or dislike, as Hobbes suggested, then virtues and vices are also matters of preference. Hobbes' powerful assertions shaped much of English moral philosophy. His successors tried either to rebut the primacy of self-interest or reconcile it with some more altruistic principle. I can give only a few examples here.

John Locke (1632–1704), for example, agreed with Hobbes that good and evil are determined by pain or pleasure or conformity to some law. He did assert that we ought to help others but only if it did not endanger our own self-interest. Shaftesbury (1671–1713) tried hard to show that self-interest and service to others were synonymous. Virtues, he said, "pay off" in self-interest because of the pleasure we get from benevolent acts. The vices, like anger, intemperance, and covetousness, on the other hand, bring pain. Shaftesbury thought that we ought to embrace virtue because we have an obligation to protect self-interest, so that affection for virtue is really affection for self-interest. Hutcheson (1694–1746) developed Shaftesbury's moral sense theory more fully, as did Hume (1711–1776). They identified virtue as that which gives the spectator of virtuous acts a feeling of approbation while vicious acts elicit disapproval. They took some of the bluntness out of Hobbes' emphasis in self-interest. But they end up agreeing that we have no ultimate obligation to virtue other than its bearing on our self-interest or happiness. Adam Smith (1723–1790) holds that virtues are those traits of character that are useful or agreeable to the moral sentiment of the agent or others. Bentham (1748–1832) argued that whatever is conducive to the general happiness always conduces the happiness of the agent. In this way his utilitarianism reconciles self-regarding and other-regarding interests by subsuming all of these interests under the principle of greatest happiness. J. S. Mill (1806–1873) went further than Bentham, positing that the greatest good of all is the source of one's own happiness. One's own self-interest, therefore, is best served by acting for the good of all. According to this view, consciously doing without happiness to achieve the greatest good of all is, paradoxically, a source of happiness.[22]

In contrast with the moral sentiment theorists and the utilitarians, the Cambridge intuitionists like Cudworth (1617–1688), Henry More (1614–1687), and Cumberland (1631–1718) tried to show that there were reasons for virtuous acts even if they conflicted with self-interest. More even postulated a "Boniform faculty," a virtue that gives us mastery over our baser impulses to serve selfish interests first.[23]

Bishop Joseph Butler (1692–1752) took issue with both Shaftesbury and Hobbes. Neither self-love nor benevolence were the only affections involved in human behavior. Altruism and self-interest do not completely exclude other desires and motivations. Nor are benevolence and self-interest mutually exclusive. Man has a conscience which enables him to order his passions so that he can do what is good not just for self. By conscience man can know how much benevolence will advance and how much will damage his self-interest. Butler was a cleric and looked to God to implant conscience in humans to point out what action is most in conformity with human nature. Thus conscience enables us to know that some things are inherently good and some inherently bad. Butler thus invoked theology implicitly if not always explicitly, though he tried, as did Hobbes, to extract his moral philosophy from reason.[24]

Enough has been said to demonstrate how the question of altruism and self-interest arose in Hobbes and Machiavelli and established two powerful strains of thought with which moral philosophy has been occupied ever since. As I pointed out earlier, the problem arose in ancient philosophy as well. In Christian moral philosophy as enunciated by Aquinas, self-preservation was built into natural law. What is owed to self and what is owed to others was ordered by the virtue of charity, which entails love for others as children of God and not for any ulterior purpose. This is the message of the Sermon on the Mount. Indeed, it may be that this is the only way in which the inherent tensions between self-interest and altruism can ever be finally resolved.

These tensions certainly have not been resolved in twentieth-century moral philosophy. The subjectivism and emotivism of Ayer, the prescriptivism of Hare, the existentialism of Sartre, all make moral judgment matters of approval or disapproval, preference or self-determination. The metaethical emphasis on language and logic of moral discourse rather than the content of moral judgments further weakened the classical notions of virtues. As a result, the definition of virtue has become either so vague as to be meaningless or so encompassing as to include every conceivable likable trait.[25]

Twentieth-century moralists have refined the eighteenth-century notion of moral sentiment and further psychologized ethics. In the light of the psychologies of Freud, or the behaviorism of Watson or Skinner, today, many moralists look to modern psychology to define the virtues and to close the gap between knowing the good and being motivated to do the good. Others look to genetics, culture, or social organization to explain altruism and self-interest.[26] Nagel, on the other hand, presents a challenge to this trend and argues for the rationality of altruism. In doing so, he rejects the Humean subordination of reason to desire or emotion.[27] Philippa Foot tried unsuccessfully to link virtue and self-interest in her work *Virtues and Vices*.

The disarray of normative ethics, including the destruction of virtue ethics, has occasioned a spate of recent attempts to resuscitate the classical and especially the Aristotelian idea of virtue. This more was initiated by Anscombe[28] and MacIntyre.[29] Their success varies. The extent to which they can reverse the dominance of self-interest in ethics begun by Hobbes is highly problematic.

Conceptual Difficulties of Virtue-Based Ethics

The second major factor in the erosion of virtue ethics is the philosophical difficulty inherent in the concept of virtue itself. First is its lack of specificity. Virtue ethics does not tell us how to resolve specific moral dilemmas. It deemphasizes principles, rules, duties, and concrete prescriptions. It only says that the virtuous person will be disposed to act in accord with the virtue appropriate to the situation. This lack of specificity leads to a distressing circularity in reasoning. The right and the good is that which the virtuous person would do, and the virtuous person is one who would do the right and the good. We must define either the right and the good or the virtuous person if we are to break out of this logical impasse. But, these are just the definitions that have defied the conceptual ingenuity of the world's best philosophers. Furthermore, virtue theory cannot stand apart from some theory of human nature and the good. The more vague our definitions of human nature and its telos, the more difficult it is to keep virtue from becoming vice and vice virtue. Since virtue ethics puts its emphasis on the character of the agent, it requires a consistent philosophical anthropology; otherwise it easily becomes subjectivist, emotivist, relativist, and self-destructive.

Further difficulties include the relations of intent to outward behavior. Is good intention a criterion of a virtuous person? How do we determine intention? Can a good intention absolve the agent of responsibility for an act which ends in harm—a physician telling a patient the truth out of the virtue of honesty, precipitating a serious depression or even suicide? Few are virtuous all the time. How many lapses moves us from the virtuous to the vicious category? How does virtue ethics connect with duty- and principle-based ethics which give the objectivity virtue seems to lack?

Classical ethics in the East and the West have usually eschewed systems of rules or principles or at least subordinated them to the notion of moral character. Where do virtue and supererogation meet? Are virtues synonymous with duties? Is supererogation merely a higher degree of virtue? Why are some people virtuous and others not? Must we turn to sociobiology for the answer, as some suggest?[30] Are virtues genetically ingrained, mere survival mechanisms designed to propagate the gene pool?

In spite of the ancient lineage of virtue ethics, these fundamental questions are yet to be answered. Because they have not been answered to everyone's satisfaction, moralists have turned to something more probable—to the question, what shall I do? How do I solve this dilemma before me now?

The Turn to Quandary Solving

This brings me to the third point I want to mention with regard to the erosion of virtue ethics, namely the turn—particularly in professional ethics—toward quandary and dilemma solving. This is the result of a number of factors operating in the last two decades. One is the concreteness and urgency of the new ethical issues arising in scientific advance and socio-political change. Medical and biological progress, for example, challenge traditional ethics, and yet, they must be confronted without the ethical compass points of a consensus on values or common religious beliefs. We are now a morally heterogeneous society, divided on the most fundamental ethical issues, particularly about the meaning of life and death. Without a common conception of human nature, we cannot agree on what constitutes a good life and the virtues that ought to characterize it. As a result, the ethics of the professions, especially of the medical profession, have turned to the analysis of dilemmas and of the *process* of ethical decision-making. For many, ethics consists primarily in a balancing of rights, duties, and *prima facie* principles and the resolution of conflicts among them. Procedural ethics has replaced normative ethics. This avoids the impasses generated when patients, clients, and professionals hold fundamentally opposing moral viewpoints.

But analysis cannot substitute for character and virtue—even though it provides conceptual clarity. Moral acts are the acts of human agents. Their quality is determined by the characters of the persons doing the analysis. Character shapes the way we define a moral problem, selects what we think is an ethical issue, and decides which principles, values, and technical details are determinative.

It makes a very great difference, therefore, whether a professional is motivated by self-interest or altruism. Given the realities of professional relationships, the character of the professional cannot be eliminated from its central position and that is why virtue ethics must be restored as the keystone of the ethics of the professions.

A fourth and final factor eroding a virtue approach in the medical profession is the legitimation in public attitudes of, and tolerance for, self-interest, in response to the economic imperatives acting so forcefully on the health care system. To this end, physicians and other providers have been encouraged to compete with each other. The availability, cost, and quality of health services have been turned over increasingly to market forces. The Federal Trade Commission has classified the professions, yours and mine, as businesses and made them subject to one ordering principle—the preservation of competition.[31] Health providers have been encouraged to become entrepreneurs, to invest in health care facilities and technologies, to be offered bonuses for keeping utilization of health care resources to a minimum. Without these incentives, it is argued, the best will not enter medicine, or will retire early. Medical progress would stop and new services would cease to be available. For the first time in medical history, self-interest has been given legal and moral legitimation and profit has been turned into a professional virtue. These trends are making the physician into a businessman, an entrepreneur, a proletarian, a gatekeeper, and a bureaucrat. Never has there been more confusion about who, and what, it is to be a physician.

Is There a Philosophical Basis for Restoring Virtue Ethics?

This brings me to my second major question—is there a sound philosophical foundation in the nature of professional activity for resolving the

tension between altruism and self-interest in favor of virtue and character? I believe there is, and I would ground my proposal in six characteristics of the relationship of professionals with those who seek their help.
Individually, none of these phenomena is unique in kind or degree. They
may exist individually in other human relationships and occupations. But,
as a moral cluster, they are, in fact, unique and generate a kind of "internal
morality"—a grounding for the ethics of the professions that is in some
way impervious to vacillations in philosophical fashions, as well as social,
economic, or political change. This internal morality explains why the
ethics of medicine, for example, remained until two decades ago firmly
rooted in the ethics of character and virtue. This was true of the medical
ethics of the Hippocratic school and the Stoics. It is found in the seminal
texts of Moslem, Jewish, and Christian medical moralists. It persisted in
the eighteenth century in the writing of John Gregory, Thomas Percival,
and Samuel Bard, who, although cognizant of the philosophies of Hobbes,
Adam Smith, and Hume, nonetheless, maintained the traditional dedication of the profession to the welfare of the patient and to a certain set of
virtues. Only in the last two decades has there been (to use Hume's terms)
a "sentiment of approbation" regarding self-interest.

The *first* distinguishing characteristic of professional relationships is
the dependence, vulnerability, and eminent exploitability of the person
who seeks the help of a physician, lawyer, or clergyman. The person in
need of help to restore health, receive justice, or rectify his relationships
with God is anxious, in distress, and driven by fear. To avoid death, dam-
nation, or incarceration, he is impelled to seek help though he wishes he
could avoid it. He is not free to pursue life's other goals until help is forthcoming.

The *second* characteristic of professional relationships is their inherent inequality. The professional possesses the knowledge that the patient or client needs. This places the preponderance of power in his hands.
He can use it well or poorly, for good or evil, for service or self-interest.
How can we speak, as some do, of the professional relationship as a contract when one party is so dependent upon the other's services?

The *third* characteristic of professional relationships is their special fiduciary character. In a state of vulnerability[32] and inequality, we are forced
to trust our physicians, lawyers, or ministers. We are ill equipped to evalu-

ate their competence. We are forced to reveal our intimate selves—baring our bodies, our personal lives, our souls and our failings to another person, who is a stranger. Without these invasions of our privacy, we cannot be healed or helped. Moreover, the professional invites our trust. Professionals begin their relationship with us with the question—how can I help you? Implicitly they are saying, "I have the knowledge you need—trust me to have it and to use it in your best interests." In the case of medicine, that promise is made in a public oath at the time of graduation when the graduate announces to all present that, henceforth, he can be trusted to serve interests other than his own. It is repeated in the codes of medicine and the other professions and the ordination rites of clergymen.

Indeed, it is the public declaration that defines a true "profession" and separates it from other occupations. The very word comes from the Latin *profiteri,* to declare aloud, to accept publicly a special way of life, one that promises that the profession can be trusted to act in other than its own interest. Businessmen and craftsmen ask to be trusted, but not at cost to themselves. *Caveat emptor* can never be the first principle of a profession.

Fourth, the knowledge of true professionals, as I have just defined them, cannot be wholly proprietary. Their knowledge is ordained to a practical end, to meeting certain fundamental human needs. Professional knowledge does not exist for its own sake. This is clearest in medicine, where society permits invasions of privacy that would otherwise be criminal, in order that physicians may be trained. Thus, medical students who are not fully skilled are permitted to dissect human bodies, attend and assist at autopsies and operations, and participate in the care of sick people. They are allowed *literally* to *practice,* albeit under supervision. Surgeons in training take many years to develop their skills. Their first operations are hardly as proficient as those which follow. Teaching with patients involves delays, diffusion of responsibility and accountability, and discomfort and even physical risk for the patient. Society permits these invasions of privacy and the risks attached to them, not primarily so physicians can make a living, but because society needs an uninterrupted supply of doctors. Medical knowledge and, analogously, legal and clerical knowledge are held in trust for those who need them. They can never be solely dispensed for the profit of the professional or on terms unilaterally set by him or her. That is why lawyers are officers of the court, and clergymen are ordained to minister in the name of God or their churches.

The *fifth* feature of the professional relationship is that the professional is the final common pathway through which help and harm must pass. The final decisions, actions, and recommendations must be made by one person, the professional, with whom the patient or client has a convenantal relationship of trust. No policy, no law, no regulation can be effective unless the physician, lawyer, or minister permits it to influence the professional relationship. Professionals are allowed wide discretion because the needs of those they serve are unique. Professionals are, thus, guardians of the patient's interest and responsible for any act in which they participate.

The *sixth* distinguishing characteristic feature of professional relationships is that the professional is a member of a moral community, that is, a collective human association whose members share the privileges of special knowledge and together pledge their dedication to use it to advance health, justice, or salvation. Together the members of the moral community make the same promises and elicit the same trust they do as individuals. They are bound by the same fidelity to the promise they have collectively made and the trust they have collectively elicited. The professional is, therefore, not a moral island. He belongs to a group which has been given a monopoly on special knowledge and holds it in trust for all who need it. Each professional is responsible to his colleagues and they are together responsible for him. Collectively, they are responsible for fidelity to the trust they have solicited from society. This is what the privilege of self-regulation means—not that each professional is his own judge of what is ethically permissible.

These features regarding human relationships are the components of the "internal morality" of the professions, the immediate moral ground for their obligations, and the source of definition of their virtues. To use Aristotle's terminology, those virtues make the work of the professions "be well done." The virtues of professional life are many, but I believe they are reducible, primarily to two—fidelity to trust and beneficence, which follows from the virtue of fidelity to trust. These two traits of character are the ethical foundations upon which the other virtues and principles of professional ethics depend. Clearly, they are incompatible with the Machiavellian and Hobbesian doctrines of self-interest. Their reality and irreducibility provide the most powerful argument for the restoration of virtue ethics in professional morality.[33]

The Practical Implications of Virtue Ethics

If there is validity in the philosophical foundations of professional morality, a number of practical implications follow which are pertinent to healing the moral malaise and confusion of today's professionals.

First, professionals cannot displace the moral failings of the professions on others—on society, other professions, government, economics, the market place, etc. No one can make the conscientious professional do what he thinks is not in the interests of his patient or client. Can anyone force doctors to follow a policy damaging to their interests? The fact that the professional is the final common pathway for all policies and decisions and actions forces him to be the guardian of the interests of his patient or client. Indeed, he invited that responsibility when he invited the patient or client to trust him.

As a result, individual practitioners must be very careful in exonerating themselves from morally dubious practices on the basis of survival. Professional ethics will have no future only if it is gradually suffocated by the moral compromises of individual professionals. There will be times when, as guardians of the patients' welfare, physicians will have a moral obligation to refuse: they will refuse to "dump" the patient who cannot pay; they will refuse to discharge the patient before he is ready; they will refuse to act as society's fiscal agents; they will refuse to be seduced by the profits of investments and ownership of health facilities or bonuses for denying or delaying needed care; they will refuse to be gatekeepers, except to protect their patients from unnecessary medical interventions or procedures.[34] The physician of character will be the one who can reliably be expected to exhibit the virtues of fidelity to trust and effacement of self-interest.[35]

The second practical implication is that the individual professional must not be expected to stand by when the well-being of his patient or client is threatened. It is an obligation of the professions as moral communities to be advocates for those they serve and to take collective action to assure that their services are available and accessible to all, to protect those in need of healing, justice, or salvation against legislation and public or institutional policies that may harm them. The professions as moral communities must also take the responsibility for each member's ethical behavior seriously enough to monitor, discipline, and even remove each other when the canons of professional morality are violated. Think of the enormous moral power the professions could exhort if they were truly the advocates of those they serve. Suppose that, in addition, all the helping professions were to join their efforts. Could any society resist? Can they do less? In the face of this power, can any of the three great professions blame society for their own moral lassitude?[36]

A third implication is that the formation of character is as important in the education of professionals as their technical education. Although this was a major concern of professional education in the past, it has now been forsaken. People have asked ever since Plato raised the question in the *Meno*—can virtue be taught? I believe it can. Obviously, the whole task of character formation cannot be left to the professional schools. Families, churches, and schools, all shape the students' character long before they enter professional schools. But these schools must also teach what it is to be a good physician, lawyer, or clergyman—what kind of person the good professional ought to be. Much can be done in character formation when a student is motivated by his desire to be a good professional even if his education prior to medical, law school, or seminary was morally neutral or deficient.

The most effective instruments of character formation are the professionals who teach in medical and law schools and seminaries. But they must be able to demonstrate that competence and character are inseparable, and that fidelity to trust and self-effacement can be, and must be, indispensable traits of the authentic profession. Unfortunately, not enough professional school faculty members are convinced of this or morally equipped to serve as models of virtue.

Paradigm cases of ethically sensitive professionals drawn from the history and tradition of each profession are also helpful. They are more effective than is generally realized. One of the tragedies of medical history is its depreciation of the lives of the great physicians. While biographies may not have much fascination for the sophisticated medical historians, they still have inspirational value for the aspirants to medicine. Other professions have their morally paradigmatic biographies as well. Most professional students enter with some ideal of service in mind which the professional school has a responsibility to re-enforce.

A fourth implication is that cure of the moral malaise of the professions requires something more than reordering the social organization or tailoring the semantic and semiotic feature of professional codes as Kultgen rather naively supposes.[37] What failings there are in the professions are failing in character and not in the language of our codes. If character and virtue are restored, the appropriate social reorganizations will follow—not the other way around.

Finally, there are theoretical reasons for a restoration of virtue, both in general and professional ethics. Happily, a renaissance of interest among moral philosophers in this subject is very much in evidence. But virtue ethics must not be seen as self-sufficient or as antithetical to principle for duty-based systems of the analysis of ethical dilemmas. The theoretical challenge is to develop the logical connections between analytical and virtue ethics, between principles and character, to close the gap between cognition of the right and good and the motivation to do it, and in the light of my whole analysis, to strike the morally defensible balance between self-interest and its effacement, which recognizes the primacy of altruistic beneficence.

The theoretical challenges will be complicated because virtue and duty-based ethics are today isolated from a more comprehensive moral philosophy which could tell us why we must be moral and what we define as the moral life. We need to reconnect ethics to some notion of the good and to a coherent philosophical anthropology. To this end it might be well to reexamine the classical medieval synthesis before ethics was torn from its roots in moral philosophy. That synthesis, amplified by our newer knowledge of human nature, derived from the biological and social sciences and reflected upon theologically, might provide the new resuscitation that an effective virtue ethics demands.

For the time being, a reflection on the nature of professional relationships can be fruitful even in the absence of a comprehensive moral philosophy of which it might be a part. The internal morality of the professions, based on the realities of professional relationships, is clear enough to help us repair the ozone hole opened in the fabric of professional ethics, even if we cannot repair the whole moral atmosphere on which our society depends for its survival.

Conclusion

I have emphasized what I believe to be some of the elements common to the moral philosophy of the three professions of medicine, law, and ministry. Many of these same features are shared by other professions. I must leave them to decide how the virtues of fidelity to trust and effacement of self-interest apply to them. Suppose all the professions were to acknowledge virtue as a ground for moral accountability. Would this not be the leaven for raising the standards of conventional morality as well?

Notes

1. See Address by S. Linowitz to Cornell Law School (April 15, 1988). This speech by a distinguished lawyer details some of the ethical lapses at the moral margin in current legal practice.

2. Aristotle, *Ethica Nichomachean* 1105b, 25–26 (W. D. Ross trans.). In *The Basic Works of Aristotle* 935 (R. McKeon ed. 1941).

3. *Id.* at 1106a, 16–17.

4. *Id.* at 1106a, 22–24.

5. J. Ladd, "The Internal Morality of Medicine: An Essential Dimension of the PatientPhysician Relationship." In *The Clinical Encounter* 209 (E. E. Shelp ed. 1983).

6. Aristotle, *supra* note 2, Bk. 9, Ch. 8. In this chapter, Aristotle distinguishes two types of self-love: reproachful and virtuous. Reproachful self-love is self-love that arises not according to a rational principle but according to passion. The person who loves self in this way desires what is advantageous, not what is noble. *Id.* at 1169a, 4–6. The person of reproachful self-love assigns to himself the greater share of wealth, honor, and bodily pleasure. The person who demonstrates virtuous self-love is inspired by the rational principle to secure for self the most noble goods. The actions of this person will benefit both himself and others.

7. Plato, *The Republic* 338C (R. W. Sterling & W. C. Scott trans. 1985).

8. W. K. C. Guthrie, *The Sophists* (1971). This is a thorough and detailed examination of the idea of self-interest and its relationship to justice in *The Republic*. It is particularly helpful in its discussion of how Hobbesian and Machiavellian strains were prefigured in the thinking of the Sophists.

9. Aristotle, *supra* note 2, at Bk. 9, Ch. 8.

10. See J. M. Cooper, *Reason and Human Good in Aristotle* (1975) for a consideration of Aristotle's view on love of self and of others.

11. Aristotle, *supra* note 2, at 1155b, 31; 1156b, 9–10; 1159a, 8–12, 28–33. See also W. F. R. Hardie, *Aristotle's Ethical Theory* 326 (1968).

12. See T. Engberg-Pedersen, *Aristotle's Theory of Moral Insight* 237–262 (1983) for a penetrating analysis of *Eudemian Ethics* Bks. 8 and 9.

13. Hardie, *supra* note 11, says that for Aristotle, "the end of the state is 'greater and more perfect' than the end of the individual and thus, the activities of the statesman are aimed at happiness 'for himself and his fellow citizens'." *Id.* at 216.

14. Plato, *supra* note 7, at 341e–347a.

15. See Cicero, *De Officiis* Bk. 3, Ch. 13 (W. Miller trans. 1913).

16. See "Oath of Hippocrates" quoted in 4 *Encyclopedia of Bioethics* 1731 (1978).

17. N. Machiavelli, *The Prince* (1970): "This is because, taking everything into account [the prince] will find that some of the things that appear to be virtues, if he practices them will ruin him, and some of the things that appear to be wicked will bring him security and prosperity." *Id.* at 87.

18. B. Mandeville, *The Fable of the Bees* (I. Primer ed. 1962).

19. F. Nietzsche, *On the Genealogy of Morals* (W. Kaufmann & R. J. Hollingdale trans. 1967).

20. Ayn Rand, *The Fountainhead* (1971).

21. T. Homes, Leviathan (C. B. MacPherson ed. 1968); see also H. Sidgwick, *Outlines of the History of Ethics* (1988). Sidgwick neatly summarizes Hobbes' paradoxical view of social duty: "a view of social duty in which the only fixed positions were selfishness everywhere and unlimited power somewhere could not but appear offensively paradoxical." *Id.* at 165.

22. See J. S. Mill, *Utilitarianism* Ch. 2 (G. Sher trans. 1979).

23. H. More, *Enchiridion Ethicum* (E. Southwell trans. 1930).

24. J. Butler, *Three Sermons on Human Nature* (1897).

25. E. L. Pincoffs, *Quandaries and Virtues: Against Reductivism in Ethics* (1986).

26. E. O. Wilson, *Sociobiology: The New Synthesis* (1975).

27. T. Nagel, *The Possibility of Altruism* (1978).

28. G. E. M. Anscombe, "Modern Moral Philosophy," *Philosophy* 33 (1958): 1–19.

29. A. C. MacIntyre, *After Virtue: A Study in Moral Theory* (1984).

30. Wilson, *supra* note 26.

31. See generally Pellegrino, "What Is a Profession? The Ethical Implications of the F.T.C. Order and Some Supreme Court Decisions," *Survey of Ophthalmology* 29 (1984): 221–225.

32. See R. E. Goodin, *Protecting the Vulnerable: A Reanalysis of Our Social Responsibilities* (1485). This author proposes vulnerability as a source of moral obligation in his analysis of our social responsibilities.

33. See E. D. Pellegrino and D. C. Thomasma, *For the Patient's Good: The Restoration of Beneficence in Health Care* (1988).

34. See C. Ansberry, "Dumping the Poor," *Wall St. J.,* Nov. 29, 1988, at 1 col. 1.

35. H. T. Engelhardt & M. A. Rie, "Morality for the Medical Industrial Complex," *New Eng. J. Med.* 319, no. 16 (1988): 1086–1089. These authors argue against the thesis that I am presenting particularly in their view that traditional standards must be tailored to conform to institutional and third-party payer's requirements.

36. J. Callahan, *Ethics and the Professional Life* (1988). This is an anthology dealing with the relationships between professional and ordinary morality, with contributions by philosophers and professionals in law, medicine and business.

37. J. Kultgen, *Ethics and Professionalism* 4 (1988).

Toward a Virtue-Based Normative Ethics for the Health Professions

If he really does think there is no distinction between virtue and vice,

why, sir, when he leaves our house, let us count our spoons.

—Samuel Johnson

Introduction

In his highly influential work *After Virtue,* Alasdair MacIntyre (1984) details the decline of virtue-based ethics since the Enlightenment and the obstacles to its restoration absent a community of shared values to sustain it. In this essay I shall start with MacIntyre's conclusions and examine the possibility of a restoration of virtue-based ethics to normative status in ethics generally and, more specifically, in the ethics of medicine and the health professions.

I will argue: (1) that virtue-based ethics has lost its normative force because the moral philosophy on which it was based for so long is no longer intact in either general or professional ethics; (2) that, for a variety of reasons, the recovery of a common moral philosophy to sustain a normative theory of virtue ethics is too remote at the moment to be a viable possibility in general ethics; but (3) that virtue likely can be restored as a normative concept in the ethics of the health professions; and (4) that even in this limited realm, virtue cannot stand alone, but must be related to other ethical theories in a more comprehensive moral philosophy than currently exists.

This essay is divided into three parts: the first traces the origins, erosion, and present-day revival of the Classical-Medieval conception of virtue with particular emphasis on the reasons for its metamorphosis and decline; the second part provides a similar analysis of the concept of virtue in the ethics of medicine and the other health professions with an emphasis on the possibilities and requirements for its restoration as a normative concept; and the third part suggests how virtue-based ethics could be related to other major contemporary ethical theories in an integrated view of the four essential elements of the moral life, namely, agent, act, circumstance, and consequence.

Origin, Decline, and Restoration of Virtue-Based Ethics

The Idea of Virtue Ethics

Virtue is the most ancient, durable, and ubiquitous concept in the history of ethical theory. This is so because one cannot completely separate the character of a moral agent from his or her acts, the nature of those acts, the circumstances under which they are performed, or their consequences. Virtue theories focus on the agent—on his or her intentions, dispositions, and motives—and on the kind of person the moral agent becomes, wishes to become, or ought to become as a result of his or her habitual disposition to act in certain ways. These phenomena are ineradicable elements of the moral life and any moral theory that ignores them fails to encompass the fullness and complexity of the challenge and struggle to be a good human being.

In a purely virtue-based ethic, the normative standard is the good person, the person upon whom one can rely habitually to be good and to do the good under all circumstances. This standard has been both the strength and the weakness of virtue-based ethics, the reason for its durability, but also for its fragility because of the circularity of its logic. The challenge is to provide a normative force for virtue outside of the circular logic that holds the right and the good to be what the virtuous person takes them to be while defining the virtuous person as the one who is and does what is right and good.

Every culture has a notion of the virtuous person—i.e., a paradigm person, real or idealized, who sets the standards of noble conduct for a culture and whose character traits exemplify the kind of person others in that culture ought to be or to emulate. These paradigm persons are celebrated in the myths and stories, poetry and ritual, of non-Western and Western cultures. The moral values and characteristics of these virtuous persons are given formal expression in the philosophy and theology of each era and culture. They are formalized in varying degrees in the works of Plato and Aristotle, the philosophy of Confucius (Cua 1978) and Lao Tse (Waley 1956; Yearley 1990), the Hindu concept of Dharma (Jhingran 1989), and the humanism of African tribal cultures (Wiredu 1992). Often the paradigm figures, such as Jesus, Buddha, or Confucius, antedated the community of values that would sustain them. In fact, frequently, the community of values and beliefs were framed on the model and through the person and personality of the paradigm virtuous person. The intricacies and the primacy of the mutual relationship between paradigm virtuous persons and communities of values have yet to be explored in depth.

The Classical-Medieval Conception — Origins

In the Western culture, the most pervasive and enduring concept of virtue, the one most formally and fully developed, is found in the thought of Plato and Aristotle, supplemented by the Stoics and Epicureans (Reale 1985; Rist 1980), and brought to full fruition by Thomas Aquinas. The fusion of those streams of thought became the Classical-Medieval synthesis that has shaped moral philosophy in the West for 2,500 years. Although it has gone through a variety of metamorphoses and decline over the centuries, the Classical-Medieval notion of virtue is re-emerging today among influential moral philosophers and is seeking its place among more recent normative ethical theories. This Classical-Medieval conception of virtue has also been the dominant one in the ethics of the health professions as professions. For this reason, it is the operative concept in this discussion of where to go "beyond virtue" in the wake of *After Virtue* (MacIntyre 1984).

The Classical-Medieval synthesis has been the subject of intense scholarly exegesis for centuries. There is still much debate about various facets of the traditional notion of virtue—whether the virtues are one or many, how the doctrine of the mean (i.e., virtue as a mean state that lies between the extremes, the "vices," of excess and deficiency) applies to them, whether they can be in conflict, what "list" of virtues should prevail, and the like. An adequate discussion of these questions is beyond the confines of this essay, however. Rather, I have selected what I take to be the elements of the Classical-Medieval synthesis that are most important for a resuscitation of virtue-based ethics in the health professions, i.e., the idea of virtue (1) as excellence in traits of character, (2) as a trait oriented to ends and purposes (that is to say, teleologically), (3) as an excellence of reason not emotion, (4) as centered on practical judgment, and (5) as learned by practice.

In and through the character of Socrates, Plato first advanced the idea of virtue as *areté*—i.e., excellence in the knowledge of the good, which made for a good and happy life. On this view, knowledge of the good disposes one to the good life and to happiness. The search for one's own good is "at the cornerstone of Socrates's moral philosophy" (Gomez-Lobo 1995, p. 108); the virtue one possesses makes one good. Vice is the result of ignorance of the good. Throughout his dialogues, Plato developed a list of the virtues: fortitude (*Laches*), temperance (*Charmides*), justice (*Republic*), and wisdom, which with self-restraint (*sophrosyne*), characterized the virtuous person. This list has survived as a list of the cardinal virtues—i.e., those that might subsume, or be the basis for, the other virtues. Socrates asks, but never satisfactorily answers, the questions that are still asked: Are the virtues one or many? How are they acquired? Can they be taught? (Plato 1961, *Meno* 70a)

Aristotle retains the idea of excellence and adds a strong emphasis on the *telos,* the orientation of virtues to the ends and purposes of human activity. He defines virtue as ". . . the state of character which makes a person good and makes that person to do his or her work well . . . " (*Nicomachean Ethics (NE)* 1106a22–24). Thus, for Aristotle, the teleological orientation of virtue is twofold—the fulfillment of the natural end of human life, namely happiness, and also the attainment of the end of human work. Aristotle links being a good person with doing well whatever one does and with achieving, to the greatest extent possible, the end of any human activity, whether it be the conduct of the whole of one's life or the conduct of a particular work related to the role or roles one plays in everyday life.

On this view, virtue is a character trait under rational control. Virtue is not a "habit" in the sense of being an unconscious reflex. Rather it is a *habitus,* a predictable disposition to choose the good whenever confronted with a choice (*NE* 1105a27–33). A virtuous person has knowledge of the good and chooses it for its own sake and from a firm character with regard to the passions (*NE* 1105b21–23). The virtuous person must not only know the good but *be* good (*NE* 1102b26, 1144b18). In contrast to Plato and Socrates, Aristotle takes account of emotion more clearly, but defines the virtuous person as one whose emotions are ordered by reason to the end of happiness.

Virtue is also practical in its orientation. For this reason, Aristotle's central virtue is *phronesis* or practical wisdom. Moral agents must consider what is appropriate to the occasion: "Virtue determines the end; practical wisdom makes us do what is conducive to the end" (*NE* 1145a5–6). Thus, *phronesis* is the virtue that enables one to deliberate well in making moral judgments and to choose the means most suited to the end of the activity in which one is engaged. Practical wisdom is a ". . . true and reasoned capacity to act with regard to the things that are good or bad for men" (*NE* 1140b5). *Phronesis* fuses the intellectual virtues, which have truth as their end—e.g., science, art, intuitive wisdom—with the moral virtues, which have the good as their end. The good person is the *phronimos,* the person of practical wisdom; the virtuous act is the act as it would be chosen by the *phronimos.*

Aristotle criticizes Plato's ethics as too general (*Politics* 1260a25) and unmindful of the emotions (*Magna Moralia* 1182a20). In keeping with his emphasis on the practical, Aristotle teaches that virtue is, itself, learned by practice. Thus, he answers in the affirmative one of the questions Meno put to Socrates (*Meno* 70a). By repeatedly acting in conformity with the ends of human life, as the man of practical wisdom would act, a person becomes habitually disposed to act virtuously. One can then depend on the virtuous person to act well in all circumstances.

Aristotle recognizes that certain things ought never be done—e.g., adultery, murder, and theft—and certain dispositions ought never be adopted—e.g., spite and envy (*NE* 1107a10–11). With the exception of those acts and dispositions that do not allow of a mean, Aristotle does not lay down rules, duties, or principles. We must be "content" with the ". . . truth roughly and in outline . . ." (*NE* 1094b20). Instead, in general, ". . . excellence is a state of choice lying in a mean related to us and in the way in which the man of practical wisdom would determine it" (*NE* 1107a1–3). Aristotle's mean is not just a mean between extremes; it is also the right amount for a given individual, determined not subjectively, but rationally, as the man of practical wisdom would determine it (Prior 1991, pp. 159–160). The morally good is what the virtuous person does; the virtuous person is one who does what is morally good.

Thomas Aquinas (1963), in his great study of Christian theology and Greek philosophy, develops a virtue-based ethics that begins with the same elements as Aristotle's (*Summa Theologiae* (*ST*) II-II, 108: 2 and *ST* I-II, 119: 8–15). He defines virtue very much as Aristotle does: "It belongs to human virtue to make a man and his work according to reason" (*ST* II-II, 108: 2). He posits truth as the end of the natural intellectual virtues and the good of humans as the end of the natural moral virtues. However, drawing on Christian theology, Aquinas adds the theological virtues of faith, hope, and charity. These virtues dispose humans to attain their supernatural end—union with God in the beatific vision. The infused virtues orient humans to their ultimate end of union with God: faith orients to that end, hope enables the Christian to stay the course, and charity attaches the Christian to God (*ST* I-II, 119: 8–15). Of the theological virtues, charity or love is the ordering virtue (Pinckaers 1985).

For Aquinas, as for Aristotle, practical wisdom is a central virtue. Prudence is analogous to *phronesis*. Its function is the actualization of the other virtues in attainment of the goals of human life (Pieper 1966, p. 33). Not only does prudence link the intellectual and the moral virtues, as it does in Aristotle, but it also links those virtues to the theological virtues. Prudence is a "*recta ration agibilium*," a right way of acting according to reason (Maritain 1949, p. 116). It disposes persons to choose means that most closely fit the *telos* of an act. Prudence is the virtue that sorts out the other virtues when they might be in conflict and provides practical judgment and discernment in complex circumstances thereby giving its possessor the capacity to select the means that will most closely approximate the end of a particular human activity.

The Classical-Medieval Conception — Decline

Both the Classical and the Medieval Christian conceptions of virtue were based on a clear moral epistemology and metaphysics. They were rooted in the conviction that there existed an objective moral order and a philosophy of human nature ascertainable by human reason, which, in turn, defined the *telos* for human activity. The virtues were traits that habitually disposed humans to act in accord with the ends of human nature—i.e., fulfillment in natural happiness for Socrates, Plato, and Aristotle and supernatural happiness in union with God for Aquinas. On this view, the virtues have normative force not because they are agreeable or admired but because they accord well with, and predispose to, the ends, the purposes, and the good of human beings as defined by an underlying metaphysics.

In the post-Medieval and post-Enlightenment periods up to the present, these metaphysical foundations for virtue ethics were seriously eroded by the confluence of a variety of forces. The possibility of a metaphysical definition of human nature or the good, the epistemological possibility of moral knowledge, and the possibility of a philosophical anthropology were all subjected to skepticism and denial. Beginning in the Enlightenment, theology, religious authority, and even reason were challenged as sources of morality. Aristotelian philosophy and the methods of scholasticism were especially suspect in science and theology. Hobbes and Locke replaced the Classical and Medieval philosophies of human nature with "realism" about the dubious nature of human motives and conduct; Hutcheson and Hume advanced moral psychology to counter the over-rationalization of Classical and Medieval ethics (Hume 1975). Virtues were replaced by a variety of competing concepts: rights for Locke, duty for Kant, moral sentiment for Hume and Smith, and consequences and utility for Bentham and Mill (Sidgwick 1988; Becker and Becker 1992).

From its inception, the concept of virtue had strong opponents who ridiculed it as a basis for morality. Glaucon, Ademantus, and, later, Thrasymachus, in Plato's *Republic* and Callicles in the *Gorgias* attacked the idea of virtue as unrealistic and vulnerable to submersion by power and self-interest. Later philosophers reinforced this anti-virtue bias. Machiavelli (1970) maintained that the virtuous person was doomed in a world in which others were not virtuous; Mandeville (1962) argued that vice was necessary for the survival of the economy and society; and Nietzsche thought virtue, especially the Christian virtues, was a mark of weakness unbecoming the Superman (Nietzsche 1954, 1967). More recently, Ayn Rand (1964), voicing the implicit ethics of the marketplace, condemned the traditional conception of virtue as inimical to the ethos of success.

The concept of virtue survived these assaults in a revised form. As the philosophical foundations of the Classical-Medieval synthesis eroded, virtue was redefined in terms of the emergent newer schools of philosophy. For present purposes, only a few of the multitudinous revisions need be mentioned as examples: Hume (1975, p. 211) sees virtue as ". . . a quality of mind agreeable to, or approved by, everyone who considers or contemplates it." For Kant (1986, Ak 394–396), virtue is the coincidence of the rational will with every duty firmly settled in the character. For Bentham (1969), as one might expect of a utilitarian, a virtue is a trait that disposes its possessor to increase the quantity of happiness. Many other definitions followed, each framed in terms of an underlying philosophical system. The result was the eclipse of virtue as a normative concept by intuition, moral psychology, maxims, rules, and principles.

In the twentieth century, the revolution against a metaphysical or theological foundation for ethics came to full fruition. The history of this revolution is complicated beyond the scope of this paper. Suffice it to say that ethics turned to meta-analysis, to the dissection of the language of moral discourse, to the intuitive grasp of the good or of *prima facie* principles discoverable by morally mature persons, or to a variety of alternatives to principles, such as casuistry, hermeneutics, feminist psychology, care theory, or narrative. At present, these theories and a revitalized virtue-based ethics are in competition with each other. They share a repudiation of the philosophical and theological groundings that have traditionally given virtue-based ethics its normative thrust. Each of the theories holds one or another of the shards of the Classical-Medieval synthesis—i.e., of virtue-based ethics—without the philosophical cement to repair the damage done.

Virtue-Based Ethics — The Revival

Despite the convolutions in the concept of virtue wrought by a succession of philosophical systems, the ideas of virtue and the virtuous person were never erased. Ethicists continued to confront the question of character of the agent. Principles, rules, maxims, intuitions, language analysis, and technical skill in solving moral puzzles did not encompass the full complexity of the moral life. The central nature of the character of the moral agent could not totally be ignored (Kuperman 1991). As a result, several decades ago, a number of contemporary moral philosophers began to revive the idea of virtue and to seek a place for it in ethical theory (Foot 1978; Frankena 1982; French, Uehling, and Wettstein 1988; Hauerwas 1981; MacIntyre 1984, 1990).

The philosophers who were most successful in doing so found it necessary first to revive, or at least to revise, the philosophical or theological substratum on which classical virtue theory had been built—either in Plato, Aristotle, Aquinas, or their commentators. It remains to be seen how successful these attempts to restore virtue will be in general ethical theory given the post-Modernist doubts about the utility of philosophical ethics or even of philosophy itself—especially in its current anti-foundationalist mind set (Baynes, Bohman, and McCarthy 1987; Rockmore and Singer 1992). It seems unlikely that a robust virtue ethics can be reconstructed since the probability of agreement on a conception of the good or the *telos* of human life is remote indeed. Such agreement is required, however, for any normative theory of virtue. Lacking it, we are left with such conflicting definitions of virtue as ". . . a corrective to the tendency to act against the good" (Foot 1978, p. 8), or any trait that ameliorates the human condition (Warnock 1971) or enhances evolutionary adaptation (Casey 1990; Wilson 1980).

MacIntyre has most successfully built on the Aristotelian notion of virtue and reformulated it in more contemporary terms, taking into account the erosion of the tradition and the moral consensus that gave the classical doctrine its normative strength. MacIntyre (1984) builds his definition on three elements; he regards virtues as dispositions or acquired qualities that are: (1) necessary to achieve the good internal to practices,[1]

(2) necessary to sustain communities in which individuals can seek a higher good as the good of their own lives, and (3) necessary to sustain traditions that provide necessary historical contexts for individual lives. Virtue, thus, is a character trait necessary to achievement of a good—a perfected excellence (MacIntyre 1988, p. 74). In this, MacIntyre adopts the teleological thrust of the Aristotelian definition of virtue and adds to it the sustaining force of a historical community of values.

This is not the place to evaluate MacIntyre's reformulation. However, he does make a genuine attempt to recapture some of the Aristotelian notion of virtue. MacIntyre (1990) clearly recognizes the difficulties that his reformulation faces in the absence of a shared notion of the good or a community of values to sustain it. In a more Platonic vein, Iris Murdoch (1992, pp. 482–484) also recognizes the need for and the difficulty of recovering a conception of the good as a foundation of moral life and of the virtues. Murdoch intimates strongly that the good has to confront religious reality as well, although she does not locate the good in a formalized religious belief system. In this, she counts virtue as ". . . the most evident bridge between morality and religion" (Murdoch 1992, p. 481).

In any case, the improbability of any recovery of the philosophical or theological substructures of virtue compounds the difficulties of a contemporary revival so far as general ethical theory is concerned. This is amply evident in the incommensurability of premises and methodologies characteristic of general theories of ethics. However, these impediments are less formidable in professional ethics, particularly in medicine and the other health professions. It is here that genuine possibilities for a restoration and reformulation of virtue ethics exist.

Difficulties Inherent in the Classical-Medieval Synthesis

Before turning to the possibility of restoring virtue ethics in the health professions, it may be well to examine the inherent difficulties of any virtue-based ethics as a normative theory. If virtue is to be restored to normative status, these difficulties must be acknowledged and addressed.

First is the circularity of justification to which I have already alluded, namely, that the good is that which the virtuous person does and the virtuous person is the person who does what is good for humans. Some grounding for virtue outside of this circular logic is necessary if the redundancy of this logic is to be avoided. Otherwise, virtue can become so intuitive and subjective as to be meaningless. What is virtue to one person's community is vice to another's. What some find "agreeable"—to use Hume's term—others find disagreeable with equal intensity.

In the Classical and Medieval construals of virtue, its grounding was in the ends and purposes derived from an underlying philosophical anthropology based in natural law. Within this anthropology, virtues could be defined, rejected, and even ordered with respect to one another. Their normative power arose not from their simple, intuitive affirmation as virtues but from the congruence of virtues with something more fundamental to which virtues and virtuous persons themselves conformed. This grounding is the antidote to the multiplicity of definitions and the proliferation of lists of the virtues—lists that sometimes grow to ridiculous proportions and include every imaginable agreeable trait from the most profound to the most trivial. Instrumental, moral, intellectual, and spiritual virtues become intermingled with "values," beliefs, preferences, tastes, and the like. Any characteristic agreeable to someone can be touted as a virtue.[2]

A second difficulty in virtue-based ethics is the paucity of the definitive action guidelines that give principles, rules, and maxims their force—at least in the abstract. A virtue-based ethics depends upon the grasp by the virtuous person of the good for humans in such a reliable way that, no matter what the act or the circumstances may be, that person will know how to attain the good. Such an open-ended guide to moral choice is sustainable only if there is, in fact, some agreement on the good for humans. A shared notion of the good gave focus to Aristotle's *Nicomachean Ethics* and *Eudemian Ethics,* to the Platonic dialogues, and to Aquinas's *Summa Theologiae.* But it is disagreement on the good that divides modern and contemporary ethical and metaphysical theory. So much is this the case that many deem futile the pursuit of a definition of the good beyond intuition (Moore 1903). With many goods being equally defensible, there will be many interchangeable virtues and vices. The contemporary inclination of philosophy is to abandon the quest for the good, to define it by intuitive grasp only, or to deny its existence altogether.

Third is the difficulty of supererogation. The classical insistence on the virtues as excellences seems to demand too much. In a legalistically shaped society—one that, in addition, emphasizes individual choices and life-styles—even the narrow idea of role-related responsibilities and duties is challenged. The only duty is not to infringe on the liberty of others. Everything else is beyond duty. In such a setting, virtue in the classical sense is too much to ask of individuals or communities and institutions.

Some would argue that the possession of virtues and the accompanying disposition to excellence is entirely fortuitous, the product of genetics, environment, or luck (Casey 1990; Wilson 1980). How, in justice, can we demand virtue from those who do not possess it innately? How do we attribute virtuous behavior to those who are genetically disposed to it? Is it not unfair to impose a demand for supererogation on those who are congenitally indisposed to even ordinary duties? Without the classical notion of virtue as an "excellence" consciously and rationally practiced, it may be difficult to see virtue as "virtuous."

Any viable normative account of virtue-based ethics must somehow engage these difficulties and objections. As I have already suggested, in our times at least, this is so formidable a task in general ethics that it likely is destined for failure. However, as I now hope to show, there is a reasonable possibility of satisfying the requirements for a normative virtue-based ethics in the more limited case of professional ethics.

Virtue-Based Ethics in Medicine — History and Revival

Origins and Metamorphosis

The history of the concept of virtue in medical ethics follows in general outline the history of the origin and metamorphosis of virtue in general ethics that I have described. However, in medicine, virtue ethics resisted erosion for a longer period of time, and change, when it did come, did so over a period of twenty-five years, rather than the five or six centuries that it took in general ethics.

Therefore, in medical ethics, as in general ethics, virtue was the dominant normative theory for a long period of time. It is the basis for the Hippocratic Oath and the deontological books of the Hippocratic corpus. In the Medieval world, as in the present, the Hippocratic ethic was joined with the ethics of the major world religions. For centuries, that ethic united physicians across cultural and national boundaries in a community of moral values based in the virtues of benevolence, respect for human life, and the vulnerability of the sick.

A quarter of a century ago, the dominance of virtue in medical ethics began to diminish for three reasons: First was the introduction of principle-based ethics (Beauchamp and Childress 1989), which appealed to health professionals as being more definitive than virtue because of its concreteness and applicability to clinical decisions. Second, socio-political change toward participatory democracy, greater public education, distrust of authority, and the character failings of some physicians focused public attention on autonomy-based, contractual relationships rather than trust-based, covenantal ones. Third, and importantly, the religious and philosophical consensus that undergirded professional ethics, at least in the West, was challenged and weakened (Pellegrino 1986).

Today, as a result, medical professional ethics is gradually being deconstructed as its conceptual substratum is progressively challenged. The Hippocratic Oath, the backbone of traditional medical professional ethics, is in danger of complete dissolution. It is already defunct in the minds of some very creditable ethicists (Veatch 1984)—done-in by the societal pressures to substitute autonomy or social justice for beneficence and to relax the proscriptions against abortion, euthanasia, assisted suicide, breaches of confidentiality, and sexual relations with patients. In any gathering today, it would be difficult to find a commonly accepted set of precepts or virtues that should characterize the "good" physician (Pellegrino 1988).

These changes are occurring in the domain of *professional* ethics—i.e., the domain of duties, obligations, and virtues entailed in the health professional's roles as a healer and as a participant in a special kind of relationship with a patient. Professional ethics centers on the generic obligations of the healing relationship, those common to physicians as physicians, nurses as nurses, and so on. Professional ethics is the realm of the ethics of the physician- or nurse-patient relationship. This realm is a domain distinct from the growing body of other ethical issues commonly subsumed under the rubric of "bioethics"—i.e., the issues of withholding or withdrawing life support, euthanasia and assisted suicide, embryo research, organ and tissue transplantation, managed care, and the like—the whole panorama of new issues growing out of medical technological advances.

These are the "content" questions of bioethics—the questions that have become so problematic as a result of the loss of consensus about the meanings, purposes, and value of human life. Given the pluralism, the relativism, and the privatization of morals, there seems to be little hope for agreement on such questions at the moment. Recovery of a normative role for virtue in such circumstances without agreement on the philosophical foundations for the virtues is quite remote. To recognize this fact is not to admit that moral truth is impossible or that virtue is no longer a viable concept, but only to suggest that a first, and more practical, step is to confine consideration of a restoration of virtue-based ethics to professional ethics. Whether this opening later will extend into the realm of specific moral choices that are of such consuming interest in bioethics is unforeseeable at this time.

I will now address the reasons that professional ethics is a promising prospect for virtue ethics; what the requirements for a viable, normative ethics might be; and how those requirements might be satisfied.

The Restoration of Virtue in Professional Ethics

The Opportunity

There are several good reasons to suppose that a return to virtue is a reasonable probability in professional ethics. Paradoxically, some of the reasons arise from the deficiencies now being perceived in the dominant school of principle-based moral guidelines; others stem from the more limited scope of professional ethics within the larger field of bioethics.

First is the growing disquiet in the last decade with some of the limitations of principle-based ethics. Principles are thought to be too abstract, too removed from the contextual and experiential complexity of clinical decision making, and too conducive to an overly rationalistic, quasi-legalistic ethics that over-emphasizes quandaries and stifles compassion and moral creativity (Clouser and Gert 1990; Carse 1991).

Second is the criticism that *prima facie* principles need to be grounded in some more fundamental philosophical system to give them the normative weight they must carry. Such a foundation is needed to resolve conflict between and among principles in more than a pragmatic and functional way—perhaps even to give them a lexical ordering in specific situations, if not generally.

Third is the persistent appreciation that moral agents—i.e., persons acting—cannot be left out of moral judgments. This fact has hovered over general and medical ethics even in the period of its most radical change. The moral life is a life peculiar to the human species. The way in which principles, rules, caring, hermeneutics, casuistry, or any other alternative theory of ethics is conducted will depend on the kind of persons carrying out the moral acts and their analyses. Intention, moral psychology, and the "story" of the agent's life cannot be separated from the agent's moral behavior. To avoid looking at virtue and intentions and to assume that the only justification for moral acts lies in principles are thought by many to favor the right over the good.

These shortcomings in principle-based ethics are reinforced on the positive side by the nature of professional ethics. Unlike general ethics, professional ethics offers the possibility of some agreement on a *telos*—i.e., an end and a good. In a healing relationship between a health care professional and a patient, most would agree that the primary end must be the good of the patient. The healing relationship, itself, provides a phenomenological grounding for professional ethics that applies to all healers by virtue of the kind of activity that healing entails. In general ethics, on the other hand, at least at present, the analogous possibility for agreement on something so fundamental as the *telos*, end, or good of human life is so remote as to be practically unattainable.

The Necessary Ingredients

At a minimum, any normative theory of the ethics of the healing relationship based in virtue will require the following: (1) a theory of medicine to define the *telos*, the good of medicine as an activity; (2) a definition of virtue in terms of that theory; and (3) a set of virtues entailed by the theory to characterize the "good" health professional.

A theory of medicine. David Thomasma and I (1981, 1988) have outlined a theory of medicine in some detail elsewhere. For the purposes of this essay, I will simply summarize that theory from which I will draw the *telos* and, thus, the virtues of the good physician or nurse (Pellegrino and Thomasma 1993). The theory is grounded in three phenomena of the healing relationship, in the realities and actualities of the clinical encounter that establish medicine and nursing as particular kinds of human activity (Pellegrino 1994): the fact of illness, the act of profession, and the act of medicine (healing).

The fact of illness. Persons become *patients* when they acknowledge that they are sufficiently concerned over a physical or psychological symptom to believe they need help. In this state, to varying degrees, they are anxious, dependent, in pain, disabled, and extremely vulnerable and exploitable. They are no longer free to pursue the things they want out of life without impediment. If they are to be helped, healed, and cared for, they must seek out a health professional, someone who possesses the knowledge to accomplish these ends for, and with, them.

The act of profession. To move from a state of health to a state of illness is an experiential and existential change in the way we perceive our humanity. In that vulnerable state of illness, the physician or nurse asks, "How may I help you?" Implicit in the question is the promise that the health professional possesses the knowledge needed to help and to heal and intends to use it in the interests of the patient and not at the expense of the patient's vulnerability. This "act of profession" is an act of implicit promise making that establishes a covenant of trust at the physician's or nurse's voluntary instigation. This self-imposed trust covenant imposes obligations on the professional from the moment it is made.

The act of healing. The promise made to the dependent patient directs the knowledge, techniques, and personal commitment of the physician or nurse to the *telos* of the relationship—helping and healing. The diagnostic, prognostic, and therapeutic acts—which are manipulative, judgmental, cognitive, and so on-must be directed to what is necessary to heal and to help *this* patient, to a technically correct and morally good decision and action. This is the immediate *telos* of the clinical encounter, which is, in turn, part of the ultimate *telos* of health care—the cultivation and restoration of health and the containment or cure of disease. To be sure, healing may occur outside of medicine and the health professions, but that which is specific to the health professions is the attainment of the *telos* of healing through the science and the art of medicine—those things specific to medicine as a particular kind of human activity.

A Definition of Professional Virtue

The second ingredient of a virtue-based normative theory of medical ethics is a definition of virtue in terms of the *telos* of the clinical encounter.

This encounter defines medicine as the kind of activity it is. A definition suited to professional activity would draw on the elements of virtue as defined by Aristotle and its adaptation to practices as defined by MacIntyre.

Drawing on these two sources, I define a virtue as a trait of character that disposes its possessor habitually to excellence of intent and performance with respect to the *telos* specific to a human activity. Virtue gives to reason the power to discern and to will the motivation asymptotically to accomplish a moral end with perfection. For any profession, there will be a specific activity that, if executed well, makes the professional good or virtuous. Healing is the activity specific to nursing and medicine. Those dispositions that impart the capacity to heal well are the virtues of medicine, nursing, dentistry, and the like. They are the virtues "internal"—in MacIntyre's (1984, p. 187) sense—to the practice. Possession of these internal virtues defines the good nurse or physician.

A List of Virtues

The third ingredient of a virtue-based normative theory of medical ethics is a list of virtues that will define the "good" physician, nurse, or other health professional. These are the virtues entailed by the phenomena of the relationship and the *telos* of medicine. They are the virtues essential to achieving the ends of medicine optimally and without which those ends would be frustrated or attained in less than optimal fashion.

Lists of virtues are notoriously difficult to compose. The following list is not meant to be inclusive of all the virtues necessary to healing. Rather, the virtues included are those most essential to the healing purposes of the clinical encounter. In that sense, they are "entailed" by the end of the healing relationship, that is, they are required if the end is to be attained. The virtues are not listed in order of preference. They reinforce each other so closely that to compromise one is to compromise the others. A lexical order among them would be difficult to defend.

Fidelity to Trust and Promise

This virtue is entailed by the ineradicability of trust in the patient-nurse or patient-physician relationship, the invitation of the professional to trust when the relationship is initiated, the importance of trust to healing, and the fact that, ultimately, the patient has no choice but to trust the professional.

Benevolence

This virtue intends the good of the patient. It is a *sine qua non* since the patient obviously seeks to be helped, not harmed. Intending every act to be in the patient's interest is the gold standard of medical ethics.

Effacement of Self-Interest

Given the exploitability and vulnerability of patients, a certain degree of self-effacement is entailed since without it the patient can become merely a means to advance the physician's power, prestige, profit, or pleasure. In these days of managed and for-profit care, the need for effacement of self-interest is urgent if the patient is to be protected against exploitation.

Compassion and Caring

If the patient is to be healed in the fullest sense, the physician or nurse must have compassion—i.e., the health professional must be able to feel something of the patient's experience of the predicament of illness. Such feeling is essential to adjusting the treatment to the particularities of *this* patient's life story, time of life, and so forth. Compassion is the prelude to caring—to concern, empathy, and consideration for the patient's plight. On this view, caring in its several meanings (cf. Pellegrino 1985) is more in the realm of virtue ethics than being an ethical theory of its own.

Intellectual Honesty

By virtue of the trust that health professionals enjoy and the power of knowledge and skill they exercise, physicians and nurses can be agents of great harm as well as great good. Acknowledging when one does not know something and being humble enough to admit ignorance is a virtue of healing. Knowing when to say "I do not know" is a virtue counseled by sources as different as the Babylonian Talmud and Galileo.

Justice

In the healing relationship *per se,* the virtue of commutative justice is implicit throughout. Commutative justice dictates that in interpersonal relationships what is owed to each is rendered to each and equals are treated equally. Taken as a principle, justice is blindfolded and applied strictly. But taking justice as a virtue in the healing relationship requires removing the blindfold and adjusting what is owed to the specific needs of the patient, even if those needs do not fit the definition of what is strictly owed.

Furthermore, when the physician is bound by a covenant of trust to *this* patient, distributive justice—what is owed to others in a more distant relationship to the physician—takes a lesser place. After all, the covenant, the promise to help, is made to an identifiable sick person, not to society at large nor to the managed care organization, nor even to other patients with similar needs. As I have argued elsewhere, this does not excuse the physician from societal justice outside of the covenant with a given patient here and now (Pellegrino 1986).

Prudence

Practical wisdom, the virtue of deliberation and discernment, was central to Aristotle's virtue theory as *phronesis* and to Aquinas's as prudence. It is equally central to any theory of virtue in the health professions since any clinical decision of note requires prudent weighing of the alternatives in situations of uncertainty and stress. Knowing how to unscramble apparent conflicts among the virtues, understanding their relationships to one another, and selecting the means by which to approximate most closely the *telos* of any particular healing relationship are essential tasks for the virtue of prudence in the health professions.

At a minimum, the foregoing seven virtues are entailed by the nature of the physician- or nurse-patient encounter. They can be supplemented by other virtues, but most others will be variants of these basic seven. One might argue that even the seven virtues could be reduced to benevolence, fidelity to trust, and prudence. Such a reduction begins to touch on Meno's question to Socrates about whether the virtues are one or many. In the end, however, it is less important to answer this question than to agree on a notion of the good for humans engaged in a healing relationship and on some list of virtues that are required to achieve the good within a community of healers (the profession) who can sustain that conception of the good.

Virtue Cannot Stand Alone

The schema of virtues for the health profession that I have outlined can give normative force to professional virtues, but, by itself, it is insufficient to constitute a comprehensive normative theory of ethics. The inherent difficulties of virtue as a normative concept are not, thereby, fully resolved. We may have gained insight into the kind of person the moral agent is, or is striving to become. We may also have given the virtues—at least those pertinent to being a good professional—the philosophical foundation they require if they are to have normative form. Still needed, however, is a description of the way in which the ethics of the agent that is expressed in a virtue-based ethics relates to the ethics of the other elements of a moral event.

Granting the undeniable fact of moral agency, no matter what theory of ethics one follows, it remains to give an account of the nature of the act, the circumstances under which it takes place, and the consequences of the act. These are realities of "moral events," i.e., specific instances of moral

Figure 1   The Moral Event

	Agent	Act	Circumstance	Consequence
Theories	virtue	deontology	particularizing theories	teleology
Foci	character	right	caring for *this* person or	outcomes
	intention	good	group in this place,	harms/goods
	desire	duty	time, etc.	pain/pleasure
	choice	rule	narrative, culture,	utility calculus
	will	maxim	uniqueness of the person	
	accountability		experience	
	caring		"situation ethics"	
			casuistry	

conduct essential to moral judgment and justification. In the act, the circumstances, and the consequences lie those additional contextual complexities that the present upsurge of alternative theories of ethics seeks to encompass. Each alternative adds to our understanding of some important facet of moral judgment. Each illuminates the other theories as well. Like virtue theory, each is necessary, but not sufficient, as a normative theory. Figure 1 depicts schematically how some families of ethical theories focus on different but interrelated elements in any moral event.

Virtue theories focus on the agent and his or her character as it is expressed in, and influenced by, intention, desire, choice, strength of will, and caring (in the sense of feeling for others). Accountability, innocence, and guilt are resultants of the interplay of these factors in the character of the agent. Many of these foci are in the realm of moral psychology. As such, they can impart understanding, but they are not *per se* normative. Moral psychology helps us to understand how and why a person might be the kind of person he or she *is,* but not the kind of person he or she *ought* to be.

Deontological theories focus on the act, itself, on whether it is right and good—in keeping with some moral standard, i.e., a principle, rule, maxim, or duty, that is, itself, derived from an underlying moral philosophy. The agent is judged by whether, and to what degree, his or her moral conduct is in accord with a universalizable norm from which specific actions, rules, or guidelines are derived. The standard may be utility, beneficence, justice, or Kant's Categorical Imperative. Deontological theories have a normative force and a specificity not shared by concepts like virtue or caring. The specificity of principles is abstract, however. With deontological theories, there is always the difficulty of closing the gap between general moral rules and their application in particular moral events.

A whole family of theories are "particularizing" in the sense that they focus upon and emphasize the moral situation, the circumstances, and the historical, cultural, and personal features that make each moral event unique. These are precisely the details on the other side of the gap that must be crossed in the application of principles or virtues. Some recent examples are: ethical theories based on narrative and story, lived experience, historico-cultural or genetic predispositions, caring for particular persons, casuistry, and hermeneutics. This family of theories fills in the rich detail of a moral event not capturable by virtue-based or deontological theories. Particularizing theories, like theories of moral psychology, are most valid for explanatory and heuristic purposes, but they are not *per se* normative. All particularizing theories suffer from being too closely enmeshed in concrete details to be normative—unless one is willing to accept situation ethics, and its conceptual liabilities, as a normative theory.

Finally, acts have consequences, and those consequences have moral force. If they produce harm, or more harm than good, they may be judged using a moral calculus of varying degrees of precision. The difficulties of such a calculus notwithstanding, consequences are ineradicable elements in any comprehensive normative theory. Like the other theories, consequences are linked to the circumstances and the nature of the acts in question. They are more or less independent of intentions—unless the character-damaging effects of immoral acts on the agent are taken into account as consequences.

In any case, what is evident is that full accounts of the moral life, particularly as it regards judgments of accountability and justification, require an integrated assessment of the four elements of a moral event—i.e., the agent, the act, the circumstance, and the consequence—in relation to each other. Today's challenge is not how to demonstrate the superiority of one normative theory over the other, but rather how to relate each to the other in a matrix that does justice to each and assigns to each its proper normative force. The necessity of such an effort becomes clearer when one realizes that there are very few moralists who consistently use only one theory in their deliberations. Rather, it is a question of primacy of one theory over the others and of when one theory may be used in preference to another. If, instead of this primacy, attention is focused on the four elements of moral events, the challenge becomes one of the interrelationships between a variety of theories, each illuminating important facets of moral judgment.

I am not suggesting a feeble eclecticism, a cafeteria-style ethics, that would add a spoonful of virtue here, a principle there, and a dash of consequence in another place. Nor do I suggest a formless syncretism based in egregious compromises for the sake of a unity that enervates conflicting theories. Rather, the strength of each theory must be preserved, drawn upon, and placed in dynamic equilibrium with the others in order to accommodate the intricacy, variety, and particularity of human moral acts.

Here, as in the restoration of the normative force of virtue-based ethics, the possibility for some success is greater in the limited field of professional ethics, in which the good of the healing relationship is more easily definable than in general philosophy or in bioethics, where the nature of the good for humans is much more difficult to grasp.

Conclusion

The conceptual perambulations of moral philosophy over the centuries notwithstanding, virtue-based ethics continues to hover over ethical theory. This is because, being a human endeavor, ethics cannot conveniently ignore the moral agent. But, if virtue ethics is to have normative force, it must break out of the circular logic that defines virtue as that which the virtuous person does and the virtuous person as one who acts virtuously. To break this circle, the concept of virtue must be defined in terms of some good, some *telos,* which the agent intends and acts to attain.

In the past, the *telos* was the good for human beings as derived from a philosophy of human nature. That *telos* and its foundation gave moral force to the virtues because the virtues disposed a person to the good. In modern times, the philosophical notion of the good, and, consequently, of the virtues, has been seriously weakened. For a variety of reasons, there is little likelihood of recovering a common notion of the good, of the virtues, or of human nature. As a result, the recovery of normative force for virtue in general ethics is remote.

In professional ethics, however, the possibility is more realistic. Here, a definition of virtue, a theory of healing, and a list of virtues related to both are more clearly conceivable. But, even in this case, virtue-based ethics cannot stand by itself as a normative theory. It needs to be conceptually related to other ethical theories in a comprehensive, integrated moral philosophy of the health professions. The elaboration of such a moral philosophy is a daunting but necessary task for the philosophy and ethics of the health professions.

Notes

1. MacIntyre defines a practice as: ". . . any coherent and complex form of so-cially established cooperative human activity through which goods internal to that form of activity are realized in the course of trying to achieve those standards of excellence which are appropriate to, and partially definitive of, that form of ac-tivity, with the result that human powers to achieve excellence, and human con-ceptions of the ends and goods involved, are systematically extended" (MacIntyre 1984, p. 187).

2. Pincoffs (1986, p. 85) expands Hume's notion of agreeableness into a bewil-dering list of likeable qualities that he considers virtuous.

References

Aquinas, Thomas. 1963. *Summa Theologiae,* Vols. 1–60. New York and London: Blackfriars/McGraw-Hill Book Company.

Aristotle. 1984. *The Complete Works of Aristotle,* ed. Jonathan Barnes. Princeton, NJ: Bollinger Series.

Baynes, Kenneth; Bohman, James; and McCarthy, Thomas. 1987. Introduction. In *After Philosophy,* ed. Kenneth Baynes; James Bohman; and Thomas Mc-Carthy, pp. 1–18. Cambridge, MA: MIT Press.

Beauchamp, Tom L., and Childress, James F. 1989. *Principles of Biomedical Ethics.* 3rd ed. New York: Oxford University Press.

Becker, Lawrence C., and Becker, Charlotte B., eds. 1992. *A History of Western Eth-ics.* New York and London: Garland Publishing.

Bentham, Jeremy. 1969. *A Bentham Reader,* ed. Mary P. Mack. New York: Pegasus Books.

Carse, Alisa L. 1991. "The 'Voice of Care': Implications for Bioethical Education." *Journal of Medicine and Philosophy* 16: 5–28.

Casey, John. 1990. *Pagan Virtue.* New York: Oxford University Press.

Clouser, K. Danner, and Gert Bernard. 1990. "A Critique of Principlism." *Journal of Medicine and Philosophy* 15: 219–236.

Cua, Antonio S. 1978. *Dimensions of Moral Creativity.* University Park and Lon-don: Pennsylvania State University Press.

Foot, Philippa. 1978. *Virtues and Vices.* New York: Oxford University Press.

Frankena, William. 1982. "Beneficence in an Ethics of Virtue." In *Beneficence and Health Care,* ed. Earl Shelp, pp. 63–81. Dordrecht: D. Reidel Publishing Com-pany.

French, Peter A.; Uehling, Jr., Theodore E.; and Wettstein, Howard K., eds. 1988. *Midwest Studies in Philosophy Volume XIII: Ethical Theory Character and Vir-tue.* Notre Dame, IN: University of Notre Dame Press.

Gomez-Lobo, Alfonso. 1995. *The Foundations of Socratic Ethics*. Indianapolis: Hackett Publishing Company.

Hauerwas, Stanley. 1981. *A Community of Character*. Notre Dame, IN: University of Notre Dame Press.

Hume, David. 1975. *Enquiries Concerning Human Understanding and the Principles of Morals*. 3rd ed. Ed. L. A. Selby-Bigge. Oxford: Clarendon Press.

Jhingran, Sarah. 1989. *Aspects of Hindu Morality*. Delhi: Barnaasidass Publishers.

Kant, Immanuel. 1986. *Ethical Philosophy*, trans. James W. Ellington. Indianapolis: Hackett Publishing Company.

Kuperman, Joel. 1991. *Character*. New York: Oxford University Press.

Machiavelli, Nicholas. 1970. *The Prince*, trans. George Bull. London: The Folio Society.

MacIntyre, Alasdair. 1984. *After Virtue*. 2nd ed. Notre Dame, IN: University of Notre Dame Press.

MacIntyre, Alasdair. 1988. *Whose Justice? Which Rationality?* Notre Dame, IN: University of Notre Dame Press.

MacIntyre, Alasdair. 1990. *Three Rival Versions of Moral Enquiry*. Notre Dame, IN: University of Notre Dame Press.

Mandeville, Bernard. 1962. *The Fable of the Bees; or Private Vices, Publick Benefits*. New York: Capricorn Books.

Maritain, Jacques. 1949. *Art and Scholasticism*. New York: Charles Scribner's Sons.

Moore, George Edward. 1903. *Principia Ethica*. Massachusetts: Cambridge University Press.

Murdoch, Iris. 1992. *Metaphysics as a Guide to Morals*. New York: Penguin Press.

Nietzsche, Friedrich. 1954. *Thus Spoke Zarathustra*, trans. Alexander Tille. New York: Macmillan Publishing Co.

Nietzsche, Friedrich, 1967. *On the Genealogy of Morals and Ecce Homo*, trans. Walter Kaufmann. New York: Vintage Books.

Pellegrino, Edmund D. 1985. "The Caring Ethic: The Relationship of Physician to Patient." In *Caring, Curing, Coping: Nursing-Physician Relationships*, ed. Anne H. Bishop and John R. Scudder, Jr. Alabama: University of Alabama Press.

Pellegrino, Edmund D. 1986. "Rationing Health Care: The Ethics of Medical Gatekeeping." *The Journal of Contemporary Health Law and Policy* 2: 23–45.

Pellegrino, Edmund D. 1988. "Medical Ethics: Entering the Post-Hippocratic Era." *The Journal of the American Board of Family Practice* 1: 230–237.

Pellegrino, Edmund D. 1994. "The Four Principles and the Doctor-Patient Relationship: The Need for a Better Linkage." In *Principles of Health Care Ethics*, ed. Raanan Gillon, pp. 353-366. Chichester, England: John Wiley & Sons.

Pellegrino, Edmund D., and Thomasma, David C. 1981. *A Philosophical Basis of Medical Practice: Toward a Philosophy of the Healing Professions*. New York: Oxford University Press.

Pellegrino, Edmund D., and Thomasma, David C. 1988. *For the Patient's Good: The Restoration of Beneficence in Health Care.* New York: Oxford University Press.

Pellegrino, Edmund D., and Thomasma, David C. 1993. *The Virtues in Medical Practice.* New York: Oxford University Press.

Pieper, Josef. 1966. *The Four Cardinal Virtues.* Notre Dame, IN: University of Notre Dame Press.

Pinckaers, Servais. 1985. *Les Sources de la Moral Chrétienne.* Fribourg: Editions Universitaires.

Pincoffs, Edmund L. 1986. *Quandaries and Virtues: Against Reductivism in Ethics.* Lawrence, KS: University Press of Kansas.

Plato. 1961. *The Collected Dialogues, Including the Letters,* ed. Edith Hamilton and Huntington Cairns. Princeton, NJ: Bollinger Series.

Prior, William J. 1991. *Virtue and Knowledge: An Introduction to Ancient Greek Ethics.* London and New York: Routledge and Kegan Paul.

Rand, Ayn. 1964. *The Virtue of Selfishness.* New York: Signet Books.

Reale, Giovanni. 1985. *The Systems of the Hellenistic Age,* trans. John Catan. Albany: State University of New York Press.

Rist, John M. 1980. *Stoic Philosophy.* Cambridge, MA: Cambridge University Press.

Rockmore, Tom, and Singer, Beth J. 1992. *Antifoundationalism Old and New.* Philadelphia: Temple University Press.

Sidgwick, Henry. 1988. *Outlines of the History of Ethics.* Indianapolis: Hackett Publishing Company.

Veatch, Robert M. 1984. "The Hippocratic Ethic Is Dead." *The New Physician* (September): 41–42, 48.

Waley, Arthur. 1956. *Three Ways of Thought in Ancient China.* New York: Doubleday-Anchor.

Warnock, Geoffrey. 1971. *The Object of Morality.* London: Methuen and Company.

Wilson, Edward O. 1980. *Sociobiology.* Cambridge, MA: Belkap Press of Harvard University Press.

Wiredu, Kwasi. 1992. "The Moral Foundations of African-American Culture" and "The African Concept of Personhood." In *African-American Perspectives on Biomedical Ethics,* ed. Harland Flack and Edmund D. Pellegrino, pp. 80–93 and 104–117, respectively. Washington, DC: Georgetown University Press.

Yearley, Lee H. 1990. *Mencius and Aquinas.* Albany: State University of New York Press.

THIRTEEN

The Physician's Conscience, Conscience Clauses, and Religious Belief

A Catholic Perspective

Introduction

Conscientious persons strive to preserve moral integrity. This requires that their external behavior be congruent with their conscience's internal dictates about what they take to be morally right and feel compelled to do. In our morally diverse world, conscientious persons may come into conflict with each other and with society's moral values. Except for the amoral sociopath, conflicts of conscience are a regular feature of the moral life. Even for extreme relativists, resolving these conflicts is a constant challenge.

Any society purporting to serve the good of its members is therefore obliged to protect the exercise of conscience and conscientious objection. However, this involves a serious dilemma for any pluralist, democratic, liberal, or constitutional state. On the one hand, such a society is committed to tolerance of religious diversity, freedom of individual choice, and "neutrality" with respect to religious belief. On the other hand, optimizing freedom of conscience for some individuals may often limit the legal rights, social entitlements, and moral beliefs of others.

This dilemma is most acute for health professionals who hold strong religious beliefs, some of which cannot be compromised in good conscience. Can conscience clauses protect Catholic and other religious health professionals' moral claims to freedom of the exercise of their conscience? To what extent can these legal measures secure rights of conscience in the face of a liberal, democratic, and secular society's commitments to moral relativism, personal freedom of choice, and an implicit social contract with its professionals? Is there some point at which religious believers are morally compelled not simply to refrain from participation, but to dissent in the public arena using the processes of a democratic society to change public policy? This essay engages some of these issues in the specific case of Roman Catholic physicians whose religious beliefs are becoming progressively counter-cultural on the so-called "human life" issues.[1] Roman Catholic physicians serve as paradigm cases for all whose religious beliefs compel them to refuse to participate in certain acts, which are legal and even "required" in their societal roles.[2] Although this essay focuses on physicians, the same issues confront nurses, social workers, allied health workers, and all others who serve any function in our health care system. Similarly, although end-of-life issues will be used to illustrate particular conflicts of conscience, similar conflicts arise in other dimensions of modern health care, such as contraception, abortion, various types of assisted reproduction, sterilization, stem cell research, and cloning. This essay will discuss only the ethical dimensions of the conflicts.

Good law should be based on good ethics; in other words, the rights and claims it protects should carry moral weight and justification. Yet, in resolving conflicts of conscience in secular societies the complexity of the legal issues reflects the complexity of the ethical issues.[3] Often they are extremely difficult to dissect. This is significant because once the ethical issues are expressed in law, the debate may be reduced to instrumental and procedural details that cannot resolve underlying moral sources of controversy.

For this reason, much more debate is required before conscience and exemption clauses can be applied in ethically defensible ways. The existence of a statutory protection does not assure the exercise of freedom of conscience. This essay seeks to examine some of the ethical desiderata behind conscience clauses in the case of Roman Catholic physicians' conflicts of conscience. It does so under five headings: first, why conscientious objection is so important in our day; second, the moral grounding for freedom in the exercise of conscience; third, the components of the physician's conscience; fourth, specific conflicts of conscience for Catholic physicians and institutions; and fifth, competing models of conflict resolution.

Why Conscientious Objection Is a Problem

Convictions about the right and wrong conduct, both as a professional and as a person, form the physician's conscience. Conscientious physicians have always had to protect each domain from the demands of tyrants, law, custom, and professional colleagues. Each era has had its own challenges to the physician's conscience. In our own time, profound changes in both the physician-patient relationship and society's construction of the ends of medicine, as well as the secularization of American society, have conspired to the physician's claim to freedom of conscience.

Most powerful perhaps is the shift in the locus of decision-making from the physician to the patient or her surrogate. Beginning in 1914,[4] extending through both the Karen Ann Quinlan cases[5] and related cases in the 1970s,[6] and the accompanying trend to micromanagement, the right to refuse care has rapidly metamorphosized into a right to demand and dictate the details of care. For some, the ends and goals of medicine are no longer defined solely by physicians, but by social convention or the demands of patients or their families.[7] On this view, the physician practices by virtue of a social contract, which grants her profession the privileges of freedom to practice in return for provision of those services that society requires or demands. What constitutes the practice of medicine is societally determined. In Oregon, for example, assisting suicide is defined as a normal part of the physician practice, whereas it is forbidden in other states.[8]

These trends are exacerbated by the de-professionalization of medicine, which views health care as a commodity, and its delivery a matter of corporate enterprise, profit, and commercialization.[9] A managed care organization now monitors and controls physicians' decisions.[10] Corporate policy circumscribes the physician's judgments of conscience about the patients' welfare. Recent professional organizations are trying to recapture professional commitment, but it may not be possible given the fact that most physicians are now employees of corporate entities.[11]

In such a society, such profoundly religious issues as the morality of abortion, euthanasia, human cloning, and stem cell research are determined on grounds of utility, general consensus, or freedom of choice. In the secular philosophy, there is no other world beyond the immediate utopianism of a man-made heaven on earth. This vision determines secular society's decisions about what is permissible and what is not.

All of this is occurring against the recent historical experience of past and present totalitarian governments subverting the uses of medical knowledge to political and economic purposes. We need not recite again the way the Soviet Union distorted the Hippocratic Oath to make it serve the purposes of Communism,[12] the Nazi physicians' acquiescence in using their knowledge in the service of genocide,[13] or the participation of physicians as instruments of torture or terrorism by so many petty dictators and warlords.[14] The laws and social conventions of pathological societies justified all these violations of the ethics of medicine.

Today's societal context poses serious conflicts of conscience for all physicians, but especially for the religious physician. The teachings of the Roman Catholic Church on medical morals and human life issues go back half a millennium.[15] Its present positions on many crucial issues are distinctly and unapologetically ethically counter-cultural.[16] Many Jewish, Protestant, and Moslem physicians share some of the same beliefs and experience equivalent challenges to their moral integrity. Clearly, for all religiously oriented physicians the question must be addressed—is it possible to maintain moral integrity and remain an active physician in a secular world? Secularists ask the same question, but with different expectations about what would be a morally defensible response.

It was against the background of these changes in the climate of American medicine and its practice that conscience clauses made their appearance. In 1973, when the United States Supreme Court removed the prohibition against abortion, a medical procedure was legalized which, at that time and since, was morally repugnant to many physicians and the public.[17] In recognition of these objections, the United States Congress passed legislation that exempted physicians and others from participation.[18] Most of the states[19] and other countries[20] also enacted exemption legislation, which allowed those who objected to abortion and a variety of other procedures to refrain from participation.

Several decades later, individual states recognized a patient's legal right to execute advance directives through a living will or a durable power of attorney for health.[21] The resulting statutes were designed to guarantee a patient's right to direct the manner and extent of end-of-life care when she had lost the capacity to make her own decisions to accept or refuse treatment.

The Americans with Disabilities Act reaffirmed this right and required hospitals to inquire on admission whether patients had executed an advance directive.[22] If they had, the hospital was bound to respect its requirements.[23] Similarly, in the case of abortion, Congress recognized that some physicians would have moral objections to participation, so they were exempt provided they transferred care to another physician.[24] In both cases, abortion and advance directives, the moral claim to freedom of conscience was given legal status in "conscience clauses."

Moral Foundation for Conscientious Objection and Conscience Clauses

Freedom of conscience, however, is a moral right.[25] The first axiom of a moral life is to do good and avoid evil. This remains true whatever theory of right and wrong one may hold, whether one is a moral absolutist or relativist, a deontologist or utilitarian, or a communitarian or a social constructionist. Every moral system undertakes to determine what is right and wrong, good and evil, and desires that its worshippers act so that one may be done and the other avoided. This remains true whatever substitute term moralists may use for good and bad, and even if they deny their existence. "Values" is now the term in favor. Values are labeled "good" or "bad," morally "wrong" or "right." Values are replacing terms like principles, duties, and virtues, thereby equating the normative with the subjective.

All humans, ethicists included, possess an inner conviction of what is right and wrong and feel compelled to act in accord with that judgment. That inner conviction is the result of an act of practical reason applied to the moral status of an act performed in the past, or yet to be performed.[26] In the Catholic tradition, conscience is called "the law of our intellect" because it is a judgment of reason deduced from natural law.[27] In the Catholic tradition, and in other moral traditions as well, the judgments of conscience are morally binding, i.e., they must be followed or the moral agent has acted immorally and accountably.[28] The act of conscience may be in error about the facts, it may reason erroneously, and it may misunderstand or misapply the moral precept it is using.[29] However, when it is convinced that it has seized upon the right thing to do, conscience impels the person to act in a certain way.[30] To ignore this "inner voice" is to induce guilt, remorse, and shame. Only the amoral sociopath escapes the grip of conscience.

Errors of conscience occur when an individual misidentifies the good.[31] The person who follows a wrongful conscience may or may not be morally culpable depending upon whether her ignorance of the good is willful or culpable.[32] Roman Catholics are bound to follow the dictates of conscience, but they are also responsible for the formation of a good conscience.[33] This requires serious education and reflection on the content of official church teachings.[34] Nominal "Catholics," who firmly believe that fidelity to conscience dictates opposition to church teachings on the issues of human life and sexuality, are arguably examples of wrongly formed conscience.[35] Their "consciences" compel them to oppose official (Magisterial) teaching, which, for Catholics, is a source of authoritative guidance for conscience formation.[36]

To act against the dictate of conscience is to act against natural law— that portion of divine law accessible to human reason. But, for Catholics, conscience is also "said to be of divine insertion, in the way in which all knowledge of the truth that is in us is said to be from God, by whom the knowledge of first principles has been placed in our nature."[37] Hence, for the Catholic, to then ignore, repress, or act against conscience for any reason is a violation of philosophical as well as theological ethics, an error in moral agency and a sin against God.[38] In an analogous way, similar gravity would attach to violations of conscience in all moral systems, religious or secular. Though the idea of a "human nature" is in disfavor today, the conclusion is inescapable: there exists in all but the most morally obtuse, an operative conscience, a sense of moral compulsion to follow its dictates, and a perception of ethical disquiet in not doing so.

In every belief system, fidelity to conscience is closely identified with the preservation of personal moral integrity. To arrive at a conclusion that something must be done or avoided, and to act accordingly, is to exhibit the kind of person one is, and wants to be. That act provides evidence that the individual is the kind of person she says she is. Not acting in accordance with this conclusion is to incur the justifiable charge of hypocrisy. Often, to act against conscience is to violate personal identity so directly as to lead to severe psychosocial and emotional sequelae.

Therefore, conscience clauses are firmly rooted in what it is to be a human person morally, intellectually, and psychologically. Every individual, by virtue of being human, has a moral claim to the free exercise of conscience. The practical question for positive law in framing legal conscience clauses is how to protect this claim in morally pluralistic societies. How can conscience clauses assure the individual right to conscience while at the same time recognizing how widely the content of conscience can vary between and among individuals in their personal, social, and professional roles? Whose conscience is to prevail in the worlds of individual relations and public policy?

This is a question that confronts all individuals in every walk of life. It is of growing significance in the profession of medicine with respect to doctors' professional and personal beliefs and practices.[39] For Roman Catholics it is so crucial that Pope John Paul II has called on physicians to be conscientious objectors with respect to pro-abortion and pro-euthanasia legislation.[40]

The Physician's Conscience

Physicians, in the course of their work as healers, must form their consciences in two inseparable dimensions of their lives—the professional and the personal. Professional conscience concerns itself with two facets of the physician's daily work. First is the ethical propriety of her conduct qua physician with references to the moral duties of the physician-patient relationship. Second is the moral obligation to practice "good" contemporary medicine, i.e., medicine that is scientifically competent and humane. Personal conscience deals with the physician's own moral beliefs of a spiritual, philosophical, cultural, and ethnic nature. Both professional and personal conscience are owed protection.

Conscience in Physician-Patient Relationships

One set of obligations relates to such matters as the construct one puts on the physician-patient relationship: is it a contract, a covenant, a commodity transaction, a service relationship—or a vocation? How much respect for patient autonomy is obligatory? Do the patient's "values" override the physician's beliefs? What is a just allotment of scarce resources in a given case? How absolute is the obligation to preserve confidences? Should physicians have sexual relationships with patients? Is the patient's good primary, or is society's? Is the physician-patient relationship simply whatever is negotiable between them?

In the past, one might have assumed that a more or less general consensus existed among physicians on these issues even though there always were individual lapses in application. The Hippocratic ethic was the moral *lingua franca* of physicians across history and cultures.[41] Today, consensus on the precepts of the Hippocratic ethic has been seriously eroded. Individual physicians and their professional organizations now hold different positions on the moral status of their relationship with patients.[42] One cannot assume any longer a common formation of professional conscience, or a shared conception of ethical physician behavior. Physicians in our day may act in accord with their consciences with drastically different and even contradictory presuppositions about what is morally permissible in their relations with patients.

Conscience in the Practice of Competent Medicine

A lesser, but nonetheless significant, element in the physician's conscience is her perception of what constitutes "good" medicine. This is a subtle combination of personal and professional morality. Its focus is on medicine as a *tekné*, an art based in skills and knowledge of how to heal well.[43] While there are skeptics who would argue that we cannot define what "good" medicine is, there is the fact that we all distinguish between doctors whose judgments and skills we trust, and those we do not. There are also the inescapable differences among physicians in terms of morbidity, mortality, and diagnostic accuracy. Doctors may also differ, as a matter of conscience, in their opinions about the worth of new and old procedures, consultants they do and do not trust, the reliability of clinical data, the use of alternative or complementary medicine, and the role of other health team members. These can be matters of conscience for the physician who wants to be a "good" clinician, surgeon, healer, or counselor to serve the best interests of the patient.

We will consider later whether or not this heuristic dissection of professional and personal ethics is sustainable in actuality or in light of conscience clauses.[44] First, let us turn to a few illustrations of the way these three sectors of the physician's conscience can conflict in her relationship with patients and then with the demands of our secular democratic societies.

Conscience in Personal Moral Beliefs

In addition to her perception of professional ethics, each physician brings to her relationship with the patient a personal set of moral beliefs. She bases these moral beliefs in religious affiliation, personal preference, or moral reflection. Here we confront such crucial issues as the licitness of abortion, euthanasia, assisted suicide, in vitro fertilization, and stem cell research—the whole Pandora's box of "human life" issues, emerging from our unprecedented control of every phase of human life.

These issues center on how we value human life itself, its purposes, quality, destiny, and utility. Conflicts of belief in this realm are more profound and deeply felt in one's conscience than other issues of professional behavior with patients. For religious individuals of many persuasions, these issues bear directly on their personal spiritual destinies and are, therefore, least subject to compromise.

In the last fifty years, secularism has come to dominate much of medical ethics, despite the fact that most Americans personally hold religious beliefs.[45] Secularism is a response to the plurality of moral and religious beliefs in our polyglot society in which there is wide disagreement on what a good conscience should dictate. Since no one moral system or religious set of beliefs is universally accepted, society reasons that none can or should be dominant. All should be free to express themselves, and each should respect the other. So goes the credo of political liberalism. On this view, decisions that must be made as a matter of public policy in areas such as abortion, euthanasia, and stem cell research should be made democratically, universally, and equally binding. Conscience or exemption clauses presumably are devised to protect the freedom of the dissenter. Without dissecting its merits or demerits, this liberal democratic policy has functioned to avoid civil strife. However, the recent erosion of the number of beliefs held in common, and the increasingly varied demography of our nation, has magnified the complexity and depth of our differences about what is morally right and wrong. The secular solution of moral or value neutrality has generated genuine conflicts of conscience.

Religious exemption laws and conscience clauses have appeared as a device to protect the physician's conscience. Their inadequacy, however, is becoming manifest. Lawmakers have currently drafted some of those clauses so narrowly that they disqualify most religious institutions from exemption, especially if they are involved in providing assistance and social services irrespective of the religious persuasions of those they help.[46] On these grounds, Catholic institutions are simply not religious enough unless they help the sick and needy for distinctly religious purposes. If they are to be classified as "religious," Catholic institutions must serve only Catholics.[47] On the other hand, if they do so, they are disqualified since they would then discriminate against, and take advantage of, the vulnerable, sick, and poor.

Moreover, secular morality, which supposedly tolerates differences, does so only within a narrow range of so-called "values" that are supposedly "free" of moral or religious taint. But secular morality is itself an orthodoxy. Its "values" are based in democratic procedures, personal preference as the basis for moral choice, commitment to a free market economy, the commodification of health care, and an eschewal of religious belief.[48] To deviate from this notion of moral "neutrality" in public policy is to be "undemocratic," prejudiced, and intolerably sectarian.

This is not the place to challenge these dicta of secularism as a ruling orthodoxy, but to spell out in more detail their implications for Catholic Christian physicians' freedom of conscience. Again, the Catholic physician is the focus, but the same conflicts would apply to any other religious or moral system with a clear and unequivocal set of precepts giving substance to the conscience of its followers. The conflicts can be divided into three groups: first, between patients and physicians,[49] second, between physicians and society,[50] and third, between Catholic institutions and society.[51]

Conflicts of Conscience for Catholic Physicians

Conflicts between Patients and Physicians

Physicians and patients may differ sharply in what their consciences tell them about the moral licitness of assisted suicide, euthanasia, the dignity and worth of human life, the relative importance of quality of life, age, or economics as criteria for withholding or withdrawing life-sustaining treatments, terminal sedation, or whether death of the whole brain and partial brain death are both equivalent to the death of the patient. The same is true of cloning, stem cell research, and fetal tissues transplantation.

Some would argue that the principle of patient autonomy should prevail in such conflicts, and that the physician, irrespective of her own beliefs, should provide whatever secular social convention legally allows.[52] On this view, medicine is bound by a social contract to provide the services patients or society deem worthwhile. This obligation is in return for society permitting them to set its own standards of education and practice. In addition, they would claim that it is a failure of the principle of beneficence not to do what the patient believes to be in her best interests. Still, others might reduce the argument to one of commutative justice, holding that the patient is entitled to the same care available to other patients whose doctors do not suffer from the Catholic doctor's scruples against abortion, euthanasia, or other human life issues.

At present, Catholic physicians may withdraw from the care of patients in these circumstances. However, one wonders how long this exemption will survive, as end-of-life and reproductive decisions become so much an individual prerogative that the ethical standard is no longer a determination of what is morally right, but rather of what can be negotiated to resolve conflicts.[53] One can foresee the day when patients may gain legal rights to demand a full range of death "services" from every licensed physician just as many today feel entitled to a full range of reproductive "services."

Already we hear ethicists suggesting that physicians must separate their personal moral beliefs from their professional lives if they wish to practice in a secular society and remain licensed as fully functioning physicians.[54] If universal health care were to be instituted and "death care" as well as birth and reproductive care were to be entitlements, would Catholic physicians be given only limited practice licenses?

This same question could logically be raised, for example, with respect to stem cell therapy. Using stem cells derived from the killing of human embryos is morally offensive to Catholic physicians. If the therapeutic potentials of stem cell research, genetic engineering, and cloning are actualized, could a conscience clause protect Catholic physicians in secular hospitals or in managed care organizations? Would they not be legally required to provide a full range of services despite moral objection? In an HMO would the commercial gains of services patients demand trump a conscience clause? Would religious physicians be hired in the first place?

Conflicts with Societal Mores

It has already been seriously suggested that Catholic physicians should not become maternal child specialists, since they cannot, in good conscience, provide the whole range of reproductive, pregnancy, and neonatal "services," such as selective abortion for genetic defects or late-term abortion.[55] The logical next step of such proposals is to withhold specialty certification for maternal medicine from Catholic physicians and others who oppose provision of any such services, which are legal. Should anyone who wishes to be a physician be permitted to narrow the range of services to her patients on the basis of moral and religious reservations? A medical education is a socially sanctioned process in which students learn by doing.[56] Some would argue that the physician's social contract requires her to provide what she has learned in accord with whatever society needs because society granted the privileges of a medical education in the first place.

These are not imaginary scenarios. Catholic and other religiously committed applicants to medical school have been asked about their views on the issues of abortion, euthanasia, ending life support, various reproductive technologies, and stem cell research.[57] Evidence that responses consistent with Catholic teaching have militated against admission is hard to come by for obvious legal reasons. Therefore, we do not know how heavily medical schools weigh the "Catholic" responses against a candidate. The fact that they asked the questions in the first place is sufficient cause for worry given the dominance of the secular viewpoint in academic circles today.

Based on personal experience on admissions committees, there is more than a mere suspicion that "conservative" Catholics, Orthodox Jews, and fundamentalist Christians may be looked upon with disfavor. Much depends on the lottery of interviewers one encounters by chance. Those who hold certain religious beliefs, it is argued, cannot provide all the services patients have a right to expect. Whether we shall ever come to the point at which religious believers who insist on following their consciences will be barred from certain specialties or from medicine itself is, therefore, a source of more than imaginary concern.

Conflicts between Catholic Institutions and Society

Organizational ethics is the newest addition to the broadening spectrum of ethical issues being subsumed under the term "bioethics."[58] While it may include business ethics, it covers much more, and already embraces such varied aspects of institutional behavior as relationships with employees, advertising, community commitments, quality of care for the poor and uninsured, and mergers with other institutions.

Organizational ethics is a systematic examination of the morality of collective actions in human institutions dedicated to some specific purposes in society.[59] The ethical "code" or commitment of a specific institution is now customarily expressed in its mission statement. This is in a way the "conscience" of the institution.[60] All who work in that institution are in some way accountable for adherence to the organizational mission, which is in effect a promise by the institution to behave in a particular way. Catholic institutions in America have for a long time had specific ethical directives that define them as Catholic hospitals.[61] They are also committed to a charitable, even preferential treatment for the sick and the poor.[62] Catholic hospitals can properly be considered to have a definable institutional "conscience," one, which given the content of the Catholic moral tradition, could and does come into conflict with secular society and its "values."[63]

The ethical content of the institutional conscience of particular hospitals is well known with respect to sterilization, abortion, euthanasia, assisted suicide, contraception, and cooperation through mergers with other institutions that accept these practices.[64] Fidelity to these prohibitions is not negotiable.[65] It applies to all who practice in these hospitals, regardless of their personal beliefs. Catholic hospitals, like Catholic physicians, do not have the option of being "value neutral" or of separating religious from professional ethical precepts.

There is growing evidence that public funding for Catholic health care and social service institutions may be in jeopardy if these institutions do not provide the "full range" of reproductive services. For example, the District of Columbia City Council recently passed a bill mandating that all employers in the city had to provide coverage for contraceptives in their prescription coverage plans.[66] The move to include a conscience clause to exempt Catholic institutions was rejected vitriolically by one member of the Council.[67] Fortunately, the mayor, a Catholic himself, gave the bill a pocket veto.[68]

This sort of challenge to institutional conscience is certain to return in one way or another. Some who oppose Catholic moral teaching vehemently and frankly admit to wanting to eliminate the Catholic health care system and at the least deny access to public funds.[69] The more moderate alternative is to interpret exemption clauses so narrowly that Catholic institutions cannot be classified as "religious" institutions since they treat all regardless of belief and provide much more than religious services.[70]

The challenge to institutional conscience promises to grow in severity as new, morally questionable therapeutic procedures emerge from the laboratories and research centers. There is a genuine probability that stem cell research of the kind that depends on the death of embryos, human cloning for therapeutic purposes, or cross species genetic manipulation will eventually be allowed.[71] Should these measures become clinically effective, the public demand for their availability will increase the pressure for conformity by all hospitals regardless of religious affiliation.

Even if Catholic hospitals are allowed the protection of exemption clauses there is still the more subtle threat to the conscience, stemming from cooperation with secular institutions through mergers. These mergers may be dictated by the need for economic survival, but such survival cannot be bought at the cost of even material cooperation of a direct kind with institutions that violate the established ethical directives for Catholic health care institutions. Already there is concern that mergers already in existence may involve Catholic hospitals too closely with activities that are morally objectionable.[72] Can these Faustian bargains survive closer moral scrutiny?

Catholic moral tradition contains a carefully nuanced set of conditions under which cooperation with those individuals or institutions that do not share Catholic moral beliefs may be licit.[73] Considerable controversy has already arisen as to whether the interpretation of these conditions in some mergers has been too lax. This is the case even where the non-Catholic partner promises to abide by the ethical directives of the Catholic bishops.[74] Commingling of funds, administrative entanglements, and other interminglings characteristic of today's complex institutional relationships raise serious questions of illicit cooperation in seemingly "safe" mergers.[75] Exemption and conscience clauses in these mergers or in the relationships with public policy may not be sufficient to permit financial viability for Catholic health care systems. Much depends on how well Catholic institutions can maintain their moral integrity and institutional conscience. Catholic health care institutions constitute a very significant sector of service for Americans, Catholic and non-Catholic.[76] If these institutions do not survive financially, the loss to the general public will be great. If they survive only by a loss of their institutional Catholic conscience, something even more fundamental will be lost, not just for Catholics, but for that sector of the American public who, for their own moral integrity, cannot accept the dictates of a secular order.

Conflicting Models of Conflict Resolution

How, in a morally pluralist society, can the moral claim to freedom of conscience owed to every person as a human being be sustained? Specifically, how can the Catholic physician or institution sustain freedom of conscience in a secular world whose culture is a-religious, if not anti-religious? What role might conscience clauses play? Several ways out of the dilemma have been suggested, none of them entirely satisfactory. They include: dissociation of the moral and professional life, abandonment of medicine as a profession, or maintaining moral integrity with judicious dissent.

It would be in keeping with secular orthodoxy to allow Catholic physicians and hospitals freedom of conscience, but to limit its overt exercise. Catholic physicians could have the right not to participate in medicine as a profession as long as they would do what is allowable by law (for example, euthanasia in Oregon, abortion everywhere, sterilization, etc.). The only thing Catholics would need to do is to provide whatever services are defined by social convention as legal medical practice. On this view, all physicians, Catholic and others, whose moral beliefs are at odds with a secular society simply need to take a "value free" stance. In this way, the autonomy of the patient is preserved and the doctor does not "impose" her beliefs.[77] This is the strong version of value neutrality as the litmus test for medical licensure or certification.

In a weaker version, Catholic physicians could be granted the right to participate in medicine as a profession as long as they would agree to what is allowable by law or defined as part of medical practice by the rest of the profession. Catholics, for example, could object to euthanasia in Oregon, sterilization, abortion, reproductive technologies, and stem cell research. They could refuse personally to participate. But in practice they would have to be "value neutral" if they entered specialties that required acts to which they had moral objection.

At the very least, they would have to commit themselves to arrange for referral to a physician they know would do what the patient wished and assist the patient in every way to achieve her purposes. On a stronger version of this form of accommodation, Catholic physicians would be compelled to make a clear choice, either fulfill the conditions of the social contract and provide what is legal or socially acceptable or drop out of any specialty which required services of which they took moral exception.

In its strongest form this model would logically exclude from medical practice, and eventually the study of medicine, all who did not see their social roles as conforming to all the services society felt necessary and required of physicians. Needless to say, such a compromise as accommodation requires even in its mildest form would be morally objectionable for several reasons.

It assumes that the Catholic physician and others who hold firm moral beliefs can separate their professional and personal lives when this means cooperation with what is morally objectionable. For a physician with deep religious commitments, a "value free" stance on certain issues is simply unthinkable.[78] Certain matters are so clearly prohibited as inherently wrong that there is no possibility of compromise without compromise of moral integrity and danger to one's spiritual well-being.

For Catholics, Orthodox Jews, and Moslems, the teachings of the Gospel, Torah, or Koran take precedence in their lives and indeed inspire their healing vocations. For these major religions, healing the sick is ultimately a religious act and it comes ultimately from God.[79] To practice medicine that contravenes religious teaching would be to subvert conscience to secular society and its "values," to act hypocritically, and to violate moral integrity intolerably.

For Catholics the secular demand that those who must refrain from certain practices must refer patients to physicians who will provide the disputed treatment or procedure would also be intolerable. To cooperate in an act which is regarded as inherently morally wrong, such as arranging for an abortion or assisted suicide, is to be a moral accomplice.[80] Respectfully, courteously, but definitively the religious physician must inform the patient of her objection while promising to care for the patient until transfer or referral can be arranged by the patient, family, or social services.

Obviously the patient cannot be abandoned, legally or morally, and must be cared for until a transfer has been effected. The doctrine of cooperation does not forbid transferring information, findings, or records to another physician or hospital.[81] Indeed, this is required in the interests of patient care. What is illicit is active cooperation in finding a physician who will provide the morally objectionable service.

The requirement of a secular society that physicians practice "value neutrality" is impossible to achieve. First, it is a psychological schism that violates the integrity of the person as a unity of body, soul, and psyche. What it amounts to is the elevation of secularism to the level of a social orthodoxy, thereby violating one of the major tenets of secularism itself—

that no ideology would have preference over any other.[82] It also violates a prized precept of the secular, democratic, constitutional social order by discriminating against a significant segment of the population, and the physicians who share certain religious beliefs.

The difficulty of a meaningful compromise between the secular orthodoxy and religious belief is illustrated in those pragmatic attempts to find a way to respect moral integrity and the right of conscientious objection. For example, Wicclair would allow for conscientious objection as long as it corresponded to "one or more core values of medicine."[83] He would use congruence with these core values as the moral test for an acceptable claim to conscientious objection.[84]

Wicclair offers a guide for assigning moral weight within recognized medical norms. For example, he gives more weight to preventing death than protecting confidentiality.[85] He takes his cue here from the integrity of the profession, rather than the integrity of the physician as a moral person.[86] In one of his examples, he clearly states that more moral weight should be given to a physician's request to preserve moral integrity as a physician than to her "moral integrity as an Orthodox Jew who happens to be a physician."[87]

In his guidelines, Wicclair clearly makes religious belief subservient to professional medical belief about what is right and wrong.[88] Its effect is to require the kind of value and belief dichotomy which is incompatible with moral integrity for a true religious person. The moral values of religious persons transcend the "values" of the profession—especially now that those values have changed so drastically. Where there might have been concurrence in the past between medically held and religiously held beliefs, that congruence has been seriously eroded today.

Indeed, consensus on the moral values of medicine is being progressively reduced to competence, refraining from harm, and the protection of confidentiality. The recent set of commitments advanced by the American Board of Internal Medicine, the American Society for Internal Medicine, and the European Federation attempts to recover the idea of professionalization.[89] However, it omits the prohibitions against abortion and euthanasia, the precepts that are most significant for many religious physicians and especially for Roman Catholics. The "moral integrity" of the profession is thus judged to be morally insufficient to justify overriding the physician's conscience.

The moral authority of professional codes does not derive from their acceptance by the profession or social convention.[90] Rather, the ethics of medicine is grounded in something more fundamental, namely the ethical obligation peculiar to what it means to be ill, to be healed, and to offer oneself as a healer.[91]

Respecting a physician's conscience claims, however, does not mean that the physician is empowered to override the patient's morally valid claim to self-determination. Both the physician and the patient as human beings are entitled to respect for their personal autonomy. Neither one is empowered to override the other. The protection of freedom of conscience is owed to both.

Therefore, patients have an uncontested moral right to informed consent and informed refusal.[92] Wicclair and May spend considerable time defending the patient's moral right to refuse treatment, prolong their life, request palliative care, or "reproductive freedom." This is not the issue here. Conscientious objection implies the physician's right not to participate in what she thinks morally wrong, even if the patient demands it. It does not presume the right to impose her will or conception of the good on the patient.

Therefore, May is correct in stating that "rights of conscience in health care must be exercised in the context of patients' rights to informed consent."[93] This does not at all imply that we should or must acknowledge limits on the physician's rights of conscience.[94] May agrees that patients do not have a right to demand "anything" they take to be beneficial.[95] Clearly the patient's moral and legal right to self-determination has limits, even in May's view.[96]

Both May and Wicclair, but especially May, spend much time on examples of conflict in choice of treatment and somewhat miss the point of religious objections, which is not whether a religious believer may impose her beliefs on a patient, but rather whether she has the moral right to refuse to be an accomplice in an act her religion teaches is wrong.[97]

The only ethically viable course for the religious physician is to maintain fidelity to moral integrity and the dictates of conscience while practicing in a secular world. Catholic physicians and institutions have the same moral claim to exercise of conscience as all other humans, even when the fruit of conscience is refusal and even resistance to accommodation of secular beliefs or the changing beliefs of their professional colleagues. This moral claim entails the right and obligation to use the methods available in a democratic society to protest morally objectionable practices by persuasion, judicious political action, and public debate, particularly in the most egregious situations.

For such a position to be tenable, Catholic physicians must make their positions publicly known, as in the case with the Directives for Catholic Health Care Institutions. Individual physicians should prepare a leaflet outlining what they can, and cannot, in good conscience do.[98] Patients should know in advance of a crisis that what they desire and believe to be morally acceptable may not be acceptable to the physicians they may be engaging.

Such advance knowledge will not be possible in emergencies or remote areas where the choice of physicians is limited. Even under these circumstances, the Catholic physician cannot violate her conscience to provide a morally objectionable procedure or treatment. Physicians must know their own belief system well enough to recognize where compromise is possible without loss of moral integrity and where it is not. Parenthetically, the Catholic physician is under serious obligation to know the content of her own faith, so that she does not impose hardship on the patient when alternative routes are morally permissible. Sadly, this is not always the case.

The dissenting physician must always treat her patient with respect, avoid moralizing condemnations, and explain the reasons for her moral objections. She must also be aware that every matter of conscience is not of equal gravity. Choosing when to take a morally dissenting stand is crucial if one's exercise of conscience is to be valid and respected.

The same prescriptions and proscriptions are applicable to the institutional conscience of Catholic health care institutions. They cannot compromise on fundamental Catholic moral teachings even if resistance might lead to their extinction. Total extinction is not likely; however, the withdrawal of public funds will probably restrict the number of persons in the community, Catholic or non-Catholic, that can be served by institutions faithful to their religious commitments. Although morally illicit, Catholic hospitals may also "cooperate" more fully with the secular mores.

Conscience clauses for physicians probably have a limited value, although they ought to be sought whenever possible. The likelihood, given the current societal mores, is that conscience clauses will be denied or progressively applied so narrowly as to be self-defeating. At the least they provide legal limits that in a democratic society should protect dissenting physicians and institutions from the grosser forms of ostracism.

Catholic institutions will probably find greater difficulty obtaining exemption clauses, especially if they accept public funds or purport to serve community needs. Survival may require formation of a Catholic health care system nationally. Mergers with non-Catholic institutions, except those that share Catholic perspectives on the human life issues, will raise an increasing number of questions about cooperation. Given the size, geographic extent, and resources, a Catholic health care system faithful to magisterial teachings is not an impossibility. Much would be lost were a secular society's dissonances to require the dissolution or "ghettoization" of Catholic health care.

All the societal and political forces of our day are converging on an actualization of the secular state. As medical technology endows humans with ever greater power over the reproduction, genetic endowment, and dying of our species, crises of conscience will surely increase for those who hold religious beliefs about human life, its creation, and ending. In democratic societies, there is a commitment to protection of the right to hold and exercise individual and institutional conscience.

Conscience clauses are straws in the wind telling all of us that public policy and individual conscience on some of the most important matters of human life may be on a collision course. How individual physicians and institutions preserve their moral integrity in such a socio-political milieu is a matter of significance for both secularists and believers.

Conscience clauses will help at least to establish a right to dissent. However, the conditions under which they will be applicable and their effectiveness are very much at issue. It will be a stringent test both of democracy and religious beliefs to see how these conflicts will be resolved.

Notes

1. U.S. Catholic Conference, Congregation for the Doctrine of the Faith, *Instruction on Respect for Human Life in Its Origin and on the Dignity of Procreation, Donum Vitae* (1987) [hereinafter *Donum Vitae*]; John Paul II, *Evangelium Vitae,* Encyclical Letter *Origins* 24 (1995): 690, 691–700 [hereinafter *Evangelium Vitae*].

2. *Donum Vitae, supra* note 1, at 14–20, 35–39.

3. Mark R. Wicclair, "Conscientious Objection in Medicine," *Bioethics* 14 (2000): 205, 210.

4. See *Schloendorf v. Soc'y of N.Y. Hosp.*, 105 N.E. 92, 93–94 (N.Y. 1914) (stating that a patient has the right to refuse treatment when doctors operate on a patient that explicitly stated that they did not want the operation).

5. See In re *Quinlan*, 355 A.2d 647, 671 (N.J. 1976) (installing father as guardian of comatose daughter "with full power to make decisions with regard to the identity of her treating physicians").

6. See, e.g., *Rizzo v. United States,* 432 F. Supp. 356, 360 (E.D.N.Y. 1977) (granting patient a preliminary injunction preventing the Food and Drug Administration from prohibiting the importation of a drug not approved for his personal use).

7. Edmund D. Pellegrino, "The Goals of Medicine: How Are They to Be Defined?" In *The Goals of Medicine* 55, 58–60 (Daniel Callahan & Mark J. Hanson, eds., 1999).

8. Compare *Or. Rev. Stat.* § 127.630, 127.635, 127.640 (1996), with *Ark. Code Ann.* § 5-10-106 (2001); Cal. Penal Code § 401 (1999).

9. Edmund D. Pellegrino, "The Commodification of Medical and Health Care: The Moral Consequences of a Paradigm Shift from a Professional to a Market Ethic," *Journal of Medicine and Philosophy* 24 (1999): 243, 244–251.

10. *Id.* at 253.

11. "Medical Professionalism in the New Millennium: A Physician Charter (Project of the ABIM Foundation, ACP-ASIM Foundation and European Federation of Internal Medicine)," *Annals Internal Med.* 136 (2002): 243, 244–246, available at http://www.annals.org/issues/v136n3/toc.html (last visited Oct. 21, 2002).

12. Edmund D. Pellegrino, "Guarding the Integrity of Medical Ethics: Some Lessons from Soviet Russia," *J. Am. Med. Ass'n.* 273 (1995): 1622, 1622–1623.

13. Henry Friedlander, *The Origins of Nazi Genocide: From Euthanasia to the Final Solution,* 216–245 (1995).

14. See generally Maxwell G. Bloche, *Uruguay's Military Physicians: Cogs in a System of State Terror* (1987).

15. David F. Kelly, *The Emergence of Roman Catholic Medical Ethics in North America* 25 (1979).

16. *Donum Vitae, supra* note 1, at 12–13, 16–20, 23–25, 32–38; *Evangelium Vitae, supra* note 1, at 691 700, 709–16; Pope Paul VI, Encyclical Letter of Pope Paul VI, Humanae Vitae: To Our Dearest Sons and Brothers, Health and Apostolic Blessing, in *Humanae Vitae and the Bishops: The Encyclical and the Statements of the National Hierarchies* 33, 37–44 (John Horgan ed., 1972).

17. See generally *Roe v. Wade,* 410 U.S. 113, 152–153 (1973) (holding that abortion is a fundamental right guaranteed by the due process clause of the Fourteenth Amendment). 18. 42 U.S.C. § 300a-7(b) (1999).

19. Wicclair, *supra* note 3, at 207 (citing L. D. Wardle, "Protecting the Rights of Health Care Providers," *J. Legal Med.* 14 [1993]: 177, 177–230).

20. M. L. DiPietro, "Evoluzione Storica dell'istituto, dell'obiezione di coscienza," *Italia Medicina e Morale* 6 (2001): 1093, 1093–1151.

21. E.g., *Ark. Code Ann.* § 5-10-106(d) (Michie 1987); *La. Rev. Stat. Ann.* § 40:2233 (West 2001); *Okla. Stat. Ann.* tit. 63, § 3101.4 (West 1997).

22. 42 U.S.C. § 1395cc(f); 28 C.F.R. § 35.130(e)(2) (2001); see also *Cruzan v. Mo. Dep't of Health,* 497 U.S. 261, 269–270 (1990) (inferring the necessity of inquiry into a patient's desire to refuse treatment as the natural corollary of the duty to obtain consent).

23. 42 U.S.C. § 1395cc(f)(1)(D); see generally *Cruzan,* 497 U.S. at 269–270 (discussing the right of a competent adult to leave express instructions declining consent to life-sustaining medical treatment).

24. 42 U.S.C. § 238n.

25. Rev. Donald W. Wuerl, "The Bishop, Conscience and Moral Teaching," in *Catholic Conscience Foundation and Formation* 123, 127–128 (Russell E. Smith ed., 1991).

26. Thomas Aquinas, "On Conscience. Disputed Question on Truth, 17." In *Thomas Aquinas Selected Writings* 217, 221–223 (Ralph McInerny ed. & trans., 1998) [hereinafter Aquinas, "On Conscience"].

27. *Id.* at 224–226; Thomas Aquinas, *The Summa Theologica of St. Thomas Aquinas* I, question 79, at art. 13 (Fathers of the English Dominican Province trans., 1920), available at http://www.newadvent.org/summa (last visited Sept. 29, 2002).

28. Aquinas, "On Conscience," *supra* note 26, at 228–233 (stating "that conscience binds means that when one does not follow it he incurs sin").

29. *Id.* at 226–228. Aquinas claims that conscience is a science that never errs, but rather, any errors occur from the application of this science to "some special act." *Id.* at 226.

30. Wuerl, *supra* note 25, at 127–128.

31. Aquinas, "On Conscience," *supra* note 26, at 226–227.

32. See *id.* at 234–236 (claiming that not following an erroneous conscience would constitute a sin, but that actively pursuing this erroneous conscience is also a sin).

33. Rev. Benedict Ashley, "Elements of a Catholic Conscience," in *Catholic Conscience Foundation and Formation, supra* note 25, at 39, 48–52.

34. *Id.* at 50–52.

35. Frances Kissling, "The Place for Individual Conscience," *J. Med. Ethics* 27 (2001) ii24, ii25–27.

36. Ashley, supra note 33, at 50–52.

37. Aquinas, "On Conscience," *supra* note 26, at 225.

38. *Id.* at 228–233; see also Wuerl, *supra* note 25, at 127–128.

39. Thomas Faunce, "Peri-Gravid Genetic Screening: The Spectre of Eugenics and Medical Conscientious Non-Compliance," *J.L. & Med.* 6 (1999): 147, 152–155, 161–166; Thomas May, "Rights of Conscience in Health Care," *Soc. Theory*

& *Prac.* 27 (2001): 111, 111–121; Richard S. Myers, "On Laws: On the Need for a Federal Conscience Clause," *Nat'l Cath. Bioethics Q.* 1 (2001): 23, 23–25; Carl A. Osborne, "How Can We Practice Veterinary Medicine Conscientiously?" *J. Am. Veterinary Med. Ass'n.* 215 (1999): 1238, 1238–1239; Jing-Bao Nie, "Chinese 'Conscientious Acceptance' of the Birth Control Policy," *Med. Human. Rev.* 13 (1999): 82, 82–85 (reviewing Cecilia Nathansen Milwertz, *Accepting Population Control: Urban Chinese Women and the One-Child Family Policy* [1997]).

40. John Paul II, "Doctors Protest Conscience Discrimination, The Holy Father's Address to the International Congress of Catholic Obstetricians and Gynecologists," *Dolentium Hominum* 48 (2001): 65, 65–66; John Paul II, "The Medical Doctor Should Respond as a Conscientious Objector to Legislation in Favor of the Crimes of Abortion and Euthanasia," *Dolentium Hominum* 15 (2000): 133, 133–135.

41. See generally Edmund D. Pellegrino, "Bioethics at Century's Turn: Can Normative Ethics Be Retrieved?" *Journal of Medicine and Philosophy* 25 (2000): 655, 655 (discussing the growth of bioethics from traditional medical ethics) [hereinafter Pellegrino, "Bioethics at Century's Turn"].

42. See, e.g., *Mich. v. Kevorkian*, 639 N.W.2d 291, 311–312 (Mich. Ct. App. 2001) (demonstrating the spectrum of physicians' interpretations of the Hippocratic Oath's medical ethics according to their conscience).

43. *Tekné* is an ancient Greek term that characterizes actions and professions as an art or craft rather than just a normal action. *Oxford Concise English Dictionary* 1471 (10th ed. 1999) (origin of the word techno-).

44. See *infra* "Conflicting Models of Conflict Resolution."

45. See Frank Shakespeare, "A View from Administration and Government," in *Catholic Conscience Foundation and Formation, supra* note 25, at 259–264 (discussing the evolution of our society into a secular state).

46. Myers, *supra* note 39, at 23–26; Msgr. Dennis Schnurr. "Mandating Employer Coverage of Contraceptives: Protecting Conscientious Objection," *Origins* 30 (2000): 161, 163–164.

47. *Cath. Charities of Sacramento, Inc. v. Super. Ct.*, 109 Cal. Rptr. 2d 176, 183 (Cal. Ct. App. 2001), petition for review granted, 31 Cal. Rptr. 2d. 258 (Cal. 2001); "Religious Refusals and Reproductive Rights," *Reprod. Rts. Update*, 2002, at 8, available at http://www.aclu.org/issues/reproduct/refusal_report.pdf (last visited Sept. 24, 2002).

48. Pellegrino, "Bioethics at Century's Turn," *supra* note 41, at 655, 663–664.

49. See *infra* "Conscience in Physician-Patient Relationships."

50. See *infra* "Conscience in the Practice of Competent Medicine."

51. See *infra* "Conscience in Personal Moral Beliefs."

52. Cf. May, *supra* note 39, at 111–112 (suggesting that there are certain situations in which a health care professional could acknowledge her moral concerns with particular treatment choices).

53. Pellegrino, "Bioethics at Century's Turn," *supra* note 41, at 656–657.

54. See Jeffrey Blustein & Alan R. Fleishman, "The Pro-Life Maternal-Fetal Medicine Physician: A Problem of Integrity," *Hastings Center Rep.* (Jan.–Feb. 1995): 22–26 (discussing the dilemma faced by physicians who must perform abortions and maintain their own integrity); Franklin G. Miller & Howard Brody. "Professional Integrity and Physician-Assisted Death," *Hastings Center Rep.* (May–June 1995): 8–17 (analyzing the relationship between professional integrity and physician-assisted suicide).

55. See Blustein & Fleishman, *supra* note 54, at 25.

56. Edmund D. Pellegrino, "Philosophy and Ethics of Medical Education." In *The Encyclopedia of Bioethics,* vol. 2, pp. 860, 863–869 (Warren T. Reich ed., 2nd ed. 1978).

57. *Id.*

58. Susan Dorr Goold, "Trust and the Ethics of Health Care Institutions," *Hastings Center Rep.* (Nov.–Dec. 2001): 26, 27–28.

59. *Id.* at 32.

60. *Id.* at 28.

61. U.S. Conference of Catholic Bishops, *Ethical and Religious Directives for Catholic Health Care Services* 9–11, 13–16, 18–22, 25–28, 30–33, 36–37 (4th ed. 2001), available at http://www.usccb.org/bishops/directives.shtml (last visited Oct. 2, 2002).

62. *Id.* at 8–11.

63. *Id.* at 12–16, 23–33.

64. *Id.* at 8–16, 23–37.

65. *Id.*

66. Schnurr, *supra* note 46, at 161–163.

67. Myers, *supra* note 39, at 23–26; Schnurr, *supra* note 46, at 164.

68. Schnurr, *supra* note 46, at 161–163.

69. Myers, *supra* note 39, at 23–26.

70. *Id.*

71. *Id.*

72. U.S. Conference of Catholic Bishops, *supra* note 61, at 34–37.

73. See generally Orville N. Griese, *Catholic Identity in Health Care: Principles and Practice* 373–416 (1987).

74. U.S. Conference of Catholic Bishops, *supra* note 61, at 34–37.

75. *Id.*

76. See *id.* at 34–36 (discussing how Catholic health care institutions are forging partnerships and ventures with many other health care providers).

77. Blustein & Fleishman, *supra* note 54, at 22–26; Miller & Brody, *supra* note 54, at 8–17; Edmund D. Pellegrino, "Commentary: Value Neutrality, Moral Integrity, and the Physician," *J.L. Med. & Ethics* 28 (2000): 78, 78–80 [hereinafter Pellegrino, "Commentary"].

78. Pellegrino, "Commentary," *supra* note 77, at 78–80.

79. Ecclesiasticus (Sirach) 38 (Jerusalem Bible).

80. Griese, *supra* note 73, at 386–390.

81. *Id.*

82. See also May, *supra* note 39, at 111 (discussing the conflict that arises when a physician's values and conscience conflict with a patient's values and autonomy rights, and noting that society increasingly and unfairly pressures physicians to disregard their personal consciences in their professional roles).

83. Wicclair, *supra* note 3, at 217.

84. *Id.*

85. *Id.* at 223.

86. *Id.* at 224.

87. *Id.* at 225.

88. *Id.*

89. "Medical Professionalism in the New Millennium: A Physician Charter," *Annals Internal Med.* 136 (2002): 243, 243–244.

90. Edmund D. Pellegrino, "Professional Codes," in *Methods in Medical Ethics* 70, 74–76 (Jeremy Sugarman & Daniel Sulmasy eds., 2001).

91. *Id.* at 78–79.

92. Wicclair, *supra* note 3, at 208.

93. May, *supra* note 39, at 127.

94. Edmund D. Pellegrino, "Bioethics as an Interdisciplinary Enterprise: Where Does Ethics Fit in the Mosaic of Disciplines?" In *Philosophy of Medicine and Bioethics: A Twenty-Year Retrospective & Critical Appraisal* 1–23 (Ronald A. Carson & Chester R. Burns, eds., 1997).

95. May, *supra* note 39, at 127.

96. *Id.*

97. *Id.*; Wicclair, *supra* note 3, at 205–211.

98. See *supra* notes 61–65 and accompanying text.

I V

HUMANISM AND HIPPOCRATES
FACING THE FUTURE

Humanities in Medicine

FOURTEEN

The Most Humane of the Sciences, the Most Scientific of the Humanities

There are no subjects in which, as a rule, practice is not

more valuable than precept.

—Quintilianus, *Institutio Oratoria* II, v, 15

Reasons of exquisite urgency impel the examination of an ancient and much labored subject: the humane education of the physician.

The physician of today works in the wake of a metaphysical rebellion, which on the one hand exalts man and on the other overshadows him in technology and mass organization. Things and services designed for the presumed benefit of man too often end up dehumanizing him. Man's most daring creations promise to annihilate him as a person unless he can decide who he is and what his existence is for and where it should lead.

The physician has had to become part of the technological apparatus of society in order to attain mastery over many of man's bodily ills. Yet, as never before, he is also compelled to remain the practitioner of the most humane of all the sciences. Is it possible to be at once a practitioner of the new biology and an advocate for the person against the dehumanizing thrust of a mass civilization? Can the doctor simultaneously attend Man the molecular aggregate and Man the person; Man the unit of a complex society and Man the ineffable?

Society can tolerate no answer except that the impossible must be achieved: medicine must become master of its technologic base and, at the same time, use that technology within a humanist framework. No other solution is equal to the tensions medicine itself creates in human values—tensions far more critical to human welfare than the cure of individual illnesses.

Few would deny that medicine today needs a more vigorous and more penetrating intercalation with humane studies than ever before. But this intercalation is too simplistically equated with larger or more sustained doses of liberal studies assembled according to a traditional formula more romantically than critically conceived. These, once taken, are expected to guard the nascent physician against the narrowness, insensitivity, and hubris his education is thought to inculcate.

This view is too firmly rooted in a romantic, nineteenth-century ideal of the educated man. It depends too heavily on a naive hope of resurrecting the Renaissance man as prototype of the physician. It propagates the myth that there is something sacred in the four-year liberal arts education for inculcating human values, hence making it a necessary prelude to specialized studies of any kind and of medicine in particular. Most fundamental of all, this conception misreads the history of the humanities and liberal studies and their meaning in contemporary life.

The prevailing conception that everyone can be, or needs to be, liberally educated before undertaking professional studies must be countered with a goal that is less pretentious, more realistic, and more consonant with both the inclinations of today's students and the need for more competently trained manpower.

The aim should be to provide liberal education a variety of ways, but probably most often by reversing the traditional order of liberal and professional studies. Medicine is the most humane of sciences, the most empiric of arts, and the most scientific of humanities. Its subject matter is an ideal ground within which to develop the attitudes associated with the humanistic and liberally educated. Pursued simultaneously with medicine or even later, the humanities can more effectively humanize practice and cultivate the mind of the practitioner.

To advance this thesis, I must examine several questions: What *precisely* is the nature of the deficiency in the physician's education that has aroused such concern? How have the humanities failed in their own purposes? What alternatives are being tried as remedies? What is a viable formula for today? What are its implications for medicine and the university?

It is a common assertion nowadays that the physician is too often an uneducated man, technically proficient but insensitive to values, ideas, and esthetics. These deficiencies are presumed to lead to neglect of the person of the patient, to disregard of the needs of the total community, and even to economic rapacity. They are to be eliminated, it is said, by a "humanistic" education prior to entering medicine and by deeper study of the humanities.

The charges are not new. In one form or another they have been popular with the literati from Molière to George Bernard Shaw and Mark Twain. They are more stridently proclaimed by the medically disenfranchised and by patients in every class of society. Medical students sensitive to any trace of hypocrisy in their teachers have added their voices and have called for changes in medical education designed to avoid replication of the same pattern in their own lives.[1]

The medical educator interested in instant education can achieve it with his university colleagues by reciting the same litany. He will often be rewarded by being called a humanist himself, thus being separated from that rude band of technicians, his colleagues.

There is considerable justification both for the criticism and for the demand that in today's world the physician must be more responsive to what society and his patients expect of him. Clearly, medicine's responsibilities have grown along with its capabilities. The physician must look at himself with uncommon candor. He does not need defense, but a clearer delineation of the reasons for the criticisms and more effective antidotes than are now available.

The questionable feature in current criticisms of the physician's humanistic education lies in the line of reasoning generally followed. Two aspects of the physician's life, that of the educated man and that of the compassionate person, are confused; lacks in either are assumed to stem from insufficient exposure to the humanities or to liberal education. Such studies are presumed automatically to confer on the physician a sense of human values and thus make him a humanitarian and a man educated in the use of the liberal arts—a humanist physician. This is too much to expect of any formal educational method, liberal arts or other. The misconception arises from a perennial vagueness in the definitions of such terms as *humanism, humanitarian, humanities,* and *liberal studies.* They are too often lumped together as a mithridatic prescription to insure a human approach by professionals to their work. Some distinctions in defining these terms are essential for development of my thesis.

Few words are as entrancing in concept or as varied in interpretation as *humanism.* It has been subjected to a wide range of definitions. Some see it as a literary concept based in a knowledge of classical languages and literature; others equate it with a mode of education. Still others see it as a democratic or socialist theory of politics, or as a form of man-centered religion, or as an instrument for the suppression of the working class, or as the antidote to vocationalism (Babbitt and More). Most commonly today it is applied to any study or endeavor which is man-centered or places primacy on man and human values. In this latter sense, it is indistinguishable from humanitarianism.

Thus, it is clear that an education which emphasizes studies of the works of man may be conducted from divergent points of view, based in differing sets of values and priorities. When critics demand a more humanistic education for physicians, they may be talking about any of these humanisms—though most will mean that they want physicians who are more interested in patients as people, an attribute which does not necessarily result from any of the *humanisms* formally defined.

Equal confusion pertains to definitions of the conglomerate of studies called the *humanities* or *liberal studies.* Professor Albert Levi has recently reanalyzed the difficulties in defining the humanities today. He illustrates well the problem of separating them from the social sciences and the natural sciences, also concerned with human values. He concludes that the humanities are best limited to three arts: communication, continuity and criticism—i.e., language and literature, history, and philosophy. These are in turn equated with liberal studies and then sharply distinguished from the sciences.[2]

Although Levi's definition is acceptable, it is apparent that the studies thus defined may or may not teach values. They might make the physician a learned or an educated man, but not necessarily a humane or compassionate one. As Levi himself points out:

The "conviction," the "faith," the "presupposition," that the humanities teach values is not enough. They must be taught with this constant aim in mind and with an experimental willingness at every point to explore the actual relationships between the content of the liberal arts and the humanitarian values and the humanistic attitude which are their reasons for existence, their card of accreditation in the spectrum of teaching and research.[3]

This point has special pertinence for liberal studies in a medical education.

Clearly society today needs physicians who, in addition to being technically competent, are compassionate and educated—physicians who can understand how their work intersects with the culture of which it is a part, physicians who can work empathetically with other humans in distress. All of these attributes rarely will be found in one man. One mode of education, even if based in humanistic studies, cannot guarantee all. This conclusion is essential to any restructuring of medical education to meet the full flavor of the criticism now leveled at it.

Other professionals are as susceptible to deficiencies in their liberal education and in their abilities to react empathetically to their clients. But such lapses have a moral tone in medicine. The physician is most intimately in touch with suffering man, with the misery and the joys of the human condition. Behind the vehemence of the criticisms is society's hope that medicine, more than other endeavors, can heal the rift between science and technology on the one hand and art and wisdom on the other. Since Descartes, man has been told he is a machine. Yet, all his strivings since have been toward becoming more of a person.

The imperative, then, becomes this: medicine must become more humane, more infused with the spirit of liberal studies, and more willing to address itself to the metaphysical dichotomy between the arts and the sciences. This is an undertaking fraught with presumptions, but no other science or art has the potential for attempting such a task successfully. Indeed, the need for drastic revision of the mode of the physician's liberal education derives intellectual impetus from the need for this synthesis. Without it, medicine can justifiably be reduced to what its severest critics say it has already become—just another technology.

The Erosion of the Humanities

Before the humanities are fixed into the framework of medical education, their state in the contemporary university needs to be ascertained. Liberal studies have been transformed by the potent influence of science and technology, the needs of education in a democratic society, and changing motivations of the student body.

Today's university is no longer essentially a training ground for an elite corps of leaders, as it was in the nineteenth century. In an egalitarian society, it has become mainly an instrument for mass education and the most effective means for socioeconomic advancement. Society expects our universities to prepare large numbers of young people for socially useful roles. It supports higher education with this expectation, not primarily to increase the number of "educated" men or scholars.

Students too have changed their perception of the university experience. They see it mainly either as a means of providing the tools for some profession, including specialized scholarship in this definition, or as a means of "finding" themselves as persons. Very few enter universities nowadays to train their intellects in the sophisticated mode advocated by Cardinal Newman. Refinement of the intellect and the cultivation of tastes and esthetic values as lifelong endowments for work and leisure are not conscious goals. Rather, these goals are consciously rejected by increasing numbers of students, who see in them the remnants of an outmoded social and economic caste system.

As universities and students have changed character, so have humanistic and liberal studies. Europe inherited from the Italian Renaissance and the Enlightenment a special ideal of the educated man. He was steeped in the Greek and Latin tongues and classics, at home in the Scriptures, knowledgeable in the history of his country, and skilled in the artful use of its language. These endowments were not considered inconsistent with competence in some profession; and indeed they enhanced professional pursuits. We in America have been most influenced by this ideal as exemplified in nineteenth-century Oxford and Cambridge and epitomized in Newman's *Idea of a University*. This ideal has suffered substantial attenuation in the past century under the impact of science and technology, the needs for mass education, and the trend toward specialization through graduate studies. Even at its height, the traditional ideal was really effective in only a few exemplary men of letters, science, and government. Today it has been deprived of meaning for the majority of students who attend universities for more pragmatic and more immediate goals. It can only be a limited formula for education in a democratic society needful of large numbers of professionals, technicians, businessmen, and bureaucrats.

The humanities themselves have been compelled to assume the stance of specialties and to adopt the research attitudes and the objectivity of the sciences. In today's universities the departments in the humanities are primarily the training ground for scholars, and, as Northrop Frye so aptly points out, scholarship is distinctly not the same thing as education.[4] The professional practitioners of the humanities now direct their major energies to the replication of research specialists in their graduate students. They have lost their capability for communication with the general undergraduate and with their colleagues in other faculties. Indeed, from being the teachers of all, they too have become specialized teachers just like all the rest.

The humanities today seem well along the road of abandoning wisdom for information. In so doing, they have become the antithesis of liberal studies, which were originally intended to free the mind and the spirit. The professional humanists still insist that their disciplines have value for all educated men, and lament early specialization in other fields. Students still hope that by some magical formula the humanities will somehow become relevant. Professional schools continue to speak piously of educating the man first and the professional second.

Medical educators, hoping to preserve medicine as a "learned" profession, are especially susceptible to these illusions. They assert that all medical students should first receive a liberal education, and the professionals believe that today's collegiate experience can provide such an education. Two annoying factors militate against the reality of these assertions. The first is the attenuation of the humanities as liberal studies. The second is the notorious imperviousness of premedical students to genuine liberal studies when those studies are obstacles that must be hurdled to enter medical school.

The clear reality is that few of the purposes of a traditional liberal education are provided in today's undergraduate experience. The fact is that most students enter professional schools without the "broad" base they are assumed to have acquired. Medical education can no longer be postponed until this dubious base has been acquired by all students.

None of this is to say that the attitudes traditionally called "liberal" are in any way less essential to an educated man and to the profession of medicine. Without them, medicine cannot be a humane science or avoid the confusion of purposes to which its unprecedented knowledge makes it so susceptible. Manifestly, we must seek some better way to free the minds of some physicians at least, so that they can see the relationship of their work to the whole fabric of culture and society. Where can one look for an approach consistent with the state of contemporary science, society, politics, and student interests? Under what conditions can the humanities be revitalized?

Some Insufficient Alternatives

In the past two decades medical educators and students have striven to fill the vacuum left by the defection of the humanists by modifying the medical curriculum several ways: adding behavioral sciences, religion, real-life experiences, and involvement. It is worth examining each briefly before turning in more detail to another possible approach.

The social and behavioral sciences—sociology, anthropology, economics, and psychology—do contribute much to understanding the person, the family, and the institutions that figure so intimately in the genesis of health and illness. They are fundamental studies for the psychiatrist, specialists in community medicine, and for all physicians who hope in some measure to understand the "whole" patient. These studies serve to sensitize students to the importance of personal and social values in diagnosis, therapeutics, and prevention. Undeniably, the social sciences introduce new and valuable data into medical education as well as into the techniques of sociomedical research.

For several reasons, the social sciences do not, however, fully compensate for the deficiency left by the defection of the humanities.

First of all, the social sciences, striving like the humanities for the objectivity of the physical sciences, have become specialized studies. The "establishment" of social scientists relies heavily on descriptive or statistical language and eschews values and philosophical insights. At the same time, the younger generation of radical sociologists rejects any hope of understanding society. Instead, they perceive their roles as activists who must destroy existing social structures and remake them according to some private and viscerally apprehended formula. Such antirationalism is fashionable with the young, who, lacking experience with the genuine article, accept these views as the basis for a "new humanism," which is, in fact, nonhumanist at its roots.

Last, medical educators expect too much of the social sciences. These studies increase our understanding of certain critical factors in the care of the patient. They do not guarantee that physicians exposed to them will act in a socially responsible or compassionate manner. They must be reinforced by the behavior of clinical teachers who actually use these data in their daily practice and teaching, and most importantly, in the care of their own patients.

Another alternative to the humanities is theology. Some medical schools have filled part of the gap in humanistic education by introducing the theologian and the minister into the clinical setting. These are admirable beginnings and hold promise for the future, providing theologians can make the transition from a doctrinaire to an evolutionary stance in treating human values. Theologians today are increasingly interested in a more existential examination of human problems and seem willing to deal with the transcendent in more contemporary terms. As they become less dogmatic and less sectarian, religion and theology might well offer a more substantial base for liberal studies in the professions than many other disciplines.

Theology is, however, only rarely represented in universities and medical school faculties. Its practitioners, as in the humanities and social sciences, are also susceptible to the pull toward specialization and scholarship. Like the social sciences, religion and theology can indeed sensitize many students to some very significant questions in medicine. But these studies also suffer from the special handicap of centuries

of misunderstanding and misuse. Although the process of the intellectual rehabilitation of theology and religion has begun, we are a long way
from reestablishing their authenticity for most of today's secular-minded
students.

In the last three or four years medical students have initiated a third
and quite imaginative method for remedying some of the insensitivity to
humane values in contemporary medicine, education and practice. They
have plunged into early and direct clinical experiences and roles of advocacy for medically disenfranchised patients and communities. These
efforts have effectively revolutionized certain aspects of the medical curriculum. In the process, even faculties and deans have become more responsive to the importance of "involvement" in the major social medical
issues of our day.

This approach, like the others, supplies only part of what is missing.
It provides direct experience with human distress and thus enables the
student to confront questions of values early in his professional education.
The emotional impact is significant, and motivation of the student to help
others is reinforced. But the cogitated assimilation of these direct experiences with human distress must still be sought if the student is to emerge
as a truly educated person in the liberal tradition.

These three approaches—via the behavioral sciences, religion, and direct clinical experiences—are partial solutions to the educational deficiencies created by the present state of the humanities. These efforts will surely
be expanded further, but to be fully effective they must be complemented
by a drastically altered view of the place of liberal studies in general and
professional education. What form might this assume?

Humanities in Medicine: A New Sequence

Every culture has expected its physicians to function at several levels.
The first is concerned with professional and technical competence—the
detection and treatment of disease by the most effective means; the second deals with the management of the personal dimensions of illness—
the promotion of health and the adjustment of the patient to those things
medicine cannot cure; the last is providing society a critique of the quality

of life from the special viewpoint the physician brings to questions of population, environmental pollution, drugs, and sociopathy, for example.[5]

Educating each physician to perform adequately at all these levels would compromise competence to the point of absurdity. We live in a complex society, moving toward equal opportunity for education and service and away from restriction of these rights to the privileged. A socially responsible and more realistic goal for medical education is to provide a sufficient number of physicians able to function at one level only, not just a small number who can meet all expectations of individuals and society. The totality of personal and technical services needed by every patient can best be provided by a judicious combining of the efforts of physicians and other health professionals. What we must seek is the appropriate organizational pattern in which the limitations of each can be complemented by the strengths of each.

Many physicians will function at more than one level, and in a properly designed structure this can be encouraged. What must not be encouraged is the dangerous pretension that some form of education can generate a host of Renaissance men, capable at all levels. Even in the Renaissance, the true polymath was a rarity.

Education must, therefore, recognize the unique capabilities of each student and match these with the most congruent level of professional function. Some will do best at the technical and craftsman tasks, some at the personal and social, others at the investigative and speculative, and still others at the public expressions of medicine. There is a special compulsion today to advance the student as expeditiously as possible to the socially useful goal which best fits his particular capabilities.

To attain this end, current insistence on a traditional "liberal" education for all students before they enter specific medical studies must be abandoned, permitting these liberal studies to be pursued in a variety of ways—before entering medicine, during medical education, after medical education, or not at all. The reality is that some physicians will assimilate the liberal attitudes completely, some partially, and some not at all. Yet, all will be useful to society.

The traditional sequence of liberal studies prior to medical studies will still profit many. But many more will not want it or perceive their need for it. Forcing every student to "take" the humanities as a tonic or as an initiation rite or as a fulfillment of retrospective dissatisfactions with education is no longer reasonable. To do so is to encourage a superficial exposure to humane studies and to engender a self-defeating, lifelong distaste for them.

The same admonition was voiced by so astute and so humanist a clinician as Peter Mere Latham in the nineteenth century: "The different professions have one way of glorifying themselves, which is common to all. It is by setting forth a vast array of preparatory studies, and pretending they are indispensable in order to fit a man for the simple exercise of the practical duties that belong to them."[6]

While some students will continue in the usual sequence, a different pattern seems more consistent for many others, perhaps the bulk of students. For them, higher education can begin with the craftsmanship of medicine, and the route to liberal education and cultural awareness can be through their professional and technical studies. These students should be allowed even to choose a field of major study within medicine and acquire special skills as soon as feasible. Such goal-oriented students are notoriously immune to humane studies until they are relieved of anxiety about getting into medical school and until they acquire some competence in their chosen craft. There is little to be gained from blunting their motivation with the illusion they somehow will be "better off" if they postpone technical studies.

Capturing student motivation by early immersion in medical studies should have a high yield in enthusiasm and application, qualities often only mechanically exhibited in the first years of a traditional medical education. This enthusiasm can also be channeled into the acquisition of a humanistic outlook, provided it is an intrinsic part of medical education. A wide variety of humane studies—sociology, ethics, history of ideas, social psychology, anthropology, philosophy—can be taught around the cases with which the student becomes involved as a physician-in-training.

There can be no real question about relevance here. The starting point for thinking is always a real human being facing a real human problem in values, hopes, and aspirations. Ample opportunities in the everyday matter of patient care exemplify most of the perennial questions of human concern. Can there be more pertinent grist for the mill of the committed humanist than these: the cancer patient facing death, pain, and loneliness; the sick and lonely aged; the disaffected; the depressed; the alcohol- and the drug-addicted; the "better off" with their less dramatic but significant neuroses? All the existential problems of being human in a terrifying mechanistic world are exemplified in the medical student's daily work. Health and disease are entry points to the whole range of personal and social concerns of mankind.

Problems that transcend individuals are abundant too: the ethics of experimentation, the justice of distribution of health resources, the human uses of technology, the social and cultural roots of dissent. All problems of human life—alienation, affection, social and cultural relationships, and even salvation—come to a focus in the existential laboratories of human problems we call hospitals. Every humanistic question takes on poignancy when embedded in the concrete situation: to discuss the value of life when deciding whether or not to abort, to relieve pain, to desist from overtreatment in hopeless situations; or to discuss the ethics of confidentiality and consent when actually facing the decision in a proposed investigation; or to discuss the question of dehumanization when patients become lost in the institutionalized underbrush of the system.

The full range of perennial questions can thus be experienced and cogitated in their contemporary form by both faculty and students. Starting with the concrete case also can instill those qualities of mind classically associated with a liberal education—the capacity to search for truth, to understand the values of others and thus evaluate one's own, to frame a personal response to the problems of existence, and to communicate clearly, if not eloquently.

Even esthetic experiences can grow out of these encounters with the concrete phenomena of human life. The seminal works of art and literature are, after all, more sensitive insights into the same world, transmuted by the special responsiveness of the artist and the poet. The most general, philosophic, and abstract considerations usually flow from the concrete and the particular. The abstract need not precede experiences, as has been insisted in academic institutions for so long.

Teaching of the humanities and of humanist values in this way demands humanist teachers with special characteristics. They must first be bona fide members of social science or humanities faculties, not merely cultivated or talented physicians with an interest in these subjects. They particularly should maintain identification with their own disciplines for two reasons: to avoid the isolation which besets the humanist in a medical setting where there is usually an insufficient "critical mass" of colleagues and to maintain authenticity in their teaching. Attaining these two essentials usually requires joint appointment to both university and medical school departments.

These teachers must also have a real commitment to communicating the sense of their disciplines to students in medicine and the other health professions. They can do this in several degrees of depth: (a) introductory seminars for all students in the health professions, taught in interdisciplinary sessions; (b) elective seminars and courses in greater depth for those medical and other students stimulated by the introductory material; and (c) research and advanced study for students of the health professions who wish to pursue scholarly work in medical social sciences and humanities or to teach in these fields. Such students can drop out of the standard curricula for extended periods, or even pursue a combined Ph.D.-M.D. option as they now do in the basic health sciences.

The social scientists and humanists should be situated for a significant part of their time in the physical milieu of the health sciences center, living, so to speak, in the laboratory of their concerns. This will foster those daily fortuitous contacts with students, faculty, and patients so rich in unanticipated opportunities for dialogue, cooperative teaching, and research. Medical students and faculty will thus be exposed in an immediate way to how humanists view their daily problems; humanists in turn will gain access to the concrete human experiences that can make their cogitations truly relevant. Some humanists in such contact with those they teach may be stimulated to resume their forgotten, nonspecialist roles as teachers of the entire intellectual community.

An additional advantage of this arrangement for social scientists and humanists is freer access to every facet of activity in the health sciences centers as subject and source for research. The philosopher studying death phenomenologically, the political scientist interested in institutional policy and decision making, and the anthropologist observing the cultural transactions in patient care—these are examples of scholars whose work is enriched by open, direct contact with daily life in hospitals and clinics. Indeed, it is doubtful that such studies can have full validity or that the health sciences centers can be fully utilized as university resources without the physical presence of some of these scholars.

There are hopeful signs that some professional social scientists and humanists already see the unnatural constrictions imposed on their disciplines by the university and are bold enough to assume teaching within the context of health sciences centers. They are motivated by the need to ground their own work in the reality of human experiences and also by a genuine desire to influence and improve the education of health professionals who are to become practitioners of the applied social sciences and humanities.

Some modifications of customary teaching modes will be demanded of those social scientists and humanists who teach in the milieu of professional education. They will need especially to adapt to the individual clinical case as the usual launching point of discussion. Interdisciplinary presentations, occasioned by the multiple problems that patients so often present, will be common. Careful planning is essential to avoid the interjection of some artificial point important in itself but not arising naturally out of the clinical situation. Such teaching will take place in unfamiliar surroundings—on hospital floors or in clinics, often with the patient present and even participating to some extent.

These teachers will no doubt be dismayed at how much has been forgotten or unperceived by their students prior to "liberal" education. But they should be equally gratified with the depth of response and the flash of recognition when some idea suddenly opens the mind of a future physician to dimensions of life and thought to which he was previously unresponsive.

Reading in the classical and seminal works of history, literature, and philosophy is relatively easy to encourage when related to daily experiences in medicine and its contiguous fields. A substantial reinforcement of liberal education can be achieved quite painlessly and enthusiastically in the postgraduate years, even in the continuing education of the practicing physician. Indeed, to perceive the social and cultural intersections of one's daily work is one of the few effective antidotes to the intellectual ennui that afflicts too many successful practitioners in their middle years.

Clarity of expression, if not felicity of style, can also be taught this way. Correction and criticism of papers and assignments prepared to meet course requirements becomes a more valuable exercise in composition or rhetoric than the usual theme-writing of freshman English courses.

The interweaving of liberal studies and humanities with professional studies affords a viable opportunity for shared education experiences among students of medicine, dentistry, nursing, pharmacy, and the other health professions. The sharp differences in preparation among these groups that exist with regard to the laboratory sciences is usually not found with regard to the social sciences or humanities. All these students can profitably engage in discussion of the values, human purposes, and problems that arise in clinical situations. As a consequence, some of the barriers to future communication between health professionals may be less firmly erected. Opportunity exists, too, for sharing these sessions with university students outside the health sciences, an interface yet to be investigated.

This approach should help to soften the growing conviction, within and without the universities, that the humanities are isolated from life and work and are meant only for the leisure use of an elite class. Ideally, if a case-oriented liberal education could be provided in medical school and reinforced through the physician's life by continuing education in the humanities, it would contribute optimally to his growth as an educated man. The taste for liberal and humane studies matures late; it is focused and enhanced by life's experiences at a time when it can no longer be cultivated in the present schema. Liberal studies which seemed trivial or irrelevant in youth may provide that margin of rationality and delectation to lift us out of the mundanity of our workday functions in later years.

This pathway to a liberal education sharply reverses the traditional sequence of studies. Its utility is, of course, yet to be proved. It can, however, scarcely be less effective than the traditional method. Taking this new pathway might at least dispel some of the illusions fabricated to protect both medicine and the humanities from facing their current shortcomings in producing educated men.

With any method of liberal education, one must be prepared to find students for whom the realm of ideas, values, and esthetics will always be foreign. With the method proposed here, if students must reject these realms, they will do so only after having a still better opportunity to experience the potential significance for man and society.

The Most Humane of Sciences: The Most Scientific of Humanities

It has always been difficult to place medicine precisely among human intellectual endeavors. Medicine is unique in being so thoroughly steeped in the practical on the one hand and so dependent upon the humane and the scientific on the other. Plato recognized medicine as an essential ingredient of the Greek culture. Varro included medicine among the humanities. In his search for infallible demonstrations, Descartes attempted to mathematize medicine and thus to ground it. Modern-day reductionists would identify it as simply a sophisticated form of chemistry and physics.

One suggestion very congenial to the present thesis is set forth by Scott Buchanan in a seminal and neglected book, *The Doctrine of Signatures*. Buchanan very perceptively saw the clinical arts of diagnosis, prognosis, and therapeusis as applications of the liberal arts: "the clinical arts are applications of the liberal arts to medicine just as observation, experimentation, and verification in the laboratory are applications of the liberal arts to physics. In fact, any body of scientific doctrine has a fringe of tentative exploration and operation which consists in the application of the liberal arts."[7]

He concluded that medicine is "the medium and perhaps the focus in which the problems of wisdom and science meet."[8] He went further and saw it as the root of a new humanism, a unifying influence for philosophy and the laboratory sciences. Buchanan's thesis is unquestionably fraught with pretension, but it offers an invigorating challenge to medicine, science, and the humanities. To the contemporary humanist, medicine offers the most concrete grounding for his discipline; for the educated physician, it can become the vehicle for intensive application of the liberal arts. Interpreted broadly as "man's study of man," medicine might well be used to teach the sciences to the nonscience major and the liberal arts to the science major.

As the most humane of sciences, medicine is an excellent focus for problems of sociology, economics, political science, law, and every other discipline which concerns itself with human beings. The ethical, philosophical, and theological questions posed by modern medical progress are of the utmost consequence to all educated men. In examining abortion, population control, behavioral modification, drug use and abuse, psychopathy, neuroses, and the myriad concerns of modern medicine, there is unparalleled opportunity to treat some of the most important issues in the social sciences and the humanities. The great advantage of starting with the medical situation lies in its concreteness, immediacy, and urgency. All students have directly or indirectly experienced the challenges of disease, disability, disaffection, and death. Questions of human values and the choice of alternatives are posed in a most direct way. The relationship of thought to action is nowhere more clearly exemplified.

Underlying its intensive concerns with human values, medicine nevertheless continues to be scientific in its method. It must proceed by the careful collection of data, the critical evaluation of evidence, and reliance on experimental and empirical solutions. Medicine is nothing less than a "humane science," potentially capable of illustrating for the profession or the general student the meeting ground of traditional wisdom and science.

But medicine is equally one of the humanities because its concerns are for all dimensions of the life of man which in any way impinge on his well-being. Medicine is not one of the humanities *sui generis;* yet more than any other science it stands at the confluence of all the humanities. Its peculiar arts of clinical evaluation and decision exemplify all the major attributes of mind we seek from the liberal arts: the search for truth and the means of identifying it, the establishing of a system of values, the orderly presentation of observed data and their artful arrangement in making a specific diagnosis and in defending the case for that diagnosis. In short, the medieval trivium of grammar, rhetoric, and logic can be reified in every informed medical action.

Medicine thus can be extremely useful, in itself, in imparting the attitudes of the liberal arts and the content of the humanities to the medical student in the course of his professional education. Its value as a cultural subject and as a vehicle for the humanities and social sciences for the college undergraduate should be explored further. With certain modifications in content and depth of detail, the most human and humane questions could be introduced through an undergraduate study of medicine in both its personal and social dimensions.

All the sciences and many of the humanities were first seeded in the soil of medicine in the medieval universities. Medicine is expanding its social and human concerns as it becomes the agency of applied biology and sociology. Its potential to alter human life and nature have occasioned a deeper interaction with philosophy and theology as well. It could well become the meeting ground for all disciplines dealing with man.

But medicine may have an even greater cultural potential yet to be realized. Is it not a practical mechanism for bridging the widening gulf between the sciences and the humanities? The need for such a bridge is epitomized in the vigorous discussion which followed C. P. Snow's Rede Lecture on "The Two Cultures."[9] Never have people been so sensitive to the need to understand themselves simultaneously as subject and object, as person and machine. The marks of Descartes' hemisection of human nature are magnified in every irruption of technology into human affairs.

The reconciliation will not come, as naively suggested by some, from teaching the humanists the beauties of science or the scientists the rationality of the humanities. To hope to "humanize" the sciences and infuse the humanities with the scientific spirit is to ignore an essential contrariety between two fundamentally divergent views of reality. This contrariety is irreconcilable, and indeed it is necessary to the full expression of man's intellectual capacities. Levi has said it rather well:

> The natural sciences, for all that they are undeniably a human enterprise, are a tribute to man's ability to expurgate all mythical, teleological, and anthropomorphic elements from his thinking. They illustrate his interest in factuality. They show him at the utmost limit of his objectivity. The humanities, for all that they employ a logic and require a structure of their own, are a demonstration that drama, purposiveness, and self-concern are inescapable and indispensable elements of the human situation and the expressiveness which it requires. They illustrate man's dramatic instinct. They show in its most elegant form the propensity for teleological interpretation in man.

> This, as I have said, is a real dualism—a clear split down the center of the intellectual life, and it is difficult to see how, with such diametrically opposed cognitive needs, it could be otherwise.[10]

This fundamental split must be recognized, and its divergencies used to balance any excess trend in either direction if man is to be best served. Medicine has great, and almost unique, cultural force precisely because it is a discipline in need of both views. It does not "belong" strictly either to the sciences or to the humanities.

But it must use the languages and cognitive methods of both in the pursuit of its object: the health of man. Medicine is a humane science since it must examine man as person and object simultaneously. On the one hand, to understand Man the object, it uses the objective, factual, experimental language and method of the sciences, necessarily "expurgating" itself of myth; on the other hand, to understand Man the person, it must examine man in all his subjective, imaginative, purposive, self-conscious, and mythopoeic activity.

Taken thus, as a unification of the ramifications of man's existence as person and object, medicine has a unique opportunity to occupy the two worlds of the intellect and provide the ontologic bridge between them. This end will be achieved if medicine works into its fabric the practice of the humanities as well as it has the practice of the sciences.

Some Implications for the University

Sir Eric Ashby recently probed the dilemma of today's academics confronting the uses of technology in the university. He notes the conflict between those who see the university as a precious haven of the free intellect and those who feel its obligations to solve pressing social problems. He proposes a new technologic humanism as the way to heal this rift; interestingly he uses medicine as a paradigm.[11]

Ashby suggests that the cultural education of the physician and others who must perform technical tasks be acquired through their vocational and special training, not separately from it. He suggests that the pertinent studies are psychology, ethics, political science, and the like, rather than the classical studies, literature, and history traditionally taught. In propounding this thesis, Ashby is reinforcing in modern terms the notion expounded by Plato that medicine is a techné—a body of knowledge aimed at the benefit of man and incomplete until put into practice.[12]

Clearly, the intercalation of medical with liberal studies and the humanities in the manner outlined here would provide an excellent example for the other university faculties of one potent way to heal the humanist-scientist dichotomy. I think medicine can thus stimulate the university to a fresher and closer examination of its fundamental purposes in society.

But the dilemma is deeper than this. The university today must regain its academic and intellectual authenticity. Its current difficulties are academic much more than political or social. Students and society now expect an education more congruent with our complex world. Most reforms have thus far been at the periphery of the life of the university and have been engineered to safeguard traditional academic concerns. Clearly, there is no general agreement on the intellectual language all educated men should share. A drastic revision of prevailing concepts of general education is urgently needed—one which confronts squarely the issues of goals, standards, and alternate routes for undergraduate education and which infuses them with new realities.

Universities, like medical schools, have rigidified formulas for general education, unmindful of the diverse expectations of today's student bodies. Some come to college because they know what they want to do; they are goal oriented from the outset and want to enter a profession as soon as possible. Others, and these seem the largest number, expect college to be primarily an experience in personal searching—finding what talents they have, achieving some identity and some purpose for the future. A subset of this group wants to use college intermittently, interspersed with work or other pursuits and spread out over more than the usual four years. Greatly in the minority are the students who come to train the intellect in Cardinal Newman's sense, as a tool, useful in itself, and capable of being applied to any data in work or leisure.

Sadly, only for the last group are the traditional modes of liberal education applicable. The others need a wholly different academic approach, a different set of academic standards, and even different faculties with a lifestyle more consistent with that of the students they teach. To maintain, as many still do, that a single mode of liberal education is essential or even beneficial is to subscribe to an outmoded conception of the uses of the university. More than that, it is a defection of academic responsibility which threatens the intellectual freedom the university rightfully cherishes. The general public and the legislatures will not long accept "reform" efforts that do not permit revision of the inner life of the university—its role as the liberalizing force in all intellectual affairs.

A tripartite system of undergraduate university education, at least, seems in order: (a) early entry into professional and technical training for those who wish it, with liberal education integrated into their special studies; (b) work-study programs, community and social experiences, interspersed with formal course work for those who are seeking self-knowledge; and (c) for the few who wish it, a truly rigorous liberal and classical education. Three different faculties, as well as different standards of performance, are needed for these alternatives.

This is not the place to expand this notion of a tripartite university education. I wish simply to indicate that the troublous state of university education today demands alternatives less protective of customary modes and standards.

As the confluence point of the sciences and the humanities, medicine has a special responsibility to explore this new territory of alternatives. In thus revising its own educational forms, it can encourage the general university faculties to more candidly appraise their responsibilities. As the existential arm of the university most acutely in contact with pressing personal and community needs, medicine can lead the university toward a more effective role in contemporary society.

Medicine can thus bring the humanities into closer relationship with the world of practical affairs and help them regain their position as guardians of human values and advocates for man—an eventuality as essential to the humanities as it is to the future of mankind.

Notes

This chapter is based on the Sanger Lecture entitled "The Most Humane Science: Some Notes on Liberal Education in Medicine and the University" which was delivered at the Medical College of Virginia of Virginia Commonwealth University, Richmond, on April 10, 1970.

1. Casey Truett, Arthur W. Couville, Bruce Fagel, and Merle Cunningham. "The Medical Curriculum and Human Values," panel discussion, 65th Annual Congress on Medical Education, *Journal of the American Medical Association,* 209(7) (Aug. 18, 1969): 1341.

2. Albert William Levi, *The Humanities Today* (Bloomington: Indiana University Press, 1970).

3. Ibid., p. 92.

4. Northrop Frye,"The Instruments of Mental Production." In *The Knowledge Most Worth Having,* ed. Wayne C. Booth (Chicago: University of Chicago Press, 1967), pp. 59–83.

5. Geoffrey Vickers, *Medicine's Contribution to Culture in Medicine and Culture,* ed. F. N. L. Poynter (London: Wellcome Institute of the History of Medicine, 1969), pp. 5–6.

6. *Aphorisms from Latham* (Peter Mere Latham), coll. and ed. William B. Bean (Iowa City: Prairie Press, 1962), p. 40.

7. Scott Buchanan, *The Doctrine of Signatures: A Defence of Theory in Medicine* (London: Kegan Paul, Trench, Trubner, 1938), p. 80.

8. Ibid., p. 94.

9. Charles P. Snow, *The Two Cultures and the Scientific Revolution* (New York: Cambridge University Press, 1959).

10. Levi, *The Humanities Today,* p. 61.

11. Eric Ashby, *Technology and the Academics* (New York: Macmillan, 1969).

12. Werner Jaeger, *Paideia: The Ideals of Greek Culture,* trans. from the German by Gilbert Highet (New York: Oxford University Press, 1944), 2:21.

FIFTEEN

The Humanities in Medical Education

Entering the Post-Evangelical Era

Introduction

Since classical times the liberal arts have been the indispensable accoutrements of educated people. As the medieval trivium they provided the intellectual tools necessary for all serious scholarship and professional work. For centuries they were the essential propaedeutic to a medical education. Even today, some aliquot of liberal education is deemed necessary in preparation for medical studies.

In the last two decades an unprecedented departure from this tradition of separation of professional and liberal studies has occurred in American medical schools. Of 125 schools surveyed, 118 either had or were initiating teaching programs in human values, ethics, or the humanities.[1] To anyone familiar with the inertia of medical curricula, as well as the positivistic bias of medical faculties, this is a remarkable development indeed.

There are two major reasons for this change: first, a deepening public and professional concern for the moral dilemmas posed by new medical capabilities, and second, an awareness of the need to guarantee the humanistic elements of medical care against erosion by its increasingly technological character. In the late 1960s and early 1970s these same concerns attracted the support of private foundations and the National Endowment for the Humanities. With commendable prescience they enabled most of the programs now in existence to become established. An era of almost evangelical expansion was ushered in.

Today the "pump-priming" funds are beginning to run out. Medical schools and universities must decide whether or not to support programs on university funds at a time when fiscal constraints are becoming a major problem for most institutions. Financial support must now be more vigorously justified. As a result, the teaching of medical ethics, human values, and the humanities must squarely confront some fundamental questions. The Post-Evangelical Period has begun.

Why should the humanities be taught in medical schools in the first place? Are they not the province of college education? How can the time, effort and expense be justified? Do they make for better patient care? In the evangelical period these questions could be answered more with exhortation and missionary fervor than conceptual clarity. Now, as future survival becomes a real problem, the answers must be more definitive.

These questions are vexing not only to medical educators. They occur at a time when the place of the humanities themselves in American life is under scrutiny. Very recently the Commission on the Humanities asserted the need for a reaffirmation of their importance to education and public life. Especially, the Commission said, "the humanities, science and technology need to be substantially connected."[2] What are those connections and how do they operate?

Recent trends seem to militate against making these connections—weakening of the teaching of the humanities in the universities, demands of the job market, bias against intellectual elitism, lowering of the standards of civilized discourse, expansion of technical information, the dominance of television, films and other non-verbal forms of learning. Yet in the face of a decline in their influence generally, the humanities have established a promising beachhead in an unpromising place, the medical school curriculum.

Some of the answer lies in the nature of medicine itself. It has always been situated halfway between science and technology on the one hand, and the needs of suffering human beings on the other. Medicine connects technical and moral questions in its clinical decisions; it is required to be both objective and compassionate. It sits between the sciences and the humanities, being exclusively neither one nor the other but having some of the qualities of both. Medicine is, in fact, an excellent paradigm of those "connections" the Commission on the Humanities is seeking. By examining the teaching of the humanities in medicine we can gain some insight on the larger issues of the way the humanities relate to public and private life in a technological society.

Why Teach the Humanities at All?

There are at least three reasons for teaching the humanities to all educated people and especially to physicians: (1) they are vehicles for teaching the liberal arts; (2) they convey a special kind of knowledge that liberates the imagination; and (3) they are sources of delectation for the human spirit.

Vehicles for Teaching the Liberal Arts

It is a common misconception that the humanities and the liberal arts are synonymous. This is an error as common to humanists as it is to the general public. The liberal arts are habits of mind, not disciplines or bodies of knowledge. They have, since classical times, consisted of the intellectual skills needed to be a free man—not only in the political sense, but more critically in the sense of being free of the tyranny of other men's thinking and opinions, free to make up one's own mind and take one's own position, free to become a person of one's own. The liberal arts comprise the skills most commonly associated with being human—the capability to think correctly and critically, to read and understand language, to write and speak clearly, to make moral judgments, to recognize the beautiful, and to possess a sense of the continuity between the present and the past which it inherits.

Philosophy, literature, language and history are the classical *Studia Humanitatum*. They can most effectively inculcate those skills that enable us to live truly human and humane lives. They are preeminently the arts of the word. Only humans use and manipulate words and symbols to express ideas. To serve that end the humanities must be taught liberally—as vehicles for the liberal arts and not as specialties, not primarily as research endeavors, not as professionalized bodies of knowledge, and not as imitations of science. That they are often not taught as vehicles for the liberal arts accounts for much of the loss of connection between the humanities and contemporary life.

Yet the liberal arts are the cognitive instruments needed in every truly human activity. They enable the trained mind to address any body of data in an intelligent and orderly way, to distinguish truth from untruth, opinion from demonstrated conclusion, and to define what is known and not known, to distinguish fact from value. While they are best taught through the humanities, the liberal arts are also essential for a full appreciation of the humanities themselves as bodies of knowledge. They are as essential to science as to the humanities. Science and the humanities are essential but different ways of knowing reality. To minimize those differences is to lose sight of the importance of a productive tension between these two ways of knowing the world.

Since they are the working tools of the educated person they are essential to the daily work of all the professions. In medicine the arts of the word are intrinsic in the arts of the clinician.[3] The physician's thinking is not solely scientific. To be sure, scientific and actuarial logic are crucial in diagnosis, prognosis, and therapeutics. But in deciding what ought to be done the physician is required often to analyze an ethical dilemma and make a moral judgment. Differential diagnosis is an exercise in dialectics; history-taking is the development of a narrative—really a biography—using a unique primary source, the patient himself; the physician-patient transaction is an exercise in communication demanding a deep perception of the meanings of words, language, and culture. The cognitive skills of the liberal arts are what make the physician's decision more than the simple application of diagnostic algorithms or decision trees. They are what distinguish the technical from the professional elements of medical practice. They are as important to being a good physician as the knowledge of the basic and clinical sciences.

Liberating the Imagination; The Content of the Humanities

The humanistic disciplines are not only vehicles for the liberal arts, but also they convey a special kind of knowledge not susceptible to the methods of the sciences. They liberate the imagination. Their specific content antedates modern science and in some ways opposes as well as complements it.

The humanities deal with the dramatic, the artistic, the meanings of language, symbol, and myth, and the history of men's ideas about reality and how men respond to the experience of living. Humanistic studies seek out the idiosyncratic, the particularities, the uniqueness in human experience. They have the power, too, to evoke vicarious experience through the artful use of language, sound, paint, stone, or design. They struggle with all the things science must eschew—the mysteries of living, dying, suffering, enjoying, with their meaning for persons and the way they are communicated between human beings. The prodigious advances of science have not eradicated mystery; wisdom is still a rare commodity; creativity is as inexplicable as ever; aesthetic experiences delight some of us and not others, The humanities wrestle in every age with the same questions and problems—who are we, why are we here—with the inextinguishable search for meanings. Science, too, searches for the meanings of natural phenomena, but the humanities focus on those experiences that are not quantifiable, testable, or instrumentally explicable. Science has values of its own. While it uses values, it does not prepare us with the methods needed to analyze, judge, and sort out competing values.

Science deals with new answers to old problems. Its content is progressive and cumulative. Scientific paradigms change. Things previously credible are no longer so. Instead, the humanities ponder the same questions, often posed in the same way, century after century. They exasperate anyone who seeks the solace of certitude because they always throw us back upon ourselves—to ascertain our own meanings. They ask us to make our own assessments and force us to realize that we cannot be fully human by merely parroting other men's opinions. They create anxieties precisely because they challenge us to be persons, to locate ourselves not just in time and place, but in relationship to ideas—other men's and our own.

Medicine is turning today to the humanities because it needs this special kind of knowledge. Being ill and being healed are complex, not wholly comprehensible phenomena, involving the person as much as his organs and tissues. The ill person is an historical entity whose experience is not wholly penetrable by even the most dedicated healer. To heal another person we must understand how illness wounds his or her humanity, what values are at stake, what this illness means and how *this* illness expresses the whole life of *this* patient. The physician who does not understand his own humanity can hardly heal another's. This is a powerful reason why the humanities are now taught in many medical schools even though they were studied in college.

Literature has proven an effective way to teach empathy for the sick, suffering, and dying. Through the creative words of George Eliot, Tolstoy, Chekhov, Camus, or Thomas Mann, the experience of being ill, being a doctor, or dying can be powerfully evoked and vicariously felt. Literature also teaches the nuances of language, the way its structure and form communicate the inner experience of another person.

Philosophy teaches the arts of logic and dialectic but also tells us what men have thought about human nature, truth, goodness, right and wrong. It challenges the physician to know his own values and to give a reasonable account of them before daring to undertake the delicate task of deciding with another person what is "good" for that person. The skills of ethics are as essential to being a competent physician as those of the basic and clinical sciences because at the heart of the clinical there is a value choice—an interaction between what the doctor decides what is good for this person and what this person thinks is good.

History traces where we have been as a species and what constraints the human past puts on each of us. It creates the sense of continuity without which individuals and societies lose their bearings. It teaches how to validate a temporal account of human events which is what the patient's own history turns out to be. In a sense the physician has an opportunity rarely afforded the historian—he is almost always in direct contact with his primary source, a unique one at that—the patient. Yet how many times do physicians, like historians, ignore the source in favor of a plethora of secondary and tertiary sources—or their own imaginations?

All the things the humanities teach, write, and think about have some relevance for the work of medicine and, parenthetically, of all the professions. That is why they are essential to good education in the first place. The need for reinforcement in medical school of what they teach is strong evidence of the pertinence of the content as well as the method of the humanities.

Sources of Delectation for the Human Spirit

The practical uses of the method and content of the humanities must not overshadow their intrinsic worth, which is to enrich and enhance the whole experience of human living. This value of humanistic learning and study transcends even their most practical applications because it enables us to live with satisfaction.

To cultivate literature, philosophy, history, painting, or music is to add special dimensions of delight to living. These pursuits delight us because they correspond so closely with those capacities that most clearly distinguish us as human—the capabilities to recognize and experience truth, beauty, and virtue. They stretch our capacity to enjoy what other men have created, or what we may create ourselves, thus allowing us to communicate something of our inner lived world to our fellows.

Medical men have always turned to the humanities and the arts to counter the aridity of too zealous a dedication to the technical demands of their daily work. Hours spent in the pursuit of humanistic studies refresh and restore. They reawaken sensitivities obtunded by the demands of time, routine, and detail that beset the conscientious practitioner. The number of physicians who write, paint, play an instrument, or read literature attests to the restorative powers of the humanities. Some become so entranced that they abandon medicine altogether and become "medical truants."[4] Others can even continue as active practitioners and lead a double life as creative artists.

It must be apparent by now that I believe that one cannot be a genuinely competent physician without imbibing the three things that, uniquely, the humanities have to give—their method, their content, and their power to enrich and restore the spirit. Indeed, I would say further that failure in the professions is as much a result of defects in humanistic education as it is in technical skill or information.

The liberal arts are, moreover, the indispensable requirements for a democratic and civilized society. Democracy itself is impossible without citizens whose minds are free enough to resist the tyranny of political demagoguery and who can discern the values that underlie public policies. Civil and international order depend upon a humane education. As

Camus put it, "And naturally, a man with whom one cannot reason is a man to be feared."[5] So, too, those pursuits that elevate the human spirit and make for civilization—the arts, music, literature, and conversation—are impossible without the humanities. The utility of the liberal arts to medicine is a subset of their indispensability for humane living within which medicine now plays so important a part.

Why Teach the Humanities in Medical School?

Let us grant that the humanities are important to the work of medicine and that they are tools needed by all educated persons. Why should they be taught in medical schools? Why not require that they be taught better or more fully in college than at present? Why take time in the packed medical curriculum for what should be done before students enter medical school? Does this not amount to remedial education? Is it not an unnecessary expansion of our already swollen and pretentious medical curriculum?

To begin with, there is no suggestion here that teaching humanities in medical schools should substitute for a liberal college education. As the intellectual tools of all educated people, the liberal arts are proper domain of college and secondary schools. However, even a good liberal arts education will need reinforcement, repetition and refurbishment in professional education for several good reasons.

First, we know from our experience with pre-medical science that exposure to college subjects does not mean that contagion or even subclinical infection will occur. College subjects, even those directly related to medicine, need repetition and connection with the daily work of physicians. It is a puzzling but persistent fact that medical students often fail to see the connections between the things they study in college and their utility in medicine. Thus, the points of "connection" need to be made clear in clinical teaching even if the student has had an authentic liberal arts education. If he has not, it is all the more important that these connections be established for the first time. They must be demonstrated to be intrinsic to being a good physician or they will not have any lasting influence on the medical student.

Moreover, college teaching in the humanities often neglects one or more of the three contributions of the humanities—to free the mind, to free the imagination, and to enrich the experience of being human. Often they are taught solely for their content as fields of special study. This is a legitimate aim for aspirants to professional scholarship but it is insufficient to encompass the fuller contribution that the liberal arts make to the clinical arts. In this sense, teaching humanities in medicine does have something of a remedial tinge to it. I wish it were not so. For the most part, however, repetition and reinforcement, and not remediation, will be the pedagogic aim.

Medical students need actual practice and demonstration in how the liberal arts apply in clinical medicine and the healing encounter. They are understandably wary of armchair ethicists. The lasting lessons in a medical education are the practical ones—the hands-on experiences under supervision in small groups. This is the special distinction of American medical education. It is particularly well suited to an exploration of the student's personal values, logic, and presuppositions. These need to be as carefully examined as his scientific logic and judgment. In this way, the close integration of value and fact in clinical decisions can be examined in individual cases, in the context which will be the clinician's habitat for all the years of his practice.

Finally, students who have enjoyed a creditable experience in the humanities in college will want to enrich it while in medical school. Some of the best students I have encountered have complained bitterly of the lack of intellectual stimulation in the usual medical curriculum. They accept the need for a plethora of facts. But they are surfeited with information unaccompanied by critical reflection on the deeper issues involved in the humane use of their increasing reservoir of facts.

Having experienced the capabilities of humanistic studies to enrich all of life's experiences, these students want to deepen their contact with them. Since medical curricula are so drastically out of phase with university calendars, they cannot take university courses in the humanities. The only alternative is to offer such courses in the medical school. The skepticism and negativity of medical faculties notwithstanding, these students can easily handle some study of the humanities along with their medical education, to the enhancement of both.

If we grant the importance of the humanities and the need to teach them in medical school, we must still avoid pretentiousness in the aims and objectives of such teaching. Certainly the medical school must not misappropriate the function of the liberal arts college, nor aim to make each student an ethicist, philosopher, literary critic, or historian. The aim must be to refurbish, renew, and implant the liberal arts in the student's experience so they can be used in medicine, clinical decision-making, and judgment. All students who intend to be clinicians ought to have enough familiarity with the skills of ethics and enough sensitivity to moral questions to know how to define a conflict of values between themselves and their patients and to resolve it. This means they should be able to analyze a critical dilemma as rigorously as they analyze a dilemma in diagnosis or prognosis. The physician should be familiar with his own values and presuppositions and know how to handle conflicts of values in a morally responsible way. He or she cannot distinguish or compromise a principle at a lesser level if he does not understand the ethical foundations of the decision. For this reason, all physicians should be able to use ethical reasoning, to understand the meaning of the terms used in ethical discourse and how they apply in clinical decision-making.

Medical students and physicians need to appreciate that the medical decision rests on several modes of reasoning—not just one. Classical and probabilistic logic are intermingled in medical decisions and both are modulated by the end of medicine—a right and good healing action for a particular patient. That end is moral as well as scientific; it requires a combination of objectivity and compassion, the capacity to stand back, and at the same time to empathize and become involved with the patient.

It is this combination of objective compassion, or "compassionate objectivity" as Temkin has termed it, that fuses the sciences and the humanities in the doctor's education.[6] In addition to the basic skills in ethics, then, at least one other humanistic study pertinent to medicine should be experienced by each student. For some it will be literature with emphasis on evocation of empathy and vicarious experience of illness or suffering, for others it might be medical history, for others philosophy or religious studies. The aim in these studies, as with teaching ethics and human values, is to expand the physician's awareness of as many of the dimensions of healing as possible. The various ways in which these objectives are being reached in different medical schools are detailed in the most recent *Human Values Teaching Programs for Health Professionals.*[7]

How Should the Liberal Arts be Taught? By Whom?

How should the humanities and human values be taught, when, and by whom? These operational questions can now be addressed on the basis of a decade of experience in the nation's medical schools. Drawing on our recent survey of some 125 schools and personal visits to some 60 of them, we can outline a profile of how the most successful programs answer these questions.

Most successful programs consist of an introductory course in the first year, followed by some integration of teaching in the clinical years, and the opportunity for elective experiences in specific humanistic disciplines throughout the medical curriculum. The emphasis in the introductory courses is on ethics and human values, as well as clinical decision-making. Teaching is most effective when conducted in seminars, small groups, or a combination of lecture and small group discussion. The optimal approach is exposure to specific clinical cases or problems, selected to illustrate the major dilemmas encountered in clinical practice.

Following the introductory experience, many schools offer more detailed elective instruction in ethics or one of the humanities related to medicine. But the most important teaching occurs in the clinical years—not by lecture, but by some form of integration with instruction at the bedside or in the clinic.

The most successful integration occurs when teaching of human values least disrupts the normal patterns of clinical instruction. One very useful method is to devote one grand rounds per month in a major clinical department to a case in which ethical or moral dilemmas figure prominently. Another is, in each clerkship, to spend one session per week discussing a current case or problem pertinent to the appropriate specialty. Most successful experiences are built on current cases in which decisions are being made as part of the day-by-day care of patients on a clinical unit. In this way the students see that the liberal arts are united to the arts of the clinician and are therefore part of being a "good" doctor.

As with all clinical teaching, cases must be selected carefully, the questions they pose clearly defined, and back-up readings offered for deeper understanding. The all-too-frequent reliance on a fortuitous clinical situation or off-the-cuff discussion is even more damaging in this kind of teaching than it is in clinical medicine *per se*. This caveat is particularly serious in teaching human values, since the amateur ethicist too easily substitutes random thought and "experience" for critical and informed reflection. Few clinicians are well enough grounded in the discipline of ethical analysis to teach ethics by themselves.

For this reason, the optimal teaching mode is a cooperative one. An experienced clinician interested in, and open to, serious discussion about ethical and value questions must work with a bona fide humanist or ethicist interested in communicating what he knows to medical students and their faculties. The technical expertise of the clinician complements the ethical expertise of the humanist. In this way the positivism of clinical medicine and the intellectual hubris of the humanist are both leavened to the advantage of student and patient.

To be successful, the humanist must respect the difficulties and urgencies of clinical decision-making, concentrate on concrete details, and restrain his natural impulse to criticize what he may perceive as moral lapse or sophomoric ethics. He must be secure in his own discipline, willing to learn and to teach in the milieu of actual decision-making. There is evidence that, given the satisfaction of these conditions, humanists are well accepted and can teach effectively in clinical settings.[8] The initial skepticism of clinicians usually yields if the humanist combines competence with authentic interest in improving the quality of clinical decisions.

Will Physicians and Patient Care Be Better?

One of the most difficult questions is whether or not teaching human values makes for better physicians or patient care. The current emphasis on evaluation and cost/benefit analyses guarantees that this will be the skeptics' trump card. Unfortunately, it cannot be answered with definitive data at present. But neither can the question be answered for individual basic or clinical sciences. Within limits, more technical knowledge should make for better decisions. By the same token, more familiarity with making ethical decisions should improve their quality.

So far as ethics and the humanities go, they undoubtedly raise the sensitivity of students and faculty to ethical and value questions. Such issues as patient autonomy, truth-telling, promise-keeping, consent, and justice in the patient-physician relationship are now openly discussed. Even a decade ago they were the private domain of each physician, not open to criticism or examination, even among one's own peers. The growing number of articles on such topics in scientific and professional medical journals is sufficient evidence of a heightened sensitivity and common concern in the profession for the moral foundations of physicians' daily work.

Almost everywhere, as a result, patients are better apprised of their part in clinical decisions, and of the value and moral issues woven into their relationships with the physician. This is a result to be desired in a society that is democratic, educated, and pluralistic in its value systems. Whatever personalizes and particularizes healing will make it more humane. The heightened sensitivity of physicians to value questions cannot fail to make some of them better persons, more competent physicians, and more efficient healers. What better justification can there be for teaching the method, content, and rewards of the humanities of physicians, while they are also learning how to be good physicians?

Some Problems for the Post-Evangelical Years

Even if the teaching of the humanities and liberal arts in medical schools can be justified, and financial support assured, there remain some significant impediments to its future viability.

Perhaps the most subtle but most critical danger is a failure to secure the intellectual foundations of this kind of teaching. It is true that a large volume of literature has appeared and this seems to be expanding at present. Close scrutiny of this literature raises some serious questions however. Most of it is in medical ethics and bioethics. This is to be expected given the preoccupation of public and profession with the urgency of many ethical dilemmas. But there are some signs that the productivity of this kind of research may be reaching a plateau. The growing evidence of repetition points to some exhaustion of the vein of bioethics *per se*.

There is promise in the still-small literature on the philosophical foundations of medical ethics. The logical, epistemological, or metaphysical problems underlying the more urgent ethical issues are receiving more attention.[9] Formal interest in fundamental questions about the nature of medicine, the concepts of health and illness, the meaning of autonomy, and the broader issues of social medical ethics are receiving more attention. So, too, is the search for some theory of medical ethics.[10]

These studies are still too sparse to tell whether a vigorous intellectual effort can be sustained. No formal theory of medicine or healing is yet available. The humanities in medicine and medical ethics can survive in the hypercritical environment of the medical schools only if the research they foster compares favorably in quality and depth to that which is occurring in the medical sciences.

Equally worrisome is the lack of models whom students can emulate—clinicians who themselves can demonstrate that the liberal arts are useful, and actually used in daily clinical medicine. Without such models, medical students quickly conclude that the few physicians who can function at the junction of medicine and the humanities are *rarae aves*—more to be observed than emulated.

The problem of faculty development will remain serious for some years to come. It cannot be approached through formal training programs. Faculties resent any suggestion that they are not "ethical" or lack something in their pedagogical armamentaria. Many will protest that they "teach medical ethics every day" in their care of patients. The most successful approach is by some form of participation, not some massive institutional program of "faculty renewal."

The mere presence, for example, of a program teaching bioethics or human values alerts a faculty to the issues and generates discussions with students and faculty colleagues. If ethical grand rounds or sessions within the clerkships are part of the program, many faculty and house staff members will be exposed. This is a non-threatening way to introduce the subject, to permit involvement when faculty members are included to do so and on their own terms.

Another effective way to involve clinical faculty members is by their participation as discussion leaders in small groups, following the more formal seminar lecture presentations. Many schools use this method, which has the advantage not only of involving the clinical faculty, but of convincing the student that the subjects have clinical relevance. To be successful, this method requires careful selection, orientation, and supervision of the participating faculty, whose teaching capabilities, sophistication, and knowledge will vary widely.

Perhaps the most hopeful sign for the future is the number of medical students manifesting an interest in a career that combines clinical medicine with bioethics or one of the humanities. Some are interested in obtaining both the M.D. and the Ph.D. degrees and hope to follow teaching careers in these fields in medical schools. While formal programs are still in their early stages, a significant number of students on their own are doing master's degree–level work in the humanities and human values and some in divinity schools. Others are taking a year out to study and do research in the humanities or ethics.

Another source for faculty development are the special institutes and seminars in bioethics, humanities and human values in medicine like those at the Kennedy Institute of Ethics at Georgetown, at various universities under auspices of the National Endowment for the Humanities, the Hastings Center, or fellowships of the Institute on Human Values in Medicine. These institutes vary in length but they have often had a significant impact on the career decision of both humanists and medical faculty members out of proportion to their brevity.

Faculty development in the humanities related to medicine parallels the development in the late 1940s when medical faculties began to educate themselves in the sciences basic to medicine. This was the group from which came today's senior clinical scientists and clinical investigators. They were succeeded by clinicians more formally educated in the biological sciences, even with M.D. and Ph.D. degrees.

Tomorrow's clinical humanists and ethicists will similarly come from the ranks of today's medical students and young faculty members now schooling themselves in the techniques and knowledge of the humanities and liberal arts as they relate to medicine and healing.

The most important assurance that these programs will not disappear from the medical curriculum is of course the continuing importance of value and the enduring nature of ethical questions in medicine. There is no question that medical, moral dilemmas will continue to confront individuals and society. The wise use of medical knowledge will demand the same intensity of engagement between medicine and the humanistic disciplines that medicine has enjoyed so fruitfully over the last century with the physical and biological sciences.

The public concerns for the humane use of medicine and other technologies is not likely to wane in the years ahead. Medicine has been too influential in contemporary life to be left to professional and technical judgment alone.

There is every indication therefore that powerful external stimuli will impel medical schools to continue their new-found teaching and research efforts in human values, ethics, and the humanities. In the Middle Ages, Greek philosophy and Christian theology confronted and influenced each other. In the last century science and medicine have had a similar mutual influence. Today, medicine and the humanities seem about to engage each other in the same way—medicine becoming the science of man *par excellence,* the humanities giving to that science its humane purposes and values.

In his latest book, Norman Cousins quotes one of the fathers of clinical science, Claude Bernard, as follows: "I feel convinced there will come a day when physiologists, poets, and philosophers will all speak the same language."[11] The national experience of the last decade or so in teaching the humanities, liberal arts, and human values in medical schools, is a beginning fulfillment of Claude Bernard's prophecy. It confirms the fact that science and the humanities, values and technology are not incompatible, that they converge in the clinical decisions, and that they are both essential, though different, ways of knowing about the realities of illness, healing, and health.

Medicine is therefore the example *par excellence* of the "connections" between the liberal arts and the humanities and everyday life. Even in the coming "post-evangelical" period, the humanities and the liberal arts can be confidently and unequivocally justified as permanent and integral parts of the education of all health professionals.

Notes

Presented at the Conference on the Humanities and the Profession of Medicine, The National Humanities Center, April 16–17, 1982.

Based on a paper presented before the Council of Graduate Schools in the United States 31st Annual Meeting, *Graduate Education in the Humanities: The Need for Reaffirmation, Connection, and Justification,* December 2, 1981.

1. Pellegrino, E. D., and McElhinney, T. K., *Teaching Ethics, the Humanities, and Human Values in Medical Schools: A Ten-Year Overview* (Washington DC: Institute on Human Values in Medicine, Society for Health and Human Values, 1982).

2. Report of the Commission on the Humanities, *The Humanities in American Life* (Berkeley and Los Angeles: University of California Press, 1980), p. 21.

3. Pellegrino, E. D., "The Clinical Arts and the Arts of the Word," *The Pharos*, 44(4) (1981): 2–8, Alpha Omega Alpha Honor Medical Society.

4. Lord Moynihan of Leeds, *Truants: The Story of Some Who Deserted Medicine Yet Triumphed* (London: Cambridge University Press, 1936).

5. Camus, Albert, *Neither Victims Nor Executioners* (New York: Continuum, 1980), p. 26.

6. Temkin, Owsei, *The Double Face of Janus* (Baltimore: The Johns Hopkins University Press, 1977).

7. McElhinney, T. K. (ed.), *Human Values Teaching Programs for Health Professionals* (Armore, PA: Whitmore Publishing Company, 1981).

8. Pellegrino, E. D., and McElhinney, T. K., *op. cit.*

9. See especially *The Journal of Medicine and Philosophy* and *Theoretical Medicine*, formerly *Metamedicine*. Also, a recent anthology gathers some of the conceptual work on health and illness: Caplan, A. L., Engelhardt, H. T., Jr., and McCartney, J. J., *Concepts of Health and Disease* (Reading, MA: Addison Wesley, 1981).

10. Examples are: Veatch, R. M., *A Theory of Medical Ethics* (New York: Basic Books, 1981); Pellegrino, E. D., and Thomasma, D., *The Philosophical Basis of Medical Practice* (Oxford: Oxford University Press, 1981); and Pellegrino, E. D., and Thomasma, D., "Toward an Axiology for Medicine: A Response to Kazem Sadegh-Zadeh," *Metamedicine* 2 (June 1981), D. Reidel, pp. 331–342, as well as the growing number of papers applying Rawls' *Theory of Justice* to the issues on bioethics.

11. Cousins, Norman (ed.), *The Physician in Literature* (Philadelphia: W. B. Saunders, 1982), p. xxiii.

SIXTEEN

Agape and Ethics

Some Reflections on Medical Morals from a Catholic Christian Perspective

Introduction

A Catholic "perspective" on morals—medical or otherwise—implies
a coherent view of the moral life that transcends purely philosophical ethics in some distinctive ways. What those ways consist in, whether they are
different in kind or degree, and whether they entail a distinctive moral life
are all important and still problematic questions.

At a minimum, any definition of a Catholic perspective must confront some of these fundamental questions: Does a Christian belief entail
a content and methodology distinct from, and closed to, philosophical
ethics? Is uncritical fideism or unrelenting rationalism the only alternative? Is ethics as a reasoned discipline reconcilable with ethics as a response to the moral imperatives of the Gospels or their authoritative
interpretation by the Official Church?

Many of these issues are engaged in contemporary theological discourse. They form the inescapable backdrop for this essay, which examines them in the limited confines of professional ethics. My principal aim
is to examine the way in which the central virtue of the Christian life—the
virtue of Charity—shapes the whole of medical morals.

This essay proceeds in two steps: In the first, it examines some of the
conceptual relationships between reason and Charity in traditional and

contemporary ethical discourse. In the second, it tries to show how Charity shapes our interpretations of: (1) the central principles of philosophical ethics—beneficence, autonomy, and justice; (2) the way we construe the healing relationship itself; and (3) the way we make some of the crucial moral choices facing health professionals and society today.

Two important caveats must be established at the outset: First, the Christian virtue of Charity is the central distinguishing feature of a Catholic and Christian perspective on the moral life. Christian ethics is by definition therefore an "agapeistic" ethics. But this is not synonymous with the situation ethics of Joseph Fletcher [12] which claims also to be agapeistic. Fletcher's form of ethics eschews principle and precept and dissociates reason and Charity in ways incompatible with a Catholic perspective.

Second, to put some emphasis on the practical consequences of an agapeistic ethics does not necessarily place orthopraxy and orthodoxy in opposition to each other [45]. Rather it is the special task of Catholic and Christian ethics to reconcile doctrine and practice and to effect a harmonious equilibrium between them. Only in that equilibrium can the moral life of the Catholic Christian become the integrated whole required by both reason and faith.

The theses I wish to argue are three: First, any medical moral philosophy ought to begin with the nature of medicine itself, as a human activity, which, on grounds of natural reason alone, imposes certain obligations on the physician and other health professionals. This is the "internal" morality of medicine itself [25]. Second, a "Catholic perspective" begins but does not end with this internal morality. It adds dimensions of insight and obligation that grow out of Christian teachings of Charity such that Charity "informs" ethical reasoning in certain specific ways. Just how Charity and reason relate is a central question for traditional and contemporary accounts of the moral life. A "Catholic perspective" for our times should try to reconcile the traditional and contemporary views.

Third, though the relationships between reason and Charity and between traditional and contemporary views of Christian ethics are still under discussion, certain moral choices are clearly more consistent with the virtue of Charity than others. It *does* make a practical difference if one professes to be a Christian as well as a physician, nurse, or administrator.

In this discussion, three topics pertinent to the Catholic perspective are consciously excluded: (1) the relationships between ethics as a reasoned discipline and the teachings of the official magisterium; (2) the place of the casuistic method in medical moral decisions; and (3) the moral dilemmas of reproductive and sexual morality. The first is amply covered in papers by Hughes, McCormick, Fuchs, and Cahill; the second is the subject of a recent study [23]; and the third is so much at the focus of Catholic moral theology today that it needs no further discussion here ([29, 7]).

Instead, my focus will be on the kind of person the Catholic physician and health professional should be. This is more consistent with a virtue-based ethic than with a focus on the solution of specific moral quandaries. Though the emphasis is on virtue-based ethics, the great importance of linking virtue, principle, obligation, and rule is clearly acknowledged. It is beyond the scope of this essay to forge those links except tangentially.

The Internal Morality of Medicine

Many prominent thinkers[1] conclude that belief in God, Creation, Redemption, and the Incarnation does not provide specific answers to general or medical moral problems. They argue that the whole of the right and the good is open to human reason since the good is intrinsic to the world God created. On this view, God asks obedience to moral law because it is good; moral law is not good simply because God asks obedience to it.

In the case of medical ethics, Fuchs summarizes this argument as follows: Medicine is a moral enterprise because it deals with human problems. The ethics of medicine derives from medicine as a human activity. Its moral nature is prior to, or at least not dependent on, faith. Medical ethics thus must accord with human understanding, and in this sense it has a certain autonomy [14].

Fr. Sokolowski follows essentially the same line of argument. He begins with the phenomenology of medicine as a special kind of human activity [51]. He focuses on the art of medicine and the way it functions in the physician-patient relationship. What is at stake is the person of the patient. He and the physician, as rational beings, each play a part in effecting the end of medicine, which is the good of the patient. In this relationship, the physician is the embodiment of the medical art whose end is the patient's good.

On this view, beneficence is a moral obligation which is programmed into the art. If the physician does harm, he violates the art. If he is faithful to the art, he becomes a good moral agent and is, himself, ennobled. Thus, the art establishes the way in which physician and patient should relate to each other. This is the "internal" morality of medicine itself, and it is derivable by reason with Christian belief. I have argued similarly for the obligations that are derivable from the fact of illness, the vulnerability of the patient, and the physician's promise to help [36].

According to Sokolowski, Christian belief affects this internal morality of medicine in several ways: it reveals more fully and truthfully the good intrinsic to the art; it corrects the tendency to reductionism and the neglect of form characteristic of modern scientific medicine; it highlights the dignity of the human persons—doctor and patient—who confront each other in the healing relationship.

Christian belief thus expands the range of insights available to ethics as a reasoned discipline.[2] As Lisa Cahill points out [6], the Catholic perspective operates best when it brings together philosophical reflection, religious images, logical interpretation, concrete human experience, and magisterial teachings. Each contributes to a fuller comprehension of the natural law and enables Christians to make moral choices in conformity with the spirit of Gospel teachings.

On this view, ethics as a reasoned discipline becomes insufficient to express the whole of the moral life. It becomes more than the application of principles and rules. It gains insights from the Gospel teachings on Charity that are not admissible into ethical discourse by those who reject those teachings.

Romano Guardini, in his meditation on the Sermon on the Mount, puts it this way:

Once we restrict ethics to its modern sense of principles it no longer adequately covers the Sermon on the Mount. What Jesus revealed there was no mere ethical code but a whole new existence, one in which an ethos is immediately evident. . . . Only in love is fulfillment of the ethical possible. Love is the New Testament. ([17], p. 79)

and Thomas Merton says similarly:

We must, of course, point out that mere ethics, as a moral philosophy, has its limitations. It needs to be completed by a higher science that apprehends other and more mysterious norms which have been revealed to man by God and which arise out of the deep personal relation of man to God in saving grace, by which man is oriented to his true and perfect finality: his ultimate fulfillment as a person in the love of God and of his fellow man in God. ([31], p. 127)

The Philosophical Status of Charity-Based Ethics

We agree with Guardini and Merton that we must go beyond "mere ethics" to fulfill the Christian commandment of love. Like St. Paul (Col. 2:8), we must be wary of the possibility of the submergence of Charity by philosophy. Both Guardini and Merton recognize that it is the complementarity between faith and reason that distinguishes the Catholic moral tradition and preserves it against the heart-over-head experiential ethics of Jansenists, Quietists, and Modernists. Nonetheless, a Charity-based agapeistic ethic poses difficult philosophical questions that remain problematic.

Frankena, for example, notes the philosophical dilemma in the double imperative of Christian ethics—to love God and one's neighbor as oneself ([12], p. 58). He argues that an agapeistic ethic could be grounded in the principle of love of neighbor but that love of God could not be derived from beneficence alone. Without faith in God's existence we could not derive the command to love God. But for the Christian this is the ground of his agapeistic ethic. The Christian loves God because God has created all that is good. Charitable beneficence is grounded in God's love for us and in His revelation of that love. It follows from faith, which is the "virtue of entry" into the Christian life and which assures us of a personal relationship of love with God.

Yet, Frankena admits ". . . there is a sense in which the law of love underlies the entire moral law even if this cannot be derived from it" ([13], p. 57). That the law and all the prophets are summed up in the love of God and neighbor is not a conclusion of reason, but neither does it violate reason.

These metaethical difficulties do not preclude the possibility of a Christian moral philosophy. Every moral philosophy rests ultimately on some ordering principle, whether it be the categorical imperative, the principle of utility, moral sentiment, love of man without God, or love of man because of God. In each philosophy, there is, at the outset, an act of faith in some ordering principle. To deny that any such principle exists is itself an ordering principle. For the Christian, the existence of God and revelation is one such starting position. It does not, on that account, have a lesser claim to coherence than moral philosophies that deny both God and revelation.

In recent years, Catholic thinkers have approached the question of a specifically Christian and Catholic ethics with renewed interest. They have examined the ways in which Charity and reason are related by linking traditional moral theology to contemporary philosophy and psychology. These attempts are not always mutually reconcilable. But they do open up possibilities for the fresh synthesis of old and new ideas that a comprehensive Catholic moral philosophy requires today.

For Catholics, the central question is how to reconcile an ethics based in reason, principles, and precepts with the fact that the fullness of the Christian ethos of charitable love is somehow beyond ethics in Guardini and Merton's sense. Is it possible to avoid the extremes of an unthinking totally experiential fideism on the one hand, and a rigid, unfeeling, legalistic rationalism on the other?

Hallett attempts an answer by linking Charity and reason through analytic philosophy [18]. He focuses on the criteria by which a Christian ethic based in Charity can be judged. He posits a system of "Christian Moral Reasoning" that purports to reconcile the traditional allegiance to reason and objective norms with the concrete particulars involved in actual moral decisions. He proposes to avoid both the absolutization of precepts he finds in traditional Christian ethics and the abandonment of objective norms in the agapeistic situation ethics of Joseph Fletcher.

Hallett thus argues for a "third position" between the extremes of preceptive and anti-preceptive ethics. This he calls "value ethics," which makes use of the insights of analytical philosophy and judges the Christian nature of an act or decision by a balance of Christian values over disvalues. Hallett's concept of Christian value maximization is provocative and deserves further examination. His proposal is, however, largely procedural. It bypasses the substantive metaethical issues. He tries to give due preeminence to Charity, even while denying the value of a specific hierarchy of values which would give the first place to Charity.

An even more ambitious attempt to re-define Christian ethics comes from the "Murray Group"—theologians thinking, in the spirit of John Courtney Murray, from a "North American" viewpoint. They examine Catholic theology "through the eyes of American philosophy" [33], by which they mean the philosophies of James, Dewey, Whitehead, Pierce, Royce, and especially Jonathan Edwards. From these sources they claim to derive a theology that is not only rational and objective but also takes into account the experiential, affective, aesthetic, and pragmatic dimensions of the moral life. They hope thus to balance the excessive rationalism they perceive in traditional Catholic moral philosophy by drawing on experience, feeling, and imagination.

This perspective is well represented by William Spohn [52]. Spohn expands on the place of discernment, and *metanoia,* in making concrete ethical decisions by what he calls the "reasoning heart." The reasoning heart does not contravene reasoning and moral principles in ethics. Rather, it operates within them, but draws also on imagination and experience to illuminate individual moral decisions. "Discernment," says Spohn,

> remains a personal search for the action of God in one's own history and in the events of the world. Although its conclusions are not morally generalizable as judgments of rationality are, the reasoning heart of the Christian finds normative guidance in the symbols and story of revelation. ([52], p. 66)

On this view, what distinguishes Christian ethics is that it is motivated, in the moment of moral choice, by a specific set of affections—those that most closely correspond to the character, affections, and goodness of

Christ. Christian ethics differs from purely philosophical ethics because it can draw on these affections which, without conversion, are closed to non-Christians.

This is not the place to enter into a detailed critique of this interesting mode of theologizing. Spohn recognizes the dangers of intuitionism and situationism in his approach. Just precisely how the balance is struck between moral sentiment and moral reason in this form of theology is not clear from Spohn's or from the other essays in the anthology. Like Hallett, Spohn is seeking a middle position between the extremes of fideism and rationalism. As with all middle positions, finding the precise point of balance is the crucial challenge.

Another linkage between Christian belief and philosophy is Pittenger's application of Whitehead's process philosophy to the understanding of religious affirmation [43]. Pittenger examines the origins of Christian faith in humans as a Whiteheadian "event" and how, in those terms, it apprehends the reality of Jesus and the way that reality opens "a window into God." Here, as with any interpretation of Christian belief in terms of a specific philosophical system, the links with more traditional ways of philosophizing need critical examination. With Whitehead, or any of the other "North American" philosophical approaches, there is always a danger of eroding the still-viable truths of the more traditional Catholic moral philosophy.

Pertinent to many of the attempts to balance affect and intellect in moral decisions are the current discussions on the relationships between moral cognition and moral motivation. Here the question is this: Does a recognition of the right and good impel to doing the right and good? Are these totally separable operations, and, if they are not separable, how are they in fact linked?

Such questions are relevant to the nature of Christian ethics and to the various meanings of discernment as it is found in St. Ignatius, Karl Rahner, or the Murray Group. Some theorists suggest that moral motivation is a function of one's sense of self, rather than a function of one's conceptualization skills on the one hand or a matter of anticipations of external bribes and rewards on the other [55]. Conversion to the Christian Faith creates St. Paul's "new man," one whose sense of self is shaped by the Christian virtues. Is this the way being a Christian makes a difference in ethics? Is it this transformation of the self that links cognition and motivation? Is this the locus for the "illumination" spoken of in the more classical moral theologians and the "discernment" preferred by their contemporary counterparts?

Each of these approaches attempts to reinterpret, in contemporary terms, the more traditional viewpoints on the relationships of philosophical and theological ethics as found in St. Thomas. They are interesting in their own right, and they force us to seek a deeper understanding of the Catholic moral tradition. Gilby reminds us that St. Thomas

> jogs us to remember that philosophical ethics is contained within *sacra doctrina,* that the discourse is drawing from sources beyond the reach of reason alone, and that from within there is a reaching out to a good beyond reasonable statement, the ultimate good, transcendent yet not abstract, the burden of all yearning which is God himself, the end beyond measure of all morality. ([15], p. 148)

St. Thomas' extended treatment of the human psychology of habit and passion gives a personalist cast to his ethics that should be reassuring to contemporary thinkers who fear the rigidity and absolutization of an exclusively preceptive moral system. As Walgrave points out, St. Thomas was

> in his own way a personalist . . . because he combined a radical methodical intellectualism with a personalistic anti-rationalism, showing the radical insufficiency of ratiocination in determining the principles and in deciding the practical issues of moral life. ([54], p. 214)

In another recent series of studies Pinckaers shows how central to Thomistic ethics was the doctrine of charitable love, as revealed in the beatitudes ([38, 39, 40]). Pinckaers traces the evolution and maturation of the idea of the good and its link with ethics from the *finis bonorum* of Cicero, through Augustine's dictum that the Sermon on the Mount provided the "perfect pattern of the Christian life" to St. Thomas' own morality. In them is to be found the sure guide to happiness sought by the pagans as by Christians. Pinckaers sees in Thomas' interpretation the possibility of once more reconciling morality and the desire for happiness, which he sees divorced in contemporary ethics.

Pinckaers also takes the view that duties and obligations are secondary in the morality of St. Thomas. They are the "crutches" of the virtues, placed at their service:

> La Morale de St. Thomas est donc une morale du bonheur et des vertus, groupant celles—ci autour de la foi, de la charité et des vertus cardinales. Ainsi s'explique le peu de place accordé dans la Somme à l'obligation morale. ([38], p. 109)

He goes on to show how during the Reformation and Counter-Reformation, both Protestantism and Catholicism divorced morality and faith, the one in the direction of rejecting reason, the other in exalting the natural law. Both are misguided, says Pinckaers. If we wish to understand Thomistic ethics, we must restore the primary place to faith. The essential fact is the internal disposition to charitable action formed by faith and helped by the Holy Spirit. This, he holds, gives freedom, not arbitrariness, to Christian ethics.

In his reflection on the methodology of St. Thomas, T. C. O'Brien distinguishes St. Thomas' vision of beatitude from Aristotle's. For Aquinas beatitude is the result of union with God, not of virtuous activity, as in Aristotle. The moral quality of human acts is, thus, measured by the degree to which they advance Charity as the prime moral principle. Beatitude is a form of friendship, and therefore of mutual love between God and man—a relationship that comes only through Grace.

> It is not, then, a question of seeing a natural moral structure, then filling it in by identifying the ultimate end as God; the vision of grace and charity is first; the moral structure is chosen to express something of its intelligibility. ([32], p. 114)

St. Thomas thus reverses the usual order of a naturalistic ethic, in which practice of the virtues can move man to his proper end of happiness. Instead, for Aquinas the only way to the fullness of beatitude is through grace and Charity. Such fulfillment is for man "above the condition of his nature but not in disregard or negation of his nature" ([32], p. 97).

One of the more promising recent re-examinations of the philosophical foundations for Christian ethics is the interesting amalgam of Thomistic realism, Christian existentialism, and phenomenological methodology that goes under the heading of "Lublinism" ([24, 26, 56]). Here Christian ethics is grounded in the personalism of an ambitious philosophical anthropology. One of its most prominent exemplars is Karol Wojtyla (John Paul II), whose personalist ethics centers on the lived experience and participation in love of the acting person [56]. On that view, the traditional values of Catholic morality are preserved and enriched by some of the creative ideas in contemporary European philosophy. This is in distinct contrast with both the analytic thrust of Anglo-American ethics and the legalistic bias of some of Catholic moral theology in the past.

These recent attempts to bridge the gap between ethics as an enterprise of reason and ethics as fulfillment of the law of love are valuable extrapolations of the traditional Catholic "perspective." They offer fresh insights into the links between philosophical and theological ethics, between contemporary and traditional ways of doing ethics, and between faith and reason, intellect and will, virtue and duties, agape and moral principles. We are far, however, from bridging all these gaps. To do so would require something of a "Summa Moralia Christiana." Pinckaers has recently offered an impressive new synthesis of the old and new sources of Christian morality that moves in this direction in an impressive way ([41, 42]).

In all of this, it is important to avoid an overly eager acceptance of the new or an overly rigid adulation of the past. Intuitionism, situationism, psychologism, and biologism are easy traps to fall into. Yet, the divisions between preceptive and non-preceptive ethics may not be as wide as their respective protagonists may feel. Those who favor existential and experiential modes of ethical thinking need a deeper and updated reacquaintance with Thomistic ethics. Those who favor the more traditional modes need to acquaint themselves with the richness of possible connections between Thomas' thought and contemporary philosophy and psychology.

The great strength of St. Augustine and St. Thomas was their capacity to engage in creative dialogue with the dominant cultural ideas of their times. Their intellects, illuminated by Faith, were able to apprehend what was congruent with the law of Charity and to discard what was not. If we can still philosophize and theologize in the spirit of Augustine and Thomas, it seems possible that a truly comprehensive Catholic medical moral philosophy will emerge. Such a philosophy would tell us more about the kinds of persons we ought to be than the rules we ought to follow. In medical morals it would call for Catholic health professionals who possess an intellectual grasp of moral principles as well as a capacity to apply them in the spirit of Charity. In this way they might fulfill that law of love which, as Guardini says, "is the New Testament" ([17], p. 79) and without which Christian ethics is not possible.

Charity, the Form of the Virtues, and the Catholic Perspective

Whatever new synthesis may be effected by the dialogue between traditional and contemporary Catholic perspectives Charity remains the ordering principle ([3, 20, 48, 49]). D. J. B. Hawkins puts it well:

> What is distinctive of the moral teaching of the gospel is not a new code of morality or a new theory of its basis, but the insistence on raising morality to the level of love. The commandments are to find their full meaning and completion in the love of God and our neighbor for God's sake. ([20], p. 28)

This is what St. Thomas teaches when he makes Charity the "form" of the virtues (*Summa Theologiae*, 2a2ae, Q23, art.8). Gilleman provides a particularly compelling account of Thomistic teaching on this point. He shows how Charity gives every virtuous act and, indeed, every virtue, a supernatural moral worth by orienting them to their final end, which is a supernatural one, i.e., union with God ([16], p. 53).

For the Christian, therefore, the moral life is conducted from several perspectives of creatureliness and incarnation ([20], p. 16). When we recognize that we are creatures, we see that everything we possess is held in trust for the Creator's purposes, not just our own. When we accept the fact of the Incarnation, we recognize that God's revelation of Himself to us makes it possible for us to lead a supernatural as well as a natural life. We are enabled to go ". . . beyond the possibilities of nature left to itself" ([20], pp. 16–17).

Clearly, in an agapeistic ethic, the motivation for being moral is explicitly different from what it is in a naturalistic ethic. The Christian knows that doing the right and the good is a means of growing closer to God the creator and Redeemer. He also has in Charity a light that illuminates the central dilemma of philosophical ethics, i.e., why some rules and principles are morally imperative and others are not. Fulfilling moral obligations is, in a sense, a way of encountering God. As John Crosby has argued, in that encounter, we conform to God's will and recognize that ". . . the binding force of moral obligation ultimately derives from divine command" ([8], p. 317).

This entails more than fulfilling duty in response to a reasoned argument about what ought to be done. Instead, the encounter with God in moral choice demands that the end of our reasoned judgment must be a right attitude of mind and heart. The virtue of Charity, therefore, consists in disposing moral judgments to their right end. It fuses the qualities of both mind and heart, of reason and faith—a fusion without meaning in a non-agapeistic ethic.

Medical Practice and the Virtue of Charity

If there is something distinctive about the Catholic perspective, it ought to be manifest in practical moral decisions. Since medicine is a praxis, an activity with its own internal goal, that goal—the good of the patient—is a moral one. A Christian perspective should therefore dispose the physician to decisions that would be, in the sense discussed above, formed by Charity. Or, to put it another way, as Fr. Sokolowski suggests, it would transform healing into an act of grace.

To be able to make choices consistent with the virtue of Charity requires a particular orientation of the capacity for deliberation in the Aristotelian or, better still, the Ignatian sense. This capacity, when shaped by a

Christian perspective, should dispose the Christian physician to select among the many particulars of a concrete moral choice those which most closely conform to the virtue of Charity. This entails a certain kind of Christian phronesis, a practical wisdom oriented and motivated by the virtue of Charity to act in a way pleasing to God in any particular situation.

Three aspects of medical moral decisions will serve to illustrate how the Christian virtue of Charity shapes moral choice: (1) in the way the dominant principles of medical ethics are interpreted; (2) in the way the physician-patient relationship is construed; and (3) in the way certain concrete choices in contemporary professional ethics are made.

Charity and the Principles of Ethics

An agapeistic ethic is by definition a virtue-based ethic. It must, therefore, confront the dilemma of how virtue relates to rules, duties, and principles. This is a prickly problem for any comprehensive philosophy of the moral life. It dates back to the post-medieval departure from virtue ethics exemplified in the overly close conjunctions of canon law with moral theology in the Catholic tradition and with the ascendance of Kant's deontology and Mill's utilitarianism in Anglo-American medical ethics.

The problem is particularly relevant for Christian ethics, for, as Plé points out, "It is not possible to love out of duty, that is, solely for the reason that authority imposes upon me the obligation of loving" ([44], p. 343). To recognize this fact is not to agree with Plé's full indictment of the morality of duty as an "obsessional neurosis" or with the primarily psychologistic line of his argument.

Principles, rules, and duties are as much a reality of the moral life as love and cannot be fully disengaged from it. What may be the essential difference in an agapeistic ethic is that rules, duties, and principles are chosen—or shaped—by Charity, i.e., by whether or not they foster its growth, a fact even Plé admits ([44], p. 344).

The primary principles of medical ethics—beneficence, justice, and autonomy—are ascertainable by human reason without resort to revelation or Sacred Scripture. They enjoy widespread acceptance today even in our morally pluralist society. What the virtue of Charity adds is a special way in which these principles are to be lived and applied in concrete situations. In a Christian moral perspective, Charity "informs" these principles. When they are in conflict, it sorts out resolutions that are in the spirit of Gospel teaching from those that are not.

Each of the principles of medical ethics is thus subject to tests of conformity with sources of moral validation—Sacred Scripture, the tradition or teaching of an official church—not acknowledged by the non-believer. As a result, a Christian or Catholic perspective may impose levels of obligation that, on purely naturalist grounds, are optional or supererogatory. Indeed, the Christian is exhorted unequivocally to perfection in Charity by the Sermon on the Mount. On reason alone such a pursuit can be accounted as unreasonable, unrealistic, or psychologically distressful.

Beneficence—acting for the good of the patient—is the central principle of medical ethics. But beneficence is interpretable at several levels, from mere non-maleficence to heroic sacrifice. Health professionals may differ sharply on precisely what degree of beneficence they consider binding. Some argue that not harming the patient is sufficient, invoking the oft-quoted principle "*primum non nocere.*" Others feel bound to a more positive interpretation, i.e., acting for the good of the patient, not just avoiding harm, thus injecting some degree of altruism. Still others feel impelled to benevolent self-effacement—that is to say, acting for the patient's good even if it means doing so at some personal cost in time, convenience, danger to self, or financial loss. Finally, for a very few, like Mother Teresa or Father Damien, beneficence means heroic sacrifice and complete dedication to the needs of the sick and dying.

It can be argued even on purely philosophical grounds that simple non-maleficence, without some degree of self-effacing beneficence, is insufficient in medical ethics given the nature of illness, the effects it produces in the patient, and the obligations the physician assumes when she/he offers to heal. I would argue that effacement of self-interest is required even on purely philosophical grounds [37]. This level of beneficence flows directly from the internal morality of medicine and is intrinsic to the traditional concept of a true profession. It is what sets true professions apart from a business, craft, or other occupation.

From a Catholic or Christian perspective, however, benevolent self-effacement is a minimum obligation consistent with the virtue of Charity. Lesser degrees of benevolence and beneficence would be inconsistent with such Scriptural exhortations as the Story of the Good Samaritan, the Sermon on the Mount, or Jesus' own healing acts. On this view medical knowledge is not proprietary or simply a means to make a living. It is a means of service to others, a mission and apostolate, a virtual ministry to those who have a special claim on the whole Christian community—the sick, disabled, poor, or retarded [22].

Thus, for the Christian the practice of medicine is transformed from a profession to a vocation, a means of gaining one's own salvation, assisting in the salvation of others, and witnessing the truth of the Gospel teaching in one's own life. Practicing medicine is inseparable from leading a life that is wholly Christian. The practice of medicine takes on meanings that go beyond even the nobler traditions of the profession. The Christian physician is impelled to act in the interests of the sick even when it may mean exposing himself/herself to danger, loss of time or income, or serious inconvenience. The moral claim of the sick person on the physician exceeds what is expected in a business relationship. Unavailability, inaccessibility, abruptness, condescension, refusal to treat for economic reasons, or fear of contagion are irreconcilable with a Charity-based ethic of medicine.

Sacred Scripture provides no algebraic formula that measures out precisely the degree of self-effacement a particular physician must practice in a specific situation. This will depend on the strength of other obligations to self, family, institutions, other patients, and the like. What is clear is that an agapeistic ethic accepts no easy justification for reducing beneficence to mere non-maleficence or to beneficence which demands nothing of the physician. It makes arguments from exigency, fiscal survival, or adherence to the canons of a competitive environment morally feeble, if not totally unacceptable.

The Christian physician is, in short, called to strive for perfection in Charity even though he or she must fail, given the ineffability of the model he/she must emulate. That Christian physicians and other health professionals do in fact fall short of the benevolent self-effacement Charity requires is obvious. But they should know when they have fallen short. They should strive to come closer always, not as an act of noble self-sacrifice but as an obedient response to a loving God (Luke 6:36) [30].

Similar considerations apply to the other two principles of medical ethics—justice and autonomy. Seen from a Catholic or Christian perspective justice becomes a charitable justice [21]. It has its origins in God, who is just to us and to whom we owe justice. Charitable justice goes beyond the strict rendering to others of what is due to them. It recognizes needs that go beyond duty. It seeks the higher good of the other person in commutative, distributive, and retributive justice.

The Christian is exhorted in the Gospels to "hunger after justice." This means more than fidelity to the natural virtue of justice as taught by Plato, Aristotle, or the Stoics. The Christian is called not only to the natural virtues but also to sanctity, to be perfect "as the father is perfect," to cooperate with God in God's work. Charitable justice is not content with rights only. It recognizes claims on us that have no grounding in legal rights but derive from a conception of the human community that enjoins the more fortunate to help the less fortunate whether they "deserve" it or not. There is thus a certain built-in tension between the strictly legal and the Christian senses of justice.

Some of these differences become clear when we examine justice in health care delivery. In a strictly legal sense it is difficult to justify a moral claim by the poor or the sick on the resources of individuals or society. Even more difficult to counter is the argument that the virtuous and the hard working should sacrifice for the poor, the outcasts, sociopaths, alcoholics, or non-compliant in the care of their own health.

Yet it is precisely to these groups that Christians, and specifically Catholic Christians, are expected to exercise a "preferential option" [9]. The recent pastoral letter of the American bishops and the social encyclicals of the popes since Leo XIII make this clear [53]. When the natural virtue of justice is formed by Charity, it goes beyond a strict calculus of duties and claims and is tempered by compassion. Charitable justice gives freely, lovingly, and without respect to strict accounting, which it leaves to God.

Charitable justice therefore fuses with beneficence in a way incomprehensible on naturalistic interpretations of these virtues. It seeks out those who may not have deserved health care or who are responsible for their own ill health. It does so because the sick, the poor, the outcast are precisely those to whom Christ himself ministered. No Christian physician can ignore that example and remain authentically Christian.

A specific example of how a Catholic Christian perspective might function is in the selection of a principle of distribution when health care resources are scarce, as in the case of kidneys for transplantation, intensive care beds, or technical procedures of great expense. Distribution theoretically could be on the basis of merit, deserts, societal contribution, needs, first-come-first-served, lottery, or equity [34]. Of these criteria, merit, deserts, societal contribution, and ability to pay are least consistent with the requirements of charitable justice while equity, need, or lottery are more so. Moreover, charitable justice requires that the underlying conditions that lead to rationing choices be eliminated or ameliorated. They cannot be left to the workings of the marketplace as so many suggest today. In a Christian community, health care is an obligation of society, more binding than if it were a legal right.

Autonomy and its accompanying virtue of respect for persons are also to be informed by Charity. Kant grounded autonomy in an *a prioristic* respect for persons. But for the Christian that respect must be grounded in the worth the Creator has given to each life—a worth only God can judge.

The antagonism some ethicists see between autonomy and beneficence is mitigated by a Christian medical ethic [4]. This is not to justify medical paternalism, which is too often confused with beneficence, but to assert that respect for persons is, in itself, a requirement of beneficence. For the Christian, this beneficence is necessary to the virtue of Charity. Humans must be free because each has worth, each is accountable to God, each must be free to follow his or her conscience in moral choices—medical or otherwise [1].

Viewed from a Christian and Catholic perspective, however, autonomy is not absolute. The Christian is obliged to use his/her God-given freedom wisely and well. Autonomy is a necessary means to doing the right and the good, to fulfilling the stewardship of our own health. This means refraining from self-destruction by suicide or deleterious life styles, or neglecting needed and appropriate medical care. But if a patient refuses to acknowledge these duties, the physician cannot impose them on him/her. Strong paternalism is uncharitable because freedom to choose and shape one's own life is intrinsic to being human. To ignore it is to violate the very humanity of the patient, a humanity given to him or her by God.

In the same way, the patient and his or her family have an obligation in Charity to respect the autonomy of the health professional or institution. The patient cannot, in the name of the absoluteness of autonomy, demand that the physician become the unquestioning instrument of the patient's will. The conscience of the religious physician or hospital cannot be overridden even if certain practices like abortion, sterilization, discontinuance of food and hydration, or euthanasia are legally sanctioned. The Christian, for example, could not accept the absolutization of patient autonomy and self-governance over life so forcefully promulgated by Judge Compton in his concurring opinion in the *Bouvia* case [5], or as argued by Engelhardt in his recent treatment of the "foundations of bioethics" [10].

In sum, a Catholic Christian perspective shapes the way we interpret and apply the principles of medical ethics in specific ways. Non-believers may interpret them the same way but they need not do so. If they do, they use different reasons. More is rightly expected of those who profess to emulate the example of Jesus' healing. For them the obligations to respect autonomy, justice, and beneficence are at the service of virtue and Charity. These principles gain their worth not *a prioristically*, but because they express what is necessary to the virtue of Charity.

Whether or not the Christian perspective calls for supererogation if examined on purely philosophical grounds is problematic. The status of supererogation in moral theory—whether it is a separate category or encompassable in Kantian deontology—is still a debatable question [2]. All we need to say at this point is that the range of interpretations of philosophical ethical principles and duties is specified in particular ways in a Charity-based ethic.

Respect for the inviolability of human conscience may bring the Christian physician or nurse into moral conflict with the autonomous decisions of patients, families, other health professionals, the hospital, and even the state. In a Charity-based ethics, he/she is obliged to handle the conflict with love and respect for those with whom one disagrees. But on the same principle the Christian health professional cannot cooperate formally or directly with an intrinsically evil act. There is the obligation to decide whether to withdraw respectfully or, if the harm being done—e.g., direct euthanasia, grossly incompetent surgery—is sufficiently great, to intervene directly. One may use those means available in democratic societies—persuasion, ethics committees, and the courts—but not violent means that violate the virtue of Charity.

Needless to say, Christian ethics cannot uncritically accept the current move from substantive to procedural ethics. Such a move is useful and doubtless necessary in a morally pluralistic society. Nonetheless, even in the interests of amicable settlement of moral conflicts, the substance of moral decisions must be defended. This means that a certain tension will exist between secular and Christian ethics.

Likewise, the substantive ethical issues are not resolved if professional ethical codes are revised to fit the needs of morally pluralistic societies. For example, refusing to treat patients with AIDS might be considered "ethical" on the grounds of the AMA principles, which permit physicians to choose whom they will treat. It is hard, however, to defend this view in any authentic interpretation of Christian medical ethics.[3]

Christian Charity and Professional Practices

If we move from principles to some concrete moral dilemmas, we can perhaps see more concretely how Charity acts as a principle of discernment and how it orders some of the moral decisions facing health professionals today. We can use as illustrations a few professional practices that have not been declared immoral by the profession as a whole, and which are even accepted, however reluctantly, on grounds of necessity or economic survival. I refer here to a range of practices—some old, some new—which compromise, endanger, or conflict with the best interests of patients. Some examples are: working in for-profit managed health care systems, medical entrepreneurship in its many forms—investing in and owning health care facilities to which one refers patients, misleading advertising, selling and dispensing medication, refusing to see Medicare or Medicaid patients, charging excessive fees, gatekeeping in its various forms, pay-as-you-go research ([46, 47]), cutting corners to contain costs or enhance profits, the many marketing artifices that ensure success in competition and the marketplace, etc. The list of morally marginal practices is spawned by the current commercialization and monetarization of health care as an industry that legitimates the financial motivations of health professionals, administrators, and owners of health care facilities.

These practices are justified on "practical" or economic grounds as means to cost containment and managerial efficiency. Many consider them salubrious to the general welfare, so long as provisions are made to avoid abuses. Even Catholic and other religiously sponsored hospitals and health professionals are enthusiastically embracing these practices.

But it is difficult to justify such practices in any truly agapeistic ethic. The possibilities of submergence of the patient's interest by the financial interests of the health professional or institution, and the downgrading of medicine from a vocation to a business, are all too obvious. Many of these practices have been condemned repeatedly as morally dubious even on non-religious grounds. How much more reprehensible are they when practiced by physicians and institutions that lay claim to the title "Christian"? It is often in the realm of the morally marginal, rather than the frankly immoral, that the more stringent requirements of an agapeistic ethic are most easily discerned.

Today many Christian physicians, nurses, administrators, and hospitals justify their compromising the virtue of Charity on grounds of exigency and survival. They thus give proof to the mordant observation of Machiavelli that "a man who wishes to act entirely up to his professions of virtue soon meets with what destroys him among so much that is evil."[4] But is not the challenge of Christian ethics to do precisely what Machiavelli thought impossible?

Charity and the Physician-Patient Relationship

Similarly, adherence to a Christian and Charity-based ethic shapes the model of the physician- or nurse-patient relationship. Certain of the models now being proposed become morally distasteful if not totally unacceptable. Thus, a genuine Christian ethic would be incompatible with health care as a commercial activity. The idea of the physician as primarily a businessman is inconsistent with the Christian ethic of medicine. Likewise, such an ethic would reject the healing relationship as primarily an exercise in applied biology or as a legal contract for services. Nor could the relationship be construed as paternalistic, or as primarily a means of livelihood, personal profit, or prestige for the physician. Equally incompatible are models which make the physician primarily a government bureaucrat, a proletarian employee of a corporation, or an agent of the state as in totalitarian regimes.

Instead, the model of physician-patient relationships most consistent with a Christian ethic is the covenant—the model in which the physician's promise to help is a binding promise to which he or she pledges fidelity ([28, 37]). That promise does not call for total, unquestioning submission to the good as defined by the patient but to the higher levels of charitable beneficence alluded to earlier in this essay. On the Christian view the idea of a profession embraces the higher ideas of a commitment to service subsumed in the idea of a Christian vocation [35].

Parenthetically, the Christian conception of the healing relationship imposes certain obligations on the patients as well. Honesty, compliance with the doctor's regimen, refraining from frivolous, frankly unjust, or injurious legal action, and respect for the humanity and moral values of the physician are logical corollaries of a covenantal relationship. A mutuality of respect by physician and patient for the virtue of Charity is therefore essential.

The physician-patient relationship—and equally the nurse-, dentist-, pharmacist-patient relationships—does not, however, call for a monastic devotion to medicine to the exclusion of other obligations to family, self, society, or country. It does not deny the fact that in some measures medicine is simultaneously a business, a craft, a science, and a technology. But what an agapeistic ethics does preeminently is to place these differing facets of medical practice into a morally defensible order, recognizing when and to what degree they must yield to the ordering principle of Charity.

This is essentially what it means to say, in medical practice, that Charity is the form of the virtues. Charity acts as a practical principle of discernment and a benchmark against which the Christian measures concretely, here and now, the moral worth of his or her practical decisions. It is often said that the Gospel gives us no categorical guidance, no set rules for resolving all the dilemmas of medical ethics. Apart from the beatitudes, this is so. Manifestly, the Gospel could not anticipate every possible moral dilemma that might arise in the history of mankind. But it gives us something more valuable. It teaches that Charity is the form of all the virtues, that Charity is the ordering principle of discernment in moral choice. And it is very specific in detailing what Charity comprises—all of the concrete examples in Christ's own life; of what he meant in concrete situations by the transcendent ethos of Charity which he preached and taught there on the Mount in full view of the Sea of Galilee and the needy of all the world.

The health professional and institution that profess Christianity must heed that Sermon every day in every encounter with the sick. It is in this sense that the Catholic Christian perspective "sees through" and beyond philosophical medical ethics to the virtue of Charity. Charity becomes an interior principle, as it were, that encompasses the philosophically derivable internal morality of medicine and, without abrogating it, transmutes healing into an act of grace.

Notes

I am grateful to the Rev. J. D. Cassidy, O.P. for his helpful criticisms and bibliographic suggestions.

1. See articles by McCormick, Fuchs, Curran, and Gustafson in Curran and McCormick (eds.), [9].

2. Others have been more specific about the differences they associate with *Catholic* belief and moral life. See Finnis [11], Hauerwas [19], and May [27].

3. Recently the AMA has clarified that Principle VI of its 1980 code does not authorize refusal to treat AIDS patients. See Council on Ethical and Judicial Affairs, "Ethical issues involved in the growing of AIDS Crisis." *Journal of the American Medical Association* 259(9) (1988): 1360–1361.

4. See chapter XV of N. Machiavelli's *The Prince* in *The Great Books*, vol. 23, Encyclopedia Britannica, Chicago, p. 22.

References

1. Abbott, W., ed. *The Documents of Vatican* II (London: Geoffrey Chapman, 1962).
2. Baron, M. "Kantian Ethics and Supererogation." *Journal of Philosophy* 84(5) (1987): 237–262.

3. Bars, H. *Faith, Hope and Charity*, trans. P. J. Hepburne Scott (New York: Hawthorn, 1961).

4. Beauchamp, T. and McCullough, L. *Medical Ethics: The Moral Responsibilities of Physicians* (Englewood Cliffs, NJ: Prentice Hall, 1984).

5. *Bouvia v. Superior Court of the State of California for the County of Los Angeles*, 225 Cal. Rep. 297.

6. Cahill, L. S. "Theological Medical Morality: A Response to Josef Fuchs." In *Catholic Perspectives on Medical Morals*, ed. Edmund D. Pellegrino et al. (Dordrecht: Kluwer, 1989), pp. 93–102.

7. Congregation for the Doctrine of the Faith. *Instruction on Respect for Human Life in Its Origin and on the Dignity of Procreation*, Vatican City, 1987.

8. Crosby, J. F. "The Encounter of God and Man in Moral Obligation." *The New Scholasticism* 60(3) (1986): 317–355.

9. Curran, C. E. and McCormick, R., eds. *The Distinctiveness of Christian Ethics: Readings in Moral Theology II* (New York: Paulist Press, 1980).

10. Engelhardt, H. T., Jr. *The Foundations of Bioethics* (New York: Oxford Press, 1986).

11. Finnis, J. "Natural Law, Objective Morality and Vatican II." In *Principles of Catholic Moral Life*, ed. W. May (Chicago: Franciscan Herald Press, 1981), pp. 113–149.

12. Fletcher, J. *Situation Ethics; The New Morality* (Philadelphia: Westminster Press, 1966).

13. Frankena, W. K. *Ethics* (New York: Prentice Hall, 1963).

14. Fuchs, J. "'Catholic' Medical Moral Theology?" In *Catholic Perspectives on Medical Morals*, ed. Edmund D. Pellegrino et al. (Dordrecht: Kluwer, 1989), pp. 83–92.

15. Gilby, T. "Philosophical and Theological Morals." In *Principles of Morality, Summa Theologiae, Vol. 18 (1a2ae 18–21) Principles of Morality* (New York: McGraw-Hill, 1966), pp. 147–150.

16. Gilleman, G. *The Primacy of Charity in Moral Theology*, trans. W. Ryan and A. Vachon (Westminster, MD: Newman Press, 1959).

17. Guardini, R. *The Lord* (Chicago: Henry Regnery, 1954).

18. Hallett, G. L. *Christian Moral Reasoning* (Notre Dame, IN: University of Notre Dame Press, 1983).

19. Hauerwas, S. and MacIntyre, A., eds. *Revisions: Changing Perspectives in Moral Philosophy* (Notre Dame, IN: University of Notre Dame Press, 1983).

20. Hawkins, D. J. B. *Christian Ethics* (New York: Hawthorn Books, 1963).

21. Hollenback, D. "Modern Catholic Teachings Concerning Justice." In *The Faith That Does Justice*, ed. J. C. Haughey. Woodstock Studies 12 (New York: Paulist Press, 1977), pp. 207–233.

22. John Paul II. *Salvifici Doloris* (1984).

23. Jonsen, A. R. and Toulmin, S. *The Abuse of Casuistry* (Berkeley: University of California Press, 1988).

24. Krapiec, M. *I-Man: An Outline of Philosophical Anthropology* (New Britain, CT: Mariel, 1983).

25. Ladd, J. "Internal Morality of Medicine: An Essential Dimension of the Patient-Physician Relationship." In *The Clinical Encounter*, ed. E. Shelp (Dordrecht, Holland: Kluwer Academic Publishers, 1983), pp. 209–231.

26. Lawler, R. D. "Personalist Ethics." *Proceedings of the American Catholic Philosophical Association LX* (1986): 148–155.

27. May, W. E., ed. *Principles of Catholic Moral Life* (Chicago: Franciscan Herald Press, 1981).

28. May, W. F. *The Physician's Covenant* (Philadelphia: Westminster Press, 1983).

29. McCormick, R. "Therapy or Tampering?: The Ethics of Reproductive Technology." *America* 153 (1985): 397–398.

30. McNeill, D., Morrison, D. A., and Nouwen, H. J. M. *Compassion, A Reflection on the Christian Life* (New York: Doubleday, 1982).

31. Merton, T. *Love and Living* (New York: Harcourt, Brace, Jovanovich, 1985).

32. O'Brien, T. C. "The *Reditus ad Deum*: A Reflection on the Methodology of St. Thomas." In *Summa Theologiae, Vol. 27*, ed. and trans. T. C. O'Brien (New York: McGraw-Hill, 1974).

33. Oppenheim, F. M., ed. *The Reasoning Heart* (Washington, DC: Georgetown University Press, 1986).

34. Outka, G. "Social Justice and Equal Access to Health Care." *Journal of Religious Ethics* 2 (1974): 11–32.

35. Pellegrino, E. D. "Professional Ethics: Moral Decline or Paradigm Shift?" *Religion and Intellectual Life* 4(3) (1987): 21–39.

36. Pellegrino, E. D. "Toward a Reconstruction of Medical Morality: The Primacy of the Act of Profession and the Fact of Illness." *Journal of Medicine and Philosophy* 4(1) (1979): 32–56.

37. Pellegrino, E. D. and Thomasma, D. *For the Patient's Good: The Restoration of Beneficence in Health Care* (New York: Oxford University Press, 1988).

38. Pinckaers, S. "Autonomie et Heteronomie en Morale Selon S. Thomas D'Aquin." In *Autonomie: Dimensions Éthiques de la Liberté: Études d'Éthique Chrétienne*, ed. C. J. P. de Oliveira (Paris: Editions du Cerf, 1983), pp. 104–123.

39. Pinckaers, S. "Le Commentaire du Sermon sur la Montagne par S. Augustin et la Morale de S. Thomas d'Aquin." In *La Teologoa Morale Nella Storia e Nella Prolematica Attaule Miscellanea*, ed. L. B. Gillon (Massimo, 1982), pp. 105–125.

40. Pinckaers, S. "La Béatitude dans L'Éthique de S. Thomas." In *Studi Tomistici*, ed. L. J. Elders and K. Hedwig (Vatican: Pontificia Accademia, 1984), pp. 80–94.

41. Pinckaers, S. *Les Sources de la Morale Chrétienne: Sa Méthode, Son Contenu, Son Histoire* (Paris: Editions du Cerf, 1985).

42. Pinckaers, S. *Universalité et Permanence des Lois Morales* (Fribourg: Editions Universitaires, 1986).

43. Pittenger, N. *Catholic Faith in a Process Perspective* (Maryknoll, NY: Orbis, 1981).

44. Plé, A. "The Morality of Duty and Obsessional Neurosis." *Cross Currents* 37 (1986): 343–357.

45. Ratzinger, J. "Magisterium of the Church, Faith, Morality." In *The Distinctiveness of Christian Ethics: Readings in Moral Theology II,* ed. C. Curran and R. McCormick (New York: Paulist Press, 1980).

46. Reade, J. M. and Ratzan, R. M. "Yellow Professionalism: Advertising by Physicians in the Yellow Pages." *New England Journal of Medicine* 316(21) (1987): 1315–1319.

47. Relman, A. S. "Practicing Medicine in the New Business Climate." *New England Journal of Medicine* 316(18) (1987): 1150 ff.

48. St. Augustine. *Faith, Hope and Charity,* trans. L. Arand (New York: Newman Bookshop, 1947).

49. St. Augustine. *The Lord's Sermon on the Mount,* trans. J. Jepson (Westminster, MD: Newman Press, 1948).

50. St. Thomas Aquinas. *Summa Theologiae* (New York: McGraw-Hill, 1974).

51. Sokolowski, R. "The Art and Science of Medicine." In *Catholic Perspectives on Medical Morals,* ed. Edmund D. Pellegrino et al. (Dordrecht: Kluwer, 1989), pp. 263–276.

52. Spohn, W. "The Reasoning Heart: An American Approach to Christian Discernment." In *The Reasoning Heart,* ed. F. M. Oppenheim (Washington, DC: Georgetown University Press, 1986), pp. 51–76.

53. U.S. Catholic Conference. *Catholic Social Teaching and the U.S. Economy: Health and Health Care: A Pastoral Letter of the American Catholic Bishops* (1981).

54. Walgrave, J. H. "The Personal Aspects of St. Thomas' Ethics." In *Studi Tomistici,* ed. L. Elders and K. Hedwig (Vatican: Pontificia Accademia, 1984), pp. 202–215.

55. Wren, T. E. "Metaethical Internalism: Can Moral Beliefs Motivate?" *Proceedings of the American Catholic Philosophical Association* 59 (1985): 58–80.

56. Wojtyla, K. *The Acting Person,* trans. A. Potocki. Analecta Husserliana 10 (Dordrecht, Holland: Kluwer Academic Publishers, 1979).

Bioethics at Century's Turn

Can Normative Ethics Be Retrieved?

Prophecy is the most gratuitous form of error.

—George Eliot, *Middlemarch*

Introduction

For more than two millennia what we now know as "bioethics" lay dormant in the chrysalis of medical ethics. It changed so little that it came to be taken as immutable. Thirty-five years ago, bioethics broke out of its pupal quiescence to enter a logarithmic growth phase whose terminus is far from clear. To predict what its adult form will be is to fall victim to the perils of prophecy. But it is important, while bioethics is still conceptually malleable, to trace some of its major trajectories which do point to the general form the adult discipline seems to be assuming.

The four trajectories I wish to examine are these: (1) the attenuation of the normative, and therefore of the ethical, nature of the bioethical enterprise; (2) the multiplication of and conflict between and among the methodologies bioethicists use to pursue their inquiries; (3) the parallel confusion and conflict between and among theories of justification; and (4) the flight from universal foundations upon which to base the directions the first three trajectories should take.

Each trajectory begets a set of questions the answers to which bioethics must address. (1) Is bioethics as a normative philosophical endeavor outmoded? (2) Are its current methodologies complementary or contradictory? (3) How are the bioethicist's conclusions to be morally justified? (4) Is a stable conceptual foundation necessary to answer the first three questions, or is the post-modern closure of the foundation question the last word?

The Question of Identity

Etymologically, "bioethics" should simply mean the systematic study of the moral issues arising in the application of biological knowledge to human affairs from agriculture and ecology to medicine and public policy. Implied in this definition is the search for the moral truth and generalized normative guidelines that have for so long characterized the ethical enterprise.

Bioethics today, however, is a multidisciplinary, interprofessional, multicultural enterprise. It has embraced virtually all of the social and behavioral sciences as well as law, politics, and economics. While it began as a critique of traditional medical ethics, it now embraces every facet of the application of biotechnology in human life. The opinions of bioethicists are sought by the media, the general public, and policymakers. Their haruspications are awaited eagerly whenever a new bit of information leaves the laboratory. Some bioethicists have come to be regarded as gurus, "philosopher kings," or have been urged to answer legal, psychological, and religious questions as well (Shalit 1997; La Puma et al. 1991; Scofield 1993).

Bioethicists have striven to accommodate the dominant cultural and social currents of multiculturalism, political liberalism, secularism, and post-modernism in its various forms. As a result, bioethics has become progressively vaguer and more amorphous in its boundaries at places, and has exceeded the perimeters of ethics formally considered to become a procedure for resolving "value" conflicts, whether those values are moral values or not. One may now legitimately wonder how much "ethics" is left in the field of "bioethics"? How much of the traditional concerns of ethics for normative questions can survive? Can bioethics, in its present state, withstand the challenges of post-modernism without slipping into moral relativism, nihilism, or chaos? Can, or should, the foundations of ethics in moral philosophy be recovered, eliminated, or modified, and in what way?

Recently, a number of contemporary American bioethicists have begun to express some concern over the need for a firmer footing for the normative claims of the field. Macklin (1999), for example, makes a case for the preservation of moral realism and objectivity based in basic human rights. Veatch (2000) argues that his long-standing commitment to moral absolutism can survive in an era of post-modernism. Beauchamp (2000) maintains that *prima facie* principlism is grounded firmly in a universal common morality. Engelhardt (1996) holds that secular ethics must recognize that we are moral strangers and that we cannot share a common moral vision, yet he also maintains that Christian bioethics is rooted in a common moral vision, one elaborated in first millennium Christianity. Meilaender (1995) and others fear that bioethics has "lost its soul," by which they mean that it has turned from moral philosophical questions to procedures and public policy. MacIntyre (1990) proposes a return to the Aristotelian-Thomist tradition as the grounding for a return to genuine moral inquiry. None seems entirely satisfied with the currently popular determinants of right and wrong, like social construction, reflective equilibrium, or dialogue, to name a few.

An even more destructive force in the erosion of the ethical component of the bioethical is the abandonment of norms of true and good, right and wrong in practical ethical decisions. What is sought is what "works" or what is "useful," i.e., what is justifiable to the parties making the decision, irrespective of whether or not the conflict resolution is true or good (Iltis 2000; Casarett et al. 1998).

This trend is furthered by the post-modernists' attack on the reliability of human reason in arriving at moral truth. With its central pediment gone, the Enlightenment project of a religion-free, metaphysics-free ethics ends in the destruction of normative ethics. The only recourse to ethical conflict is negotiation, since reason itself is now so discredited.

Much of this trend is discernable in the popular reduction of applied ethics to a matter of reconciling "values" or arriving at what is a "comfortable" decision, but feelings and values are not norms. They do not carry the moral weight of norms. Norms are guidelines to be followed at risk of censure because they rest on some notion of the true, the good, the right, the wrong. Norms have some degree of objectivity. They are not self-justifying. They can be argued about; they occupy interpersonal space. Values, on the other hand, like feelings of comfort, are subjective and internal to the one who values. They are not arguable since the one who gives a thing value has already established its weight as a priority. To reduce moral conflict to a conflict of values is to make ethics an exchange of opinions. Only "values clarification" or compromise are possible. For one value to trump another it must derive moral status from something other than itself. Lacking as we do a genuine axiology which could link values and norms, the only acceptable norm is respect for other people's values simply because they are their values. As a result, conflicts between and among values can only end in an impasse that at best forestalls decision, or at worst, results in violent confrontation.

But where decisions must be made, at the bedside or in the policy area, such an impasse is not tolerable. Barring some apocalyptic reversal of human affairs, today's unprecedented expansion of biological knowledge and of social change will continue. The need for normative direction will be ever more urgent if new techniques and realms of knowledge are to be used wisely and within boundaries set by ethics rather than those imposed by biological opportunism or commercial interests. The use of biotechnology within ethical constraints will continue to be one of human kind's gravest moral challenges for a long time to come.

This need is exacerbated by the fact that normative constraint must now extend beyond national boundaries. New knowledge and technology cannot be confined, given the ubiquity of electronic and other forms of communication. Further, the lure of profits, the relatively low cost of labor, and differences in legal and ethical constraints make crossing of national boundaries commonplace. The obstacles to global ethical agreements are formidable, given the world's cultural, religious, and ethical differences.

Yet failure to establish some normative consensus on the limits of biotechnology could in its own way be as disastrous as failure to agree on restraints on the use of atomic weaponry. In the absence of ethical constraints, even the less aggressive nations could feel justified in the name of survival, national interests, or commerce to transgress the boundaries of morality.

Clearly, the present trend to reduce normative ethics to a procedure for conflict resolution, or a social convention, poses dangers at the individual, policy, and international levels. A central challenge for bioethics is how to preserve and recover its ethical credibility, that is to say, its normative content, one with universal applicability and acceptability. This challenge cannot be met by abandoning ethics as it has been understood traditionally and replacing it with other disciplines in the humanities or social sciences. Nor is the seductive substitute of "discourse ethics" likely to recover normative ethical content.

To be sure, one of the important contributions of bioethics has been to enrich its grasp of the moral life by closer connection with these other disciplines. This makes the question of identity even more difficult and acute. How can bioethics as an inquiry into norms of good and right human conduct advance its enterprise without being absorbed or attenuated by the very disciplines which can enrich it?

Relationship with the Humanities and Social Sciences

Bioethics enters the new millennium as a mere infant among the social and intellectual movements of the twentieth century. It is barely more than a quarter century old and its history is just beginning to be reliably documented. Like any embryonic organism, however, bioethics has undergone significant metamorphoses even from its earliest days. As each stage unfolds successively, we gain a better idea of the divergent possibilities built into its primordial conception.

But we also become aware of the need for some order and prioritization among those possibilities. According to the popular account (Reich 1999), bioethics was "baptized" in 1972 virtually simultaneously at the Kennedy Institute of Ethics at Georgetown University and at the University of Wisconsin. As a result, bioethics had two conceptual *anlagen*, reflective of the differences in its places of birth. Each *anlage* was the primodium for a different vision of the place of ethics as a discipline in the larger fledgling enterprise of bioethics.

At the Kennedy Institute, ethics was pursued primarily as a branch of philosophy and an extension of the ancient field of medical and professional ethics. Its major orientation was to normative ethics, particularly as it applied to medical practice. At Wisconsin, bioethics was conceived as a more broadly scientific and interdisciplinary pursuit. It had broader biological roots extending from ecology and populations to molecular biology. Following this model, bioethics has become a quasi-utopian promise of a new biologically based ethic.

The Georgetown and the Wisconsin versions of bioethics represented two ends of the spectrum. In between, a variety of combinations of disciplines and approaches have evolved. The Hastings Center, the University of Texas at Galveston, and the Pennsylvania State University, for example, pursued intermediate programs that combined elements of both approaches. They point, perhaps, to what is becoming the predominant pattern. If this trend continues, we must eventually face the central question that occupies me here: how essential are moral norms and normative ethics to the enterprise of bioethics? When, if ever, does an interdisciplinary discipline become so inclusive as to lose its identity? When does it dilute the normative thrust of ethics so thoroughly that ethics, itself, is so etiolated as to become unidentifiable?

It is interesting in this respect to note that a decade before bioethics received its name, it was preceded by a serious interdisciplinary effort under the rather diffuse title of "Humanities, Human Values, and Ethics." This term covered a movement among medical educators to remedy the dehumanization they feared in the growing technological emphasis of medical education. Between 1960 and 1970, a dozen or so medical schools began to devise courses and curricula combining the humanities, the humanistic end of the social sciences, and medical ethics (Pellegrino 1999). In this movement, the word "values" was preferred over "norms," "principles," or "precepts."

Out of this movement, the Society for Health and Human Values (now subsumed in the new American Society for Bioethics and Humanities) was born. Under the society's auspices, the *Journal of Medicine and Philosophy* was established, as well as the Institute on Human Values in Medicine. As a result, normative ethics and the philosophy of medicine (in the *Journal*) were intermingled with the humanities and social sciences.

These strands of conceptual difference in the history of bioethics have interacted with each other and with the changing societal context. In the first decade (the sixties), the educational needs of medical students had the strongest influence; in the next decade (the seventies), philosophical ethics took the lead since the issues of physician-patient relationships and the resolution of practical clinical dilemmas presented urgent normative challenges. To meet these practical issues at the bedside, clinical ethics emerged as a branch of normative ethics with a strong emphasis on *prima facie* principles (Beauchamp and Childress 1994). In the eighties, the reaction against principlism, philosophical ethics, and the perceived abstractness of philosophical ethics set in. Virtually every discipline and profession entered into bioethical discourse. Each made a claim to be a remedy for too formal or too philosophical an approach to the moral life. Each promised a richer, fuller account of that life.

This proliferation of disciplines, professions and techniques does, indeed, give fuller expression to the richness and complexity of the moral life. On the whole, this has been salubrious, and it has enriched our understanding of the complexity of moral choices. But it also creates a significant confusion of identity. How do ethics and moral philosophy relate to the other disciplines that now claim a seat at the table?

For one thing the humanities and the social and physical sciences are necessary sources of detail. They are relevant to the full comprehension of the moral dimension of human life. Those disciplines are the substance of descriptive ethics. They provide methodologies crucial to the concrete description of moral dilemmas. Knowledge of the particularities of moral life is essential to any informed ethical opinion. Ethics without recourse to fact is precarious. But facts, observations, insights, stories, and perceptions are not norms. Without normative guidelines, ethics does not exist. In the end, ethical discourse, decision, and reflection involve a dialogue and dialectic about what "ought" to be done. To be sure, verifiable data about the moral situation are derivable from the many disciplines that study human life. Experience with these data has helped bioethics to mature. But experience *per se* is not sufficient for moral maturity. It must be reflected upon critically, formally, and from the perspective of good, bad, right, or wrong human conduct.

As bioethics matures further into the next century, it will need to retrieve its connection with philosophical and theological ethics as the source of normative principles, rules, guidelines, precepts, axioms, middle level principles, etc. (cf. Pellegrino 1997). It will also need to continue its newly forged connections with the other disciplines but without capitulating to any one of them. Ethics will need to recapture its identity as a discipline characterized by a method of analysis and a body of literature whose specific end is ascertaining moral right and wrong, good and evil in human conduct. Ethics cannot replace economics, literature, psychology, etc., but neither can they replace ethics.

Clearly, and at the most minimal level of shared peaceable interdisciplinary co-existence, moral differences must be confronted respectfully but not by granting each difference the same deference. Thousands of flowers may bloom but a thousand flowers do not make a garden. A garden implies some organizing principles. Ethics, to be a discipline, must be a garden even if one prefers the ordered disorderliness of the English garden, to the formalized orderliness of the Italian or French.

This calls for certain wariness about impassioned attacks on the supposed "rationalism," "abstractions," or syllogistics of philosophical ethics. Such excesses do exist. They are largely the result of the excesses and abuses of analytic and linguistic approaches to metaethics. The current taste for Pyrrhonian moral skepticism has exacerbated the problem. The resulting trend to normative nihilism or relativism cannot erase the fact that human beings seek and need reasons for differentiating right from wrong. We need norms, action guides, and *moral compass points*. Currently, moral skepticism and deprecation of reason are fashionable. They serve bioethics badly if they act as "solvents" of its normative ethical components.

In short, the first item on the agenda of the bioethicist for the next century will be to decide whether bioethics will be authentically an enterprise of ethics, or instead, it will become an amorphous expanding universe of preferences, opinions, feelings, or value choices filled with exquisite existential detail but enfeebled by a lack of normative content. For ethics to remain at the center of bioethics, it need not require rejection of the other disciplines and professions. They have shown how essential they are to the conduct of ethical reflection. However, when they replace ethics, or attenuate its normative thrust, they destroy the enterprise to which they want genuinely to contribute.

The Question of Methodologies

Closely linked to the identity question is the confusion and competition between the ways of practicing bioethics, i.e., the methods used to pursue the normative enterprise. Much of the scholarly literature of bioethics today consists of descriptions, defenses, or applications of one or the other of those methodologies. As with the many disciplines that may contribute to moral discourse, each of these methodologies has something valuable to contribute. The challenging question is how to relate them to each other and to the normative quest that remains central if bioethics is to maintain its claim to be "ethics" in any genuine sense of the word.

I am using the term "methodology" here to signify the conceptual, theoretical, or dialectical instruments that bioethicists use to pursue their perception of what bioethics is about. The theoretical substructures relating a particular methodology to ethics are developed to varying degrees. But if any method is to serve ethics *qua* ethics, it must be given some convincing account of the normative dimensions of ethics. Currently, the normative power of different methodologies is an insufficiently engaged issue.

For example, for many centuries, long before contemporary bioethics was conceived, Roman Catholic moral theologians systematically examined some of the questions engaging today's bioethicists, particularly those questions related to marriage, sexuality, and reproduction. Some employed the method of casuistry, the discernment of moral right and wrong by comparison of the case in question with certain paradigm cases. Paradigm cases are those in which general normative agreement seems assured. Beneath the casuist methodology, there was a long tradition of theology and practical, pastoral experience in hearing confessions. This was summarized in confessional manuals that were, in their centuries, the counterparts of today's textbooks of medical ethics or bioethics.

Jonsen and Toulmin (1988) have proposed casuistry as an appropriate method for contemporary usage in a secular society. It has great appeal because of its focus on concrete cases as opposed to "abstract" principles. It is rich in details and description of the moral life. It appeals to medical practitioners who like its "common sense" and practicality. But in a secular society, unfortunately, casuistry is stripped of its formal theological underpinnings. However one may judge that theology, it gave validity to the *praxis* of moral judgment. But a *praxis* without some deeper foundation, as we will reemphasize later in this essay, loses its credibility among competing notions of right and wrong. As a result, ethical discourse is reduced to consensus formation, mistaking a virtue of political practice as a ground for moral choice.

The dominant and immensely popular methodology is "principlism," as is called the application of four *prima facie* moral truths and moral guidelines and rules (Beauchamp and Childress 1994). The concreteness, conciseness, and practicality of this method gave it wide acceptance among clinicians, policymakers, and even the general public. This method has now been subjected to wide critical examination. As a result, principlism has spawned a number of "alternative methodologies" to make up for its presumed shortcomings. Largely, the problem with principles is the need for a ground for something more fundamental than simple consensus, or a vague, inconsistent "common morality." Without firmer grounding, the resolution of conflicts between principles is without guidance or becomes simply procedural.

There is also the tendency to make absolute one or the other of the four principles. In liberal democratic societies, for example, autonomy and personal choice are given *prima facie* dominance. Without a deeper grounding for principles, balancing the autonomy relationship (e.g., between doctors and patients) becomes impossible when there is conflict (Pellegrino 1994b; Schneider 1998; Bergsma and Thomasma 2000). Doctor and patient both being human and worthy of respect as persons, each has a *prima facie* claim to respect for their autonomy. Some principle beyond autonomy must guide resolution of the conflict. If, for example, this principle were to be justice, then the justification of why it should take precedence over autonomy would have to be addressed.

In the last several decades, the classical notion of virtue has been reinstated in moral discourse in a variety of contemporary forms, secular and religious (MacIntyre 1984). Here, the guide to "doing ethics" is discernment of what the good or virtuous person would do. The character traits of such a person are defined as "virtues," i.e., dispositions that habitually do the right and good thing. Ultimately, the character of moral agents is, indeed, central to moral choice. Every methodology, theory, principle, etc. is interpreted in the moment of moral decision and action by a singular human being. But even virtuous persons differ in their discernment of what they take to be right and good or of which virtue should be chosen over another.

Virtue ethics lacks specific action guidelines. Its logic is circular. While essential to any comprehension of the moral life, virtue ethics does not stand alone. Like the other methodologies, it must be related to other forms of justification. Most important, virtue ethics, at least as classically conceived, requires an orientation to ends. Virtuous persons are habitually disposed to act with the good always as their end. Yet even the ends or purposes of medicine are debatable and left to societal construction (Hanson and Callahan 1999), a method based in consensus and not in the perceptions of a moral truth. On this view, virtues are social constructs, not habitual character traits.

Another effort to capture the richness of detail, particularities, and concrete contexts in which the moral life is rooted is in the method of narrative. To understand the moment and direction of moral decision in any person's life, we need as much knowledge as possible of the internal and external forces that have shaped that person's life story. A clinical case history or a moral dilemma is always part of a larger life story, an act or a scene in the complex drama of a life. Certainly, to understand the moral experience of any person, familiarity with the story of that person's life is enormously helpful. But, as with the paradigm case in casuistry, the narrative itself cannot be normative. We must still distinguish between a good and a bad case, or a good and a bad life story. Narrative can enhance empathy and sympathy with a person's moral plight but that plight is not self-justifying. It could only be normative if it had intrinsic moral authority, something we reserve for the Hebrew and Christian Bible or the Koran.

Hermeneutics is extremely popular today in European bioethical circles. Its focus is the interpretation on the meanings of the moral experience. Contemporary hermeneutics derives from the older discipline of the interpretation of ancient scripture and texts. This idea is translated into ethics by seeing the moral agent, the moral situation, and the decision as "texts" to be interpreted. This "hermeneutical" method helps the ethicist and all those who participate in decisions to understand themselves and their response to the moral issue.

There can, of course, be many interpretations of a text and, therefore, many meanings of an ethical experience. This does not vitiate the idea of hermeneutics or make it entirely relativistic but raises the question of how we tell an appropriate from an inappropriate interpretation. The question remains of how to make the judgment about right and wrong, which is essential if hermeneutics is to have normative force. A hermeneutical interpretation of our own moral experiences or that of another may be illuminating and conducive to intersubjectivity and communication. It also may be useful procedurally but it is not *per se* normative.

The phenomenological method is also another useful and informative methodology. Like hermeneutics it is more popular in Europe than in Anglo-America in ethical discourse. Clear and concise definitions of phenomenological methodology are not easily available. It is often characterized as a turn from the "natural attitude" to the phenomenological, a turn from our most basic starting point and stance with respect to the world, the one we are in originally, to the phenomenological. The phenomenological perspective is the one we take when we reflect on the "natural attitude" itself, on everything in it. This is accomplished by suspending judgment about things in the "natural attitude" so that we can contemplate them, or, as Sokolowski puts it, so that we can "look *at* what we normally look *through*" (Sokolowski 2000).

So far as ethics goes, phenomenology, as with the other methodologies, gives us insights into our consciousness of the moral world, which can deepen our comprehension of its meanings and essence. But again, as with the other methodologies, this phenomenological perspective must have reference to some source of normativity to qualify as ethics. Clinical ethics may find that source in the phenomena of the clinical encounter (Pellegrino 2000). The phenomenological method is useful in uncovering the moral relationships in our lives. But it does not suffice without some source of norms by which what is uncovered is judged right or wrong, good or bad.

Contemporary methodologies applied to the moral life, its experience, and decisions can enhance our understanding by giving us a firmer grasp of the particularities of that life. Each methodology, including caring (Benner and Wrubel 1989), reveals insights into the real world of moral experience not grasped by the others.

All have some methodologic utility. All, in one way or another, enhance the public and personal pursuit of ethics. Unfortunately, these methodologies are in conflict. Can they complement and supplement each other? Or as astute observers like Engelhardt and MacIntyre insist, are they ultimately incompatible and incommensurable? (Engelhardt 1996; MacIntyre 1989). The possibility of linking these diverse methodologies, dealing with their conflicting perspectives, and making the contribution of each effective in ethical *praxis* is surely a significant item on the agenda of bioethics in the future.

The Question of Justification

The significance of some agreement on ethical theory becomes apparent in the practice of applied ethics, i.e., the justification of moral decisions as right and good. Each ethical theory in one way or another prescribes what persons ought to believe and ought to use as guides to action. These beliefs vindicate our moral choices and are used to evaluate the choices of others. They are in that sense "foundational" even though that claim may be hotly debated in theoretical ethics.

Traditionally, applied ethics has proceeded deductively and in syllogistic form. Some norm, axiom, principle, or belief is taken as the major premise. The minor premise is non-moral, defining the facts or circumstances of a particular case. The conclusion affirms what the major premise requires if this particular decision is to be right and good.

Casuists reason more analogically by starting with paradigm cases. They derive rules, beliefs, or intuitions from prior particular judgments in such cases. These become the major premises of moral syllogisms. Casuists may start with *a posteriori* intuitions, but they end up reasoning deductively. In fact, each moral theory uses some moral norm as a premise: for principlism, it is one of the *prima facie* principles; for Kantian deontology, the Categorical Imperative; for utilitarianism, the net good of the consequences; for natural law, the good for humans; and for virtue, what the good man would do.

To be universally applicable, *a priori* methods of justification would require agreement on the major normative premises of their syllogisms. In contemporary bioethics this is precisely the central issue. Without agreement on a background theory to validate a norm as a major premise, the deductive approach to justification is left behind. In its place a number of non-deductive, procedure-oriented methods of justification are proposed to circumvent the inadequacies of moral theory.

Only two examples will be mentioned here. They will not be given the consideration that they deserve. They are described simply to indicate the trajectories along which they are propelling bioethics today. One example is reflective equilibrium (Goodman 1965; Rawls 1971) and the other is specified principlism (Richardson 1995; Degrazia 1992). The latter system uses certain aspects of reflective equilibrium in its case analyses.

Reflective equilibrium aims to harmonize considered moral principles and considered particular moral judgments by a process of adjustment in which principles may modify judgements and vice versa. Neither principles nor any particular judgment has priority. Justification is a matter of striking a state of coherence between a particular moral belief and one's other moral beliefs. To be "coherent" is to eliminate contradictions and inconsistencies.

Reflective equilibrium has undergone evolution since it was first introduced in Rawls' classical study of justice. The adjustment process has been expanded to include philosophical theory and sociopolitical factors. In another form of reflective equilibrium, certain fixed moral points are taken into account and affect the adjustment process, though they themselves are not subject to revision.

In a more recent work (*Political Liberalism*) Rawls seeks a greater degree of moral neutrality. Justice becomes the product of social construction. It is a proposition of practical reason and independent of any truth claim. Nonetheless, here and in the other forms of reflective equilibrium, Rawls' conception of justice is shaped by his concepts of persons as free and equal in a fair society. Despite his efforts to do so, in his process of seeking coherence with other beliefs, Rawls seems not to have avoided background beliefs.

Casuistry is a more determined departure from theory (Jonsen and Toulmin 1988), as is specified principlism (Richardson 1995; DeGrazia

1992). These methods concentrate on the efficiency of making moral choices and acting in concrete cases. They abandon the search for moral truth in particular choices; they seek in its place to find a choice that gains the approval of the disputants or those making the decisions. The logical extension of this attitude is that this is what bioethics is all about (Iltis 2000, p. 283). Both casuistry and specified principlism employ the methods of coherentism, an adjustment characteristic of reflective equilibrium.

Lively debate centers on the proper relationship between these methods of practical decision making (Iltis 2000). These methods purport to come closer to real cases, concrete details, and practical decisions. But they have problems of their own because the details of the specification of principles in particular cases is still vague and heavily freighted with the moral beliefs of the person who does the specifying. There is no assurance that what is agreeable to decision makers is really in the best interest of a patient, particularly in the case of infants. There is no way to judge whether what emerges from the process of coherence among beliefs is right or good. To abandon the quest for the right and good decision is to abandon normative ethics in favor of the legal model of arbitration of disputes.

In any case, deduction is not escapable. Human moral reasoning cannot eliminate syllogisms. What these anti-deductive theories of justification seem to be most about is the substitution of sources of moral premises other than those found in standard theories. This in itself is not wrong. It may expand the range of moral premises. But the premises so derived must be judged by something other than themselves. There may be excellent "coherence" between eminently wrong moral beliefs. Coherence by itself seems a weak substitute for a robust moral proposition. It is a logical requirement of defensible moral reasoning, but not a quality of the moral rectitude of the conclusion of that reasoning procedure.

In any case, adjustment by coherence assumes that the "other" moral beliefs with which coherence is sought are themselves in some way justifiable. Then the question becomes how these other beliefs or whole systems of the beliefs can be justified. Ultimately there must be some end to this infinite series of adjustments in something beyond coherence. The question of foundations is simply inescapable despite the convictions of the post-Enlightenment and post-modern projects.

Those who want to limit bioethics to a procedure for resolving practical problems always cite Aristotle's insistence on ethics as a practical discipline aimed at action and not knowledge (*Nicomachean Ethics*, 1103b 26–30). They neglect to mention, however, that Aristotle devoted the first nine chapters of Book I to a discussion of the good for man. The Stagirite had the kind of appreciation of both the theoretical and the practical, of the universal and the particular case we must somehow recapture as the confusion grows in bioethics about identity, methodology, and justification. These three questions cannot be resolved without reference to the question of foundations.

The Question of Foundation

The three trajectories along which bioethics is now traveling are carrying it away from normative ethics except as an exercise of procedure or social construction. Given the inherent difficulties of agreement on the "ought" dimensions of human life, or of justifying our actions, it is understandable that some would like to abandon old notions and ethics and move "ahead" (Taylor 1970). But the old questions will not go away. They are confronted either directly as a background theory or they slip in from the periphery in the process of coherentism. The distant fixed moral points of our "other" beliefs cannot forever be denied.

If normative ethics is not to be lost, the perennial questions have to be faced again—what is the source of moral norms? How do we ground our moral assertions and judgments? Is this choice or decision that we are making right and good just because it follows a procedure "beyond" meta-ethics? Are the right and the good determined by humans alone, by nature, or the gods? In the end will we locate the right and the good like Protagoras in human custom, like the Stoics in nature and a non-personal god, like Aquinas and Aristotle in God and human nature, or like Nietzsche in the will of the "over man"?

In his Gifford lectures a decade ago, Alasdair MacIntyre (1990) cast the question in terms of three rival forms of moral enquiry. The first he called "*encyclopedic*," i.e., the view that philosophy is primarily a rational discipline progressively freed of religious and metaphysical presuppositions. The second he called "genealogical," i.e., the view equally committed to a religion- and God-free, anti-metaphysical ethic, in which reason is disciplined by the "*will* to power" of Nietzsche. The third rival is grounded in theology and metaphysics as represented by Aristotle and Aquinas.

MacIntyre clearly recognized the incommensurability of these points of view but he did not equate incommensurability with the impossibility of debate. He hoped for such a debate which might show that one or the other viewpoint could ". . . fail on its own terms and by its own standards" (MacIntyre 1990, p. 5). He was, however, discouraged by the response he received to his suggestions at Edinburgh and Yale. Academia seems disinclined to reopen those insistent questions as yet unsusceptible to easy resolution. The urgency of such a debate for academia as well as in public policy increases daily. The bypassing of the foundation question exposes humanity to submergence in its own technical proficiency. It will not be sufficient to justify our choices in the use of technology by a procedure or consensus formation. Decisions on how, when, or if ever such things as cloning, stem cell research, fetal tissue transplantation, extending the human life span, robotics, nano-engineering and germ-cell engineering should be undertaken, must be made. No system of ethics can survive without some "stop" signs. Where will they be placed in the years ahead?

The driving powers behind these and other decisions on the use of biotechnology are now profit and the ethos of the market place. The influence of the biotech industry on government regulations is already a reality. The impulse of some bioethicists to be "practical" and "reasonable" in light of the promised utility has already led them to endorse highly questionable and morally insupportable uses of biotechnology. There is no innovation in biotechnology that does not find some ethicist willing to bless it.

But this problem goes beyond the use of biotechnology. Under the spurious ethics of freedom of choice, almost every facet of health care is open not only to revision, but to distortion. The physician-patient relationship, the commodification of health care, the acceptance of inequities in distribution of care, the moral status of the embryo and even the infant or persons in permanent vegetative states are now revised to serve some utilitarian purpose or satisfy some personal desire. The new foundation for academic bioethics resembles what has recently been christened as the "Bobo" culture, an amalgam of gentle Bohemianism and bourgeois sensibilities (Brooks 2000). The result is a tolerant morality whose only limits are gross manifestations of moral violence. This culture fits well with the current taste for pragmatic, procedure-oriented, value-balancing forms of moral justification. On this view "reasonable" people should be able to compromise with all but the most extreme ethical aberrations.

At its worst, this trajectory of contemporary bioethics tends toward the gradual abandonment of the idea of normative ethics and moral truth of any kind. At its best, it could be the stimulus to re-examine where bioethics has come from, not to eradicate all of the new ideas it has propounded but to recover what has been left behind. At least the confidence might be retrieved that humans have the capabilities to discover moral truths beyond those they manufacture themselves by plebiscite.

This task calls for the kind of dialogue and dialectic MacIntyre proposed and academia seems to have rejected. Engelhardt (1996) has clearly shown how difficult such a dialogue can be without a common moral vision. Yet there is no alternative if the divergent pathways on which bioethics is traveling are to avoid the moral divisiveness that converts pluralism into polarization.

Engelhardt has done a genuine service by repeatedly emphasizing the consequence of the lack of shared moral vision. The post-modernists have argued that there can be no rational basis for a shared vision in the first place. They go beyond Engelhardt to undermine the intellectual credibility of any vision based in an idea of moral truth. On their view, any moral justification arrived at by the use of reason is an illusion since reason itself, and the moral philosophy that it produces, is impossible to justify rationally.

A less sophisticated and more polemical attack on moral reasoning is mounted by Posner (1999). He excoriates "academic bioethicists" because they are unable to change behavior, and extols "moral entrepreneurs" who do influence behavior by polemics, advocacy, and passion. Here, too, as with Engelhardt and the post-modernist, a frontal attack which uses reason to deny reason nonetheless serves to underscore the obstacles to reasonable dialogue in bioethics.

Of these and other adverse assessments of bioethics, post-modernism makes the clearest case. And it is the one case that lays out the alternatives most cogently. Post-modernism is a term of many meanings. It is stirring in every aspect of our culture from literature, architecture, social science, theology, and painting to moral philosophy. Its proponents are many, and their versions of the post-modernist attitude of mind are quite divergent. Several themes, however, seem common to most versions of philosophical post-modernism: a distrust of Enlightenment rationality, a rejection of overarching "foundational" theories, an emphasis on contextualization of philosophic thought, an opposition to existentialism and realism, and a commitment to epistemological and moral skepticism. These attributes notwithstanding, post-modernist philosophers deny they are skeptics, nihilists, or relativists. They seem loathe to extrapolate their assault on traditional philosophy to its ultimate logical antidote—i.e., to a need for a transcendental metaphysics. In this they resemble Nietzsche (1977) who denied that a transcendental metaphysics was possible.

The major tenets of post-modernism would appear to make a dialogue with any traditional form of philosophy well nigh impossible. Yet, paradoxically, the energetic assault of post-modernism on the autonomous rationality of the Enlightenment, and especially as exemplified in the most influential shapers of modernism, Descartes, Hume and Kant, provides some possible openings for a dialogue with its antitheses, i.e., with ancient and medieval philosophy and ethics (Hancock 1999).

This is because the post-modernist movement has effectively shown the irrationality of philosophy that results when it is torn from its roots in a realist metaphysics. This is not to suggest that the post-modernists themselves would accept classical or medieval metaphysics. But they have also challenged all "modern" philosophy, and philosophy itself, with a fatal *a priori*-ism which only a grounding in realist metaphysics could cure. They have carried the Enlightenment project so far into its logical conclusions that the alternatives are now unmistakable. Either we engage the so-called "deeper issues"—meaning the metaphysical and even the theological questions behind ethical choices—or we succumb to the moral nihilism that Nietzsche outlined. Post-modernism cannot, by itself, repair the fatal flaw it has exposed in the structure of modernism (Hancock 1996;

Bottum 1994). But it would provide a provocative partner in dialogue with traditional moral philosophy.

The possibilities of this dialogue are not as fanciful as they might appear. The most likely partner is classical and medieval philosophy, that which predates the "modernism" against which the post-modernist critique has been so squarely leveled. This is not to minimize the chasm that now separates post-modernism from the classical medieval tradition. Rather, it is to see the possibilities opened up by the post-modernist critique of modern philosophy.

Presuppositions against such a dialogue notwithstanding, evidence is appearing of a more positive approach both from scholars in the Aristotelian-Thomist tradition and from contemporary thinkers. One example is the serious reflection on the challenges of post-modernism in a collection of essays issued under the aegis of the Maritain Society (Ciapalo, 1997). Here one can find serious engagement by Thomists with post-modern notions of realism, gender, and prudence, and between the philosophies of Thomas Aquinas and Martin Heidegger to mention a few.

A more specific example is the implication for ethics of some degree of reconciliation between post-modern contextualization and Thomistic universalization of reason. The contingency of cognitive human acts is shown not necessarily to entail a rejection of necessity, timelessness, and universality of the objects of those acts (Reichberg 1997, p. 183). This is a connection important to ethics where the universality of moral truths and the singularity of specific human acts are in need of reconciliation (Reichberg 1997, p. 190).

While granting the inadequacies of deconstruction, Bourgeois (1998) and Caputo (1993), among others, discover positive engagements for ethics with the deconstructionist element of post-modernism. This is not the place to multiply examples, but rather to indicate that beyond the destructive nihilist, skeptical, and relativist bias of post-modernism, positive elements may be retrievable that can illuminate certain aspects of more traditional philosophical ethical approaches.

The opportunity for this type of dialogue is also clearly recognized in the recent encyclical of Pope John Paul II (1998), *Fides et Ratio* (*Faith and Reason*). John Paul, himself a distinguished philosopher, urges Catholic Christian philosophers and theologians to enter into serious dialogue with contemporary philosophy, including post-modernist thinking. He sees philosophy as the basis for genuine dialogue with those who do not share his faith. He calls on Catholic philosophers to find points of contact with contemporary philosophy on key issues. He defends the autonomy of philosophy but with a healthy skepticism for eclecticism, scientism, and pragmatism. He argues for the need of a metaphysical and anthropological grounding for moral truth (cf. sections 86, 88, 91, 104, and 106). In this, John Paul II is following in the tradition of St. Thomas, who engaged ancient Greek, Jewish, and Muslim philosophy as a Christian theologian.

One can hope for an equally serious and sincere effort on the part of contemporary philosophers to engage the rich body of reflection and speculation embodied in the secular classical medieval tradition. The kind of dialogue that would be most productive is not nostalgic immersion in the past but recognition of a cultural heritage that belongs to all humans, and is stored in a perennial philosophy constantly renewed and revitalized, but not eradicated, by new thought. It is as Thomas Merton (1961) put it, "What is really new is what was here all the time. This really new is that which may every moment spring freshly into existence" (p. 107).

Out of this kind of dialogue with all philosophical traditions (Jewish, Muslim, and others) conducted in the spirit of finding the truth where it may lie, modern bioethics may be able to recapture some of its normative content and ground that content in a philosophical anthropology more clearly explored than at present. Lacking this, the predictions of moral chaos by Dostoevsky and Nietzsche may well turn out to be the "real tomorrow," a prospect that a morally responsible person would not want to contemplate seriously.

Contemporary bioethics is a young organism freshly sprung from its chrysalis. What its next stage of metamorphosis will look like is unclear. What is clear are the trajectories along which it is traveling. They point to a troubled future for normative ethics at least in the sense of a guide to moral truth. What the actual future will be depends on the resolution of the four questions of identity, methodology, justification, and foundations. If society is to avoid a teratological species of morality, some recovery of stable moral truths is mandatory. This is a project for which the traditionalists, the modernists, and the post-modernists must share responsibility.

References

Aristotle. 1998. *The Nicomachean Ethics,* David Ross (trans.), revised by J. L. Ackrill and J. O. Urmson. New York: Oxford University Press.

Barzun, Jacques. 1999. *Dawn to Decadence: 500 Years of Triumph and Defeat.* New York: Harper Collins.

Beauchamp, Tom L. 1999. "The Failure of Moral Theories of Personhood." *Kennedy Institute of Ethics Journal* 9: 309–324.

Beauchamp, Tom L. 2000. "Universal Morality." In *Bioethics and Culture,* ed. Rihito Kimura. Tokyo, Japan: Waseda University Press and Westport, CT: Greenwood Press.

Beauchamp, Tom L. and James F. Childress. 1994. *Principles of Biomedical Ethics,* 4th ed. New York: Oxford University Press.

Benner, Patricia and Judith Wrubel. 1989. *The Primacy of Caring.* Menlo Park, CA: Addison Wesley.

Bergsma, Jurit and David C. Thomasma. 2000. *Autonomy and Clinical Medicine.* Dordrecht, Holland: Kluwer Academic Publishers.

Bottum, J. 1994. "Christians and Postmodernism." *First Things* (Feb.): 28–32.

Bourgeois, Patrick L. 1998. "Ethics at the Limit of Reason: Ricoeur and the Challenge of Deconstruction." *American Catholic Philosophical Quarterly* LXXII (1): 1–21.

Brooks, David. 2000. *Bobos in Paradise: The New Upper Class and How They Got There.* New York: Simon & Schuster.

Buttiglione, Rocco. 1997. *Karol Wojtyla: The Thought of the Man Who Became Pope John Paul II,* Paolo Guietti and Francesca Murphy (trans.), 117–173. Grand Rapids, Michigan: William B. Eerdmans.

Capaldi, Nicholas. 1999. "What is Bioethics without Christianity?" *Christian Bioethics* 5(3): 246–262.

Caputo, John. 1993. *Against Ethics: Contributions to a Poetics to Obligation with Constant Reference to Deconstruction.* Bloomington, IN: Indiana University Press.

Casarett, David J., Frona Daskal, and John Lantos. 1998. "The Authority of the Clinical Ethicist." *Hastings Center Report* 28(6): 6–11.

Ciapalo, Roman T., ed. 1997. *Postmodernism and Christian Philosophy (With an Introduction by Jude P. Dougherty).* Washington, DC: Catholic University of America Press.

DeGrazia, David. 1992. "Moving Forward in Bioethical Theory: Theories, Cases, and Specified Principlism." *Journal of Medicine and Philosophy* 17: 511–539.

Engelhardt, H. Tristram. 1996. *Foundations of Bioethics,* 2nd ed. New York: Oxford University Press.

Fan, Ruiping. 1999. "The Memoirs of a Pagan Sojourning in the Ruins of Chris-tendom." *Christian Bioethics* 5(3): 232–237.

Goodman, Nelson. 1965. *Fact, Fiction, and Forecast.* Cambridge, Massachusetts: Harvard University Press.

Hancock, Curtis. 1996. "Epilogue." In *Postmodernism and Christian Philosophy (With an Introduction by Jude P. Dougherty),* ed. Roman T. Ciapalo, 281–287. Washington, DC: Catholic University of America Press.

Hanson, Mark J. and Daniel Callahan, eds. 1999. *The Goals of Medicine: The For-gotten Issue in Health Care Reform.* Washington, DC: Georgetown University Press.

Iltis, Ana Smith. 2000. "Bioethics as Methodological Case Resolution: Specifica-tion, Specified Principlism and Casuistry." *Journal of Medicine and Philosophy* 25(3): 271–284.

Jonsen, Albert R. and Stephen Toulmin. 1988. *The Abuse of Casuistry: A History of Moral Reasoning.* Berkeley, California: University of California Press.

La Puma, John and David L. Schiedemayer. 1991. "Ethics Consultation: Skills, Roles and Training." *Annals of Internal Medicine* 114: 155–160.

Lyotard, Jean-François. 1984. *The Post-Modern Condition,* G. Bennington and B. Massoni (trans.). Manchester, England: Manchester University Press.

MacIntyre, Alasdair. 1984. *After Virtue,* 2nd ed. Notre Dame, IN: University of Notre Dame Press.

MacIntyre, Alasdair. 1990. *Three Rival Versions of Moral Enquiry: Encyclopedia, Genealogy, and Tradition.* Notre Dame, IN: University of Notre Dame Press.

Macklin, Ruth. 1999. *Against Relativism: Cultural Diversity and the Search for Eth-ical Universals in Medicine.* New York: Oxford University Press.

McCool, Gerald. 1994. *The Neo-Thomist.* Milwaukee, WI: Marquette University Press.

Meilaender, Gilbert. 1995. *Body, Soul and Bioethics.* Notre Dame, IN: University of Notre Dame Press.

Merton, Thomas. 1961. *New Seeds of Contemplation.* Norfolk, CT: New Direc-tions.

National Bioethics Advisory Commission. 2000. *Ethical Issues in Human Stem Cell Research,* Vol. 2. Rockville, MD: National Bioethics Advisory Commis-sion.

Nietzsche, Friedrich. 1977. *A Nietzsche Reader.* B. J. Hollingdale (trans.). New York: Penguin Books.

Pellegrino, Edmund D. 1994a. "Patient Autonomy and the Physician's Ethics." *An-nals of the Royal College of Physicians and Surgeons of Canada* 27(3): 171–173.

Pellegrino, Edmund D. 1994b. "Patient and Physician Autonomy: Conflicting Rights and Obligations in the Physician-Patient Relationship." *The Journal of Contemporary Health, Law, and Policy* 10: 47–68.

Pellegrino, Edmund D. 1997. "Bioethics as an Interdisciplinary Enterprise: Where Does Ethics Fit in the Mosaic of Disciplines?" In *Philosophy of Medicine and Bioethics: A Twenty-Year Retrospective and Critical Appraisal* (Philosophy and Medicine Series #50), ed. Ronald A. Carson and Chester R. Burns, 1–23. Dordrecht, the Netherlands: Kluwer Academic Publishers.

Pellegrino, Edmund D. 1999. "The Origins and Evolution of Bioethics: Some Personal Reflections." *Kennedy Institute of Ethics Journal* 9(1): 73–88.

Pellegrino, Edmund D. 2000. *The Lived World of Doctor and Patient: A Phenomenological Perspective.* New Haven, CT: Yale University Press.

Pope John Paul II. 1998. "Encyclical Letter: *Fides et Ratio.*" *Origins* 28(19), October 22.

Posner, Richard A. 1999. *The Problematics of Moral and Legal Theory.* Cambridge: Harvard University Press.

Rawls, John. 1971. *A Theory of Justice.* New York: Oxford.

Rawls, John. 1996. *Political Liberalism.* New York: Columbia University Press.

Reich, Warren T. 1999. "The Wider View: Andre Helleger's Passionate, Integrating Intellect and the Creation of Bioethics." *Kennedy Institute of Ethics Journal* 9(1): 25–51.

Reichberg, Gregory M. 1997. "Contextualizing Theoretical Reason: Thomas Aquinas and Post-modernity." In *Postmodernism and Christian Philosophy,* ed. Roman T. Ciapalo. Washington, DC: Catholic University of America Press.

Richardson, Henry S. 1995. "Beyond Good and Right: Toward a Constructive Pragmatism." *Philosophy and Public Affairs* 24:108–141.

Rie, Michael. 1999. "What Is Christian about Christian Bioethics?" *Christian Bioethics* 5(3): 263–266.

Schneider, Carl E. 1998. *The Practice of Autonomy: Patients, Doctors, and Medical Decisions.* New York: Oxford University Press.

Scofield, Giles R. 1993. "Ethics Consultation: The Least Dangerous Profession?" *Cambridge Quarterly of Health Care Ethics* 2: 417–448.

Shalit, Ruth. 1997. "When We Were Philosopher Kings, the Rise of the Medical Ethicist." *The New Republic* (April 28): 24–28.

Sokolowski, Robert. 2000. *Introduction to Phenomenology.* Cambridge: Cambridge University Press.

Taylor, Richard. 1970. *Good and Evil: A New Direction.* New York: Macmillan.

Veatch, Henry B. 1971. *For an Ontology of Morals: A Critique of Contemporary Ethical Theory.* Evanston, IL: Northwestern University Press.

Veatch, Robert M. 2000. "Moral Absolutism and Postmodernism: Are They Compatible?" In *Bioethics and Culture,* ed. Rihito Kimura. Tokyo, Japan: Waseda University Press and Westport, CT: Greenwood Press.

Wojtyla, Karol. 1979. *The Acting Person,* Andrzej Potocki (trans., in collaboration with Anna-Teresa Tymieniecka). Dordrecht, the Netherlands: Kluwer Academic Publishers.

Hippocratic Tradition

Toward an Expanded Medical Ethics

The Hippocratic Ethic Revisited

Good physicians are by the nature of their vocation called upon to practice their art within a framework of high moral sensitivity. For two millennia this sensitivity was provided by the oath and the other ethical writings of the Hippocratic corpus. No code has been more influential in heightening the moral reflexes of ordinary individuals. Every subsequent medical code is essentially a footnote to the Hippocratic precepts, which even to this day remain the paradigm of how good physicians should behave.

The Hippocratic ethic is marked by a unique combination of humanistic concern and practical wisdom admirably suited to physicians' tasks in society. In a simpler world, that ethic long sufficed to guide physicians in their service to patient and community. Today, the intersections of medicine with contemporary science, technology, social organization, and changed human values have revealed significant missing dimensions in the ancient ethic. The reverence we rightly accord the Hippocratic precepts must not obscure the need for a critical examination of their missing dimensions—those most pertinent for contemporary physicians and society. The need for expanding traditional medical ethics is already well established. It was first underscored by the shocking revelations of the Nuremberg trials.

A spate of new codes has appeared which attempt to deal more responsibly with the promise and the dangers of human experimentation; the inquiry is well under way.[1] More recently, further ethical inquiries

401

have been initiated to reflect the change in moral climate and medical attitudes toward abortion, population control, euthanasia, transplanting organs, and manipulating human behavior and genetic constitution.[2] In actual fact, some of the major proscriptions of the Hippocratic Oath are already being consciously compromised: confidentiality can be violated under certain conditions of law and public safety, abortion is being legalized, dangerous drugs are used everywhere, and a conscious but controlled invasion of the patient's rights in human experimentation is now permitted.

This essay will examine some important dimensions of medical ethics not included in the Hippocratic ethic and, in some ways, even obscured by its too rigorous application. To be considered here are the ethics of participation, the questions raised by institutionalizing medical care, the need for an axiology of medical ethics, the changing ethics of competence, and the tensions between individual and social ethics.

An analysis of these questions will reveal the urgent need for expanding medical ethical concerns far beyond those traditionally observed. A deeper ethic of social and corporate responsibility is needed to guide the profession to levels of moral sensitivity more congruent with the expanded duties of the physician in contemporary culture.

The normative principles which constitute what may loosely be termed the Hippocratic ethic are contained in the oath and the deontological books: *Law, Decorum, Precepts,* and *The Physician.* These treatises are of varied origin and combine behavioral imperatives derived from a variety of sources—the schools at Cos and Cnidus intermingled with Pythagorean, Epicurean, and Stoic influences.[3]

The oath speaks of the relationships of the student and his teacher, advises the physician never to harm the patient, enjoins confidentiality, and proscribes abortion, euthanasia, and the use of the knife.[4] It forbids sexual commerce with the women in the household of the sick. The doctor is a member of a select brotherhood dedicated to the care of the sick, and his major reward is a good reputation.

Law discusses the qualities of mind and the diligence required of the prospective physician from early life. *The Physician* emphasizes the need for dignified comportment, a healthy body, a grave and kind mien, and a regular life. In *Decorum,* we are shown the unique practical wisdom rooted in experience which is essential to good medicine and absent in the quack; proper comportment in the sickroom dictates a reserved, authoritative, composed air; much practical advice is given on the arts and techniques of clinical medicine.[5] *Precepts* again warns against theorizing without fact, inveighs against quackery, urges consideration in setting fees, and encourages consultation in difficult cases.[6]

Similar admonitions can be found scattered throughout the Hippocratic corpus, but it is these few brief ethical treatises which have formed the character of the physician for so many centuries. From them, we can extract what can loosely be called the Hippocratic ethic—a mixture of high ideals, common sense, and practical wisdom. A few principles of genuine ethics are often repeated and intermingled with etiquette and homespun advice of all sorts. The good physician emerges as an authoritative and competent practitioner devoted to his patient's well-being. He is a benevolent and sole arbiter who knows what is best for the patient and makes all decisions for him.

There is in the Hippocratic corpus little explicit reference to the responsibilities of medicine as a corporate entity with responsibility for its members and duties to the greater human community. The ethic of the profession as a whole is assured largely by the moral behavior of its individual members. There is no explicit delineation of the corporate responsibility of physicians for one another's ethical behavior. On the whole, the need for maintaining competence is indirectly stated. There are, in short, few explicit recommendations about what we would today call "social ethics."

These characteristics of the Hippocratic ethic have been carried forward to our day. They are extended in the code of Thomas Percival which formed the basis of the first code of ethics adopted by the American Medical Association in 1847.[7] They were sufficient for the less complex societies of the ancient and modern worlds but not for the contemporary twentieth-century experience. The Hippocratic norms can no longer be regarded as unchanging absolutes but as partial statements of ideals in need of constant reevaluation, amplification, and evolution.

Without in any way denigrating the essential worth of the Hippocratic ethic, it is increasingly apparent that the ideas conveyed about the physician are simplistic and incomplete for today's needs. In some ways, it is even antipathetic to the social and political spirit of our times. For example, the notion of the physician as a benevolent and paternalistic figure who decides all for the patient is inconsistent with today's educated public. It is surely incongruous in a democratic society in which the rights of self-determination are being assured by law. In a day when the remote effects of individual medical acts are so consequential, we cannot be satisfied with an ethic which is so inexplicit about social responsibilities. Nowhere in the Hippocratic Oath is the physician recognized as a member of a corporate entity which can accomplish good ends for humanity that are more than the sum of individual good acts. The necessity for a stringent ethic of competence and a new ethic of shared responsibility which flows from team and institutional medical care is understandably not addressed.

It is useful to examine some of these missing ethical dimensions as examples of the kind of organic development long overdue in professional medical ethical codes.

The central and most admirable feature of the oath is the respect it inculcates for the patient. In the oath, the doctor is pledged always to help patients and keep them from harm. This duty is then exemplified by specific prohibitions against abortion, use of deadly drugs, surgery, breaches of confidence, and indulgence in sexual relations with members of the sick person's household. Elsewhere, in *The Physician, Decorum,* and *Precepts,* the physician is further enjoined to be humble, careful in observation, calm and sober in thought and speech. These admonitions have the same validity today that they had centuries ago and are still much in need of cultivation.

But in one of these same works, *Decorum,* we find an excellent example of how drastically the relationship between physician and patient has changed since Hippocrates' time. The doctor is advised to "Perform all things calmly and adroitly, concealing most things from the patient while you are attending him." A little further on, the physician is told to treat the patient with solicitude, "revealing nothing of the patient's present and future condition."[8] This advice is at variance with social and political trends and with the desires of most educated patients. It is still too often the modus operandi of physicians dreaming of a simpler world in which authority and paternalistic benevolence were the order of the day.

Indeed, a major criticism of physicians today centers on this very question of disclosure of essential information. Many educated patients feel frustrated in their desire to participate in decisions which affect them as intimately as medical decisions invariably do. The matter really turns on establishing new bases for the patient's trust. The knowledgeable patient can trust the physician only if he or she feels the latter is competent and uses that competence with integrity and for ends which have value for the patient. Today's educated patient wants to understand what the physician is doing, why he or she is doing it, what the alternatives may be, and what choices are open. In a democratic society, people expect the widest protection of their rights to self-determination. Hence, contemporary patients have a right to know the decisions involved in managing their cases.

When treatment is specific, with few choices open, the prognosis good, the side effects minimal, disclosing the essential information is an easy matter. Unfortunately, medicine frequently deals with indefinite diagnoses and nonspecific treatments of uncertain value. Several alternatives are usually open; prognosis may not be altered by treatment; side effects are often considerable and discomfort significant. The patient certainly has the right to know these data before therapeutic interventions are initiated. The Nuremberg Code and others were designed to protect the subject in the course of human experimentation by insisting on the right of informed and free consent. The same right should be guaranteed in the course of ordinary medical treatment as well.

So fundamental is this right of self-determination in a democratic society that to limit it, even in ordinary medical transactions, is to propagate an injustice. This is not to ignore the usual objections to disclosure: the fear of inducing anxiety in the patient, the inability of the sick patient to participate in the decision, the technical nature of medical knowledge, and the possibility of litigation. These objections deserve serious consideration but will, on close analysis, not justify concealment except under special circumstances. Obviously, the fear of indiscriminate disclosure cannot obfuscate the invasion of a right, even when concealment is in the interest of the patient.

Surely physicians are expected by patients and society to use disclosure prudently. For the very ill, the very anxious, the poorly educated, the too young, or the very old, doctors will permit themselves varying degrees of disclosure. The modes of doing so must be adapted to the patient's educational level, psychological responses, and physiologic state. It must be emphatically stated that the purpose of disclosure of alternatives, costs, and benefits in medical diagnosis and treatment is not to relieve the physician of the onus of decision or displace it on the patient. Rather, it permits the physician to function as technical expert and adviser, inviting the patient's participation and understanding as aids in the acceptance of the decision and its consequences. This is the only basis for a mature, just, and understandable physician-patient relationship.

The most important human reason for enabling patients to participate in the decisions which affect them is to allow consideration of their personal values. Here, the Hippocratic tradition is explicitly lacking, since its spirit is almost wholly deontological; that is, obligations are stated as absolutes without reference to any theory of values. Underlying value systems are not stated or discussed. The need for examining the intersection of values inherent in every medical transaction is unrecognized. The values of the physician or of medicine are assumed to prevail as absolutes, and an operational attitude of noblesse oblige is encouraged.

A deontologic ethic was not inappropriate for Greek medicine, which did not have to face so many complex and antithetical courses of action. But a relevant ethic for our times must be more axiologic than deontologic; that is, based on a more conscious theory of values. The values upon which any action is based are of enormous personal and social consequence. An analysis of conflicting values underlies the choice of a noxious treatment for a chronic illness, the question of prolonging life in an incurable disease, or setting priorities for using limited medical resources. Instead of absolute values, we deal more frequently with an intersection of several sets and subsets of values: those of the patient, the physician, sciences, and society. Which shall prevail when these values are in conflict? How do we decide?

The patient's values must be respected whenever possible and whenever they do not create injustice for others. Patients are free to delegate the decision to their physicians, but they must do this consciously and freely. To the extent that they are educated, responsible, and thoughtful, modern individuals will increasingly want the opportunity to examine relative values in each transaction. When patients are unconscious or otherwise unable to participate, the physician or the family acts as their surrogate, charged as closely as possible to preserve their values.

The Hippocratic principle of *primum non nocere,* therefore, must be expanded to encompass the patient's value system if it is to have genuine meaning. To impose the doctor's value system is an intrusion on the patient; it may be harmful, unethical, and result in an error in diagnosis and treatment. Further, the concept of "health" as a positive entity is as vague today as in Hippocrates' time. Its definition is highly personal. The physician's view of health may be quite at variance with that of the patient or even of society. Doctors understandably tend to place an ideological value on health and medicine. Society should expect this from them as experts, but their views must not prevail unchallenged. Indeed, society must set its own priorities for health. The amelioration of social disorders like alcoholism, sociopathy, drug addiction, and violence can have greater value for a healthy human existence, for example, than merely prolonging life in patients with chronic disabling disorders. Indeed, the patient and society now demand to participate in making the choices. The configuration of value choices each of us makes defines concretely our uniqueness and individuality. Hence, each patient has a slightly different definition of health. Physicians are also individuals with sets of values which invariably color their professional acts. Their views of sex, alcohol, suffering, poverty, race, and so forth can sharply differ with those of their patients. Their advice on these matters, as well as their definition of cooperation, often has a strong ideologic or moralistic tinge. Physicians must constantly guard against confusing their own values as the "good" to which all must subscribe if they desire to be treated by them.

Disclosure is, therefore, a necessary condition if we really respect each patient as a unique being whose values, as a part of his or her person, are no more to be violated than his or her body. The deontologic thrust of traditional medical ethics is too restrictive in a time when the reexamination of all values is universal. It even defeats the very purposes of the traditional ethic, which are to preserve the integrity of the patient as a person.

Another notably unexplored area in the Hippocratic ethic is the social responsibility of the physician. Its emphasis on the welfare of the individual patient is exemplary, and this is firmly explicated in the oath and elsewhere. Indeed, in *Precepts* this respect for the individual patient is placed at the very heart of medicine: "Where there is love of one's fellow man, there is love of the Art."[9]

As Ford has shown, today too the physician's sense of responsibility is directed overwhelmingly toward his or her own patient.[10] This is one of the most admirable features of medicine, and it must always remain the central ethical imperative in medical transactions. But it must now be set in a context entirely alien to that in which ancient medicine was practiced. In earlier eras the remote effects of medical acts were of little concern, and the rights of the individual patient could be the exclusive and absolute base of the physician's actions. Today, the growing interdependence of all humans and the effectiveness of medical techniques have drastically altered the simplistic arrangements of traditional ethics. The aggregate effects of individual medical acts have already changed the ecology of humanity. Every death prevented or life prolonged alters the number, kind, and distribution of human beings. The resultant competition for living space, food, and conveniences already imperils our hope for a life of satisfaction for all.

Even more vexing questions in social ethics are posed when we attempt to allocate our resources among the many new possibilities for good inherent in medical progress and technology. Do we pool our limited resources and manpower to apply curative medicine to all now deprived of it or continue to multiply the complexity of services for the privileged? Do we apply mass prophylaxis against streptococcal diseases, or repair damaged valves with expensive heart surgery? Is it preferable to change cultural patterns in favor of a more reasonable diet for Americans or develop better surgical techniques for unplugging fat-occluded coronary arteries? Every health planner and concerned public official has his or her own set of similar questions. It is clear that we cannot have all these things simultaneously.

This dimension of ethics becomes even more immediate when we inquire into the responsibility of medicine for meeting the urgent sociomedical needs of large segments of our population. Can we absolve ourselves from responsibility for deficiencies in distribution, quality, and accessibility of even ordinary medical care for the poor, the uneducated, and the disenfranchised? Do we direct our health care system to the care of the young in ghettos and underdeveloped countries or to the affluent aged? Which course will make for a better world? These are vexing questions of the utmost social concern. Physicians have an ethical responsibility to raise these questions and, in answering them, to work with the community in ordering its priorities to make optimal use of available medical skills.

It is not enough to hope that the good of the community will grow fortuitously out of the summation of good acts of each physician for his or her own patients. Societies are necessary to insure enrichment of the life of each of their members. But they are more than the aggregate of persons within them. As T. S. Eliot puts it, "What life have you if you have not life together? There is no life that is not in community."[11]

Society supports doctors in the expectation that they will direct themselves to socially relevant health problems, not just those they find interesting or remunerative. The commitment to social egalitarianism demands a greater sensitivity to social ethics than is to be found in traditional codes. Section ten of the American Medical Association Principles of Medical Ethics (1946) explicitly recognizes the profession's responsibility to society. But a more explicit analysis of the relationships of individual and social ethics should be undertaken. Medicine, which touches on the most human problems of both the individual and society, cannot serve human beings without attending to both their personal and communal needs.

This is not to say that medical codes or physicians are to set social priorities. Clearly, individual physicians cannot quantitate the remote effects of each of their medical acts. Nor should they desert their patients to devote themselves entirely to social issues. They cannot withhold specific treatment in hope of preventing some future perturbation of human ecology. Nor can society relegate solely to physicians such policy questions as how and for whom the major health effort will be expended.

In these matters physicians serve best as expert witnesses, providing the basis for informed public decisions. They must lead in pointing out deficiencies and raising the painful matter of choices. At the same time, each doctor must honor his or her traditional contract to help his or her own patient. Doctors cannot allow the larger social issues to undermine that solicitude. Ethically responsive doctors will thus find themselves more and more at the intersection of social and individual ethical values, impelled to act responsibly in both spheres. The Hippocratic ethic and its later modifications were not required to confront such paradoxes. Today's conscientious physicians are very much in need of an expanded ethic to cope with their double responsibility to the individual and to the community.

The institutionalization of all aspects of medical care is an established fact. With increasing frequency, the personal contract inherent in patient care is made with institutions, groups of physicians, or teams of health professionals. Patients now often expect the institution or group to select their physician or consultant and to assume responsibility for the quality and quantity of care provided.

Within the institution itself, the health care team is essential to the practice of comprehensive medicine. Physicians and nonphysicians now cooperate in providing the spectrum of special services made possible by modern technology. The responsibility for even the most intimate care of the patient is shared. Some of the most important clinical decisions are made by team members who may have no personal contact at all with the patient. The team itself is not a stable entity of unchanging composition. Its membership changes in response to the patient's needs, and so may its leadership. Preserving the traditional rights of the patient, formerly vested in a single identifiable physician, is now sometimes spread anonymously over a group. Competence, confidentiality, integrity, and personal concern are far more difficult to assure with a group of diverse professionals enjoying variable degrees of personal contact with the patient.

No current code of ethics fully defines how the traditional rights of the medical transaction are to be protected when responsibility is diffused within a team and an institution. Clearly, no health profession can elaborate such a code of team ethics by itself. We need a new medical ethic which permits the cooperative definition of normative guides to protect the person of the patient served by a group, none of whose members may have sole responsibility for care. Laymen, too, must participate, since boards of trustees set the overall policies which affect patient care. Few trustees truly recognize that they are the ethical and legal surrogates of society for the patients who come to their institutions seeking help.

Thus, the most delicate of the physician's responsibilities, protecting the patient's welfare, must now be fulfilled in a new and complicated context. Instead of the familiar one-to-one unique relationship, physicians find themselves coordinators of a team, sharing with others some of the most sensitive areas of patient care. Physicians are still bound to see that group assessment and management are rational, safe, and personalized. They must especially guard against the dehumanization so easily and inadvertently perpetrated by a group in the name of efficiency.

Doctors must acquire new attitudes. Since ancient times, they have been the sole dominant and authoritarian figures in the care of their patients. They have been supported in this position by traditional ethics. In the clinical emergency, their dominant role is still unchallenged, since they are well trained to make quick decisions in ambiguous situations. What they are not prepared for are the negotiations, analysis, and ultimate compromise fundamental to group efforts and essential in nonemergency situations. A whole new set of clinical perspectives must be introduced, perspectives difficult for the classically trained physician to accept, but necessary if the patient is to benefit from contemporary technology and organization of health care.

A central aim of the oath and other ethical treatises is to protect the patient and the profession from quackery and incompetence. In the main, competence is assumed as basic in fulfillment of the Hippocratic ideal of *primum non nocere*. In places, more specific admonitions are to be found. Thus, in *Law*, "Medicine is the most distinguished of all the arts, but through the ignorance of those who practice it, and those who casually judge such practitioners, it is now of all arts by far the least esteemed."[12] The author of this treatise thus succinctly expressed the same concerns being voiced at greater length and with more hyperbole in our own times. In the treatise on fractures, specific advice is given to prevent curable cases from becoming incurable, to choose the simpler treatment, to attempt to help, even if the patient seems incurable, and to avoid "unnecessary torment."[13] Consultation is clearly advised in *Precepts*.[14] In *Decorum*, frequent visits and careful examination are enjoined.[15]

The Hippocratic works preach the wholly admirable commonsense ethos of the good artisan: careful work, maturation of skills, simplicity of approach, and knowledge of limitations. This was sound advice at a time when new discoveries were so often the product of speculation untainted by observation or experience. The speculative astringency of the Hippocratic ethic was a potent and necessary safeguard against the quackery of fanciful and dangerous "new" cures.

With the scientific era in medicine, the efficacy of new techniques and information in changing the natural history of disease was dramatically demonstrated. Today, the patient has a right to access to the vast stores of new knowledge useful to medicine. Failure of the physician to make this reservoir available and accessible is a moral failure. The ethos of the artisan, while still a necessary safeguard, is now far from being a sufficient one.

Maintaining competence today is a prime ethical challenge. Only the highest standard of initial and continuing professional proficiency is acceptable in a technological world. This imperative is now so essential a feature of the patient-physician transaction that the ancient mandate "Do no harm" must be supplemented: "Do all things essential to optimal solution of the patient's problem." Anything less makes the doctor's professional declaration a sham and a scandal.

Competence now has a far wider definition than in ancient times. Not only must physicians encompass expertly the knowledge pertinent to their own field, but they must be the instrument for bringing all other knowledge to bear on their patient's needs. They now function as one element in a vast matrix of consultants, technicians, apparatus, and institutions, all of which may contribute to a patient's well-being. They cannot provide all these things themselves. To attempt to do so is to pursue the romantic and vanishing illusion of the physician as Renaissance man.

The enormous difficulties of its achievement notwithstanding, competence has become the first ethical precept for the modern physician after integrity. It is also the prime humane precept and the one most peculiar to the physician's function in society. Even the current justifiable demands of patients and medical students for greater compassion must not obfuscate the centrality of competence in the physician's existence. The simple intention to help others is commendable but, by itself, not only insufficient but positively dangerous. What is more inhumane or more a violation of trust than incompetence? The consequence of a lack of compassion may be remediable, while a lack of competence may cost the patient a chance for recovery of life, function, and happiness. Clearly, medicine cannot attain the ethical eminence to which it is called without both compassion and competence.

Within this framework, a more rigorous ethic of competence must be elaborated. Continuing education, periodic recertification, and renewal of clinical privileges have become moral mandates, not just hopeful hortatory devices dependent upon individual physician responses. The Hippocratic ethic of the good artisan is now just the point of departure for the wide options technology holds out for individual and social health.

The one-to-one patient-to-physician relationship so earnestly extolled for centuries makes patients almost totally dependent upon their physician for entry into the vast complex of potentially useful services. We cannot leave to fortune or statistics the possibility that patients' choice of a physician might impede their access to all they need for optimal care. We must surround this one-to-one relationship with the safeguards of a corporate responsibility in which the whole profession dedicates itself to protecting the patient's right to competent care.

The whole of the Hippocratic corpus, including the ethical treatises, is the work of many authors writing in different historical periods. Thus, the ethical precepts cannot be considered the formal position of a profession in today's sense. There is no evidence of recognition of true corporate responsibility for larger social issues or of sanctions to deter miscreant members. Indeed, in *Law* there is a clear lament for the lack of penalties to restrain or punish the unethical physician: "medicine is the only art which our states have made subject to no penalty save that of dishonor. And dishonor does not wound those who are compacted of it."[16] Again, in *Precepts,* "Now no harm would be done if bad practitioners received their due wages. But as it is, their innocent patients suffer, for whom the violence of their disorder did not appear sufficient without the addition of their physician's inexperience."[17]

The Greek physician seems to have regarded himself as the member of an informal aristocratic brotherhood in which each individual was expected to act ethically and to do so for love of the profession and respect for the patient. His reward was *doxa,* a good reputation, which in turn assured a successful practice. There is notably no sense of the larger responsibilities as a profession for the behavior of each member. Nowhere stated are the potentialities and responsibilities of a group of high-minded individuals to effect reforms and achieve purposes transcending the interests of individual members. In short, the Greek medical profession relied on the sum total of individual ethical behaviors to assure the ethical behavior of the group.

This is still the dominant view of many physicians in the Western world who limit their ethical perspectives to their relationships with their own patients. Medical societies do censure unethical members with varying alacrity for the grosser forms of misconduct or breaches of professional etiquette. But there is as yet insufficient assumption of a corporate and shared responsibility for the actions of each member of the group. The power of physicians as a polity to effect reforms in quality of care, its organization, and its relevance to the needs of society is as yet unrealized.

Yet many of the dimensions of medical ethics touched upon in this essay can only be secured by the conscious assumption of a corporate responsibility on the part of all physicians for the final pertinence of their individual acts to promote better life for all. There is the need to develop, as it were, a functioning ethical syncytium in which the actions of each physician would touch upon those of all physicians and in which it is clear that the ethical failings of each member would diminish the stature of every other physician to some degree. This syncytial framework is at variance with the traditional notion that all physicians act as individuals and are primarily responsible only to themselves and their patients.

This shift of emphasis is dictated by the metamorphosis of all professions in our complex, highly organized, highly integrated, and egalitarian social order. For most of its history medicine has existed as a select and loosely organized brotherhood. For the past hundred years in our country, it has been more formally organized in the American Medical Association and countless other professional organizations dedicated to a high order of individual ethics. A new stage in the evolution of medicine as a profession is about to begin as a consequence of three clear trends.

First, all professions are increasingly being regarded as services, even as public utilities, dedicated to fulfilling specific social needs not entirely defined by the profession. Professionals themselves will acquire dignity and standing in the future, not so much from the tasks they perform, but from the intimacy of the connection between those tasks and the social life of which the profession is a part. Second, the professions are being democratized, and it will be ever more difficult for any group to hold a privileged position. The automatic primacy of medicine is being challenged by the other health professions whose functions are of increasing importance in patient care. This functionalization of the professions tends to emphasize what is done for a patient and not who does it. Moreover, many tasks formerly performed only by physicians are now being done by other professionals and nonprofessionals. Last, the socialization of all humanity affects the professions as well. Hence, the collectivity will increasingly be expected to take responsibility for how well or poorly the profession carries out the purposes for which it is supported by society.

These changes will threaten medicine only if physicians hold to a simplistic ethic in which the agony of choices among individual and social values is dismissed as spurious or imaginary. Physicians are the most highly educated of health professionals. They should be first to take on the burdens of a continuing self-reformation in terms of a new ethos—one in which the problematics of priorities and values are openly faced as common responsibilities of the entire profession. We must recognize the continuing validity of traditional ethics for the personal dimensions of patient care and their inadequacy for the newer social dimensions of health in contemporary life. It is the failure to appreciate this distinction that stimulates so much criticism of the profession at the same time that individual physicians are highly respected.

What are some of the ethical problems and social responsibilities which are best assured by a corporate posture? We mention but a few as examples, especially those outlined earlier in this essay.

In a technical society with knowledge increasing exponentially, all members of a profession cannot attain the same degree of competence. The whole body of physicians must assume responsibility for guaranteeing to society the highest possible competence in each member. A most effective way to assure this is for each professional group to require, as some already have, the periodic demonstration of continued proficiency as a first condition for continuing membership in the profession. Physicians should take leadership in requiring relicensure and recertification, set the standards of performance, and insist on a remedial and not a punitive approach for those who need refurbishment of their knowledge to qualify for recertification. Implicit in this idea is the possibility that at some point each of us may fail to qualify for reasons such as age, illness, or loss of interest. A profession sensitive to its ethical responsibilities cannot tolerate fading competence, even for reasons beyond the physician's control. Instead, it must provide opportunities for remediation or for alternate, more suitable functions within medicine. Surely the wide range of uses of a medical education will assure a useful place for almost all physicians.

A most potent way to assure competence is to insist that all physicians practice within a context of competent colleagues and peer surveillance. It is an ethical responsibility of the whole profession to see that every licensed physician is a member of a hospital staff. The privilege of using a hospital is primarily a privilege for the patient, not the doctor. To deprive any licensed physicians, because of training, economics, race, or other reasons, of hospital privilege is to deprive their patients and to perpetrate a social injustice. We also thereby lose the best chance to help physicians improve themselves by contact with their colleagues and with institutional standards as well as the informal network of teaching that links physicians together when they can discuss their cases with one another. No rationalization based on economics or professional prerogatives can excuse our profession from its ethical responsibility to enable every practitioner to participate in the mainstream of medical care, in the hospital and the medical school as well. This responsibility should extend to the osteopathic as well as the allopathic physician.

Once every physician is on a hospital staff, there is much the profession can do to develop a context within which competence becomes a value of prime importance. Some institutional mechanisms for review of certain aspects of competence already exist in tissue and utilization committee, though these first steps are not universally applied with sufficient vigor. A well-functioning drug information center in every hospital, a rigorous pharmacy and therapeutics committee, critical reviews of diagnostic accuracy and work-up, comparison of practices against national standards—these are examples of further institutional devices we should insist upon as ethical imperatives. Ultimately, all physicians should have available for their own edification a computerized record of their diagnostic acumen, therapeutic practices, complications, and autopsy correlations. The essential matter is not the specific mechanisms used, but acceptance of the dictum that the competence of each member of the group is, in some real sense, the responsibility of all.

These measures can easily be discounted as repressive, regimentalizing infringements of professional freedom. Or, in a more enlightened ethical view, they can be the practical expression of corporate acceptance of the necessity of workable mechanisms to ensure competence in a technological society. Is there a real ethical choice? The patient, after all, has no means whereby he or she can judge the competence of the services rendered. Individual physicians and the profession owe the patient every possible safeguard. When these are not forthcoming, they will be imposed by a public demanding more accountability in medicine and every other sphere of life.

One of the gravest and most easily visible social inequities today is the maldistribution of medical services among portions of our population. This is another sphere in which the profession as a whole must assume responsibility for what individual physicians cannot do alone. The civil rights movement and the revolt of the black and minority populations have punctuated the problem. Individual physicians have always tried to redress this evil, some in heroic ways. Now, however, the problem is a major ethical responsibility for the whole profession; we cannot dismiss the issue. We must engender a feeling of ethical diminution of the entire profession whenever there are segments of the population without adequate and accessible medical care. This extends to the provision of primary care for all, insistence on a system of coverage for all communities every hour of the day, proper distribution of the various medical specialties and facilities, and a system of fees no longer based on the usual imponderables but on more standardized norms.

Fulfilling such ethical imperatives is sure to cause discomfort for the doctor as well as some loss of privileges and even of remuneration. But unless there is corporate concern translated into corporate action and self-imposed responsibilities, restrictive legislation to achieve these ends seems certain. To an ethically perceptive profession, such legislation should not only be unnecessary, it should be a scandal. It is intrinsic to the very purposes of medicine that physicians exhibit the greatest sensitivity to any social injustice directly related to their mandate in society. The lack of this corporate sensitivity has been acutely perceived by some of today's students and has seriously disaffected them with medical education and practice.[18] We hope, when they assume leadership of the profession, that they will feel these ethical discontinuities as clearly as they do now. If tomorrow's physicians practice what they now preach to their elders, they will indeed expand the ethical responsibilities of our profession into new and essential dimensions. To do so, they will need to supplement traditional medical ethics with a corporate ethical sense as we have just described it.

There are, perforce, reasonable limits to the social ills to which the individual physician and the profession can be expected to attend as physicians. Some have suggested that medicine concern itself with the Vietnam War, the root causes of poverty, environmental pollution, drugs, housing, and racial injustice. It would be difficult to argue that all of these social ills are primary ethical responsibilities of individual physicians or even of the profession. To do so would hopelessly diffuse medical energies and manpower from their proper object—the promotion of health and the cure of illness. The profession can fight poverty, injustice, and war through medicine.

A distinction, therefore, must clearly be made between physicians' primary ethical responsibilities, which derive from the nature of their profession, and those ethical responsibilities which do not. All physicians must strike for themselves an optimal balance between professional and civic responsibilities. This will depend upon their energy, capabilities, the nature of their specialty, their family responsibilities, and other factors. The extremes of this choice are dangerous: a narrowly technical life, or a free-floating social concern which at best is neurotic and ineffectual and at worst can seriously compromise competence. Ever present is the seductive hubris to which physicians are especially susceptible—the assumption of some special authority or capability in the resolution of all social issues.

It becomes a matter of prime ethical concern for each physician consciously to establish some hierarchy of values and priorities which will define his or her individual and social ethical postures. The ethical responsibilities of the professional group should be broad; those of the individual may of necessity be narrow. Is there some reasonable order of values in the maze of conflicting duties thrust upon physicians today? We will examine this question from the point of view of the clinician.

Surely the first order of responsibility for clinicians must remain with the patients they undertake to treat. Here, the moral imperatives are clear: competence of the highest order, integrity, compassion.

These are continued in traditional medical ethics and can be made more relevant to our times by extension in some of the directions indicated earlier in this essay. To fail in this realm is to violate the trust underlying the personal relationship which characterizes medical care. Nothing is more unconscionable or socially unacceptable.

Only when this first order of ethical requirements has been met can individual physicians address themselves to a second order of responsibilities. These are generally of two kinds: those which arise from medical progress—like human experimentation and genetic and behavioral modification—and those which bear directly on the condition of life of the community—population control, eradicating malnutrition, assurance of accessibility, comprehensive health care for all citizens, abortion, drugs, and so on. Of the two sets, the latter are more directly related to the daily work of the practitioner and pose ethical issues of an immediate nature, since they flow so directly from his or her first-order responsibilities.

In these matters, physicians can indeed act as leaders, sensors of unmet needs, and expert witnesses in constructing feasible solutions. They can mobilize their county and state society to assume corporate responsibility for distributing physicians, for mandating coverage of all communities, perhaps experimenting with use of nonphysicians. Physicians can use their authority as clinicians to underline needs for improvement of services and facilities in their community. If they clearly focus on patient and community health and not on their own prerogatives, there can be no more effective voice in initiating reforms.

The third order of responsibilities—those more properly related to the physician—are among the most crucial for modern individuals. Yet they are usually outside the physician's prerogatives and distant from his or her direct function in society. Important as they are, these issues—poverty, war, racism—require knowledge doctors must acquire. If these are doctors' major concerns, they should make no pretense at also being clinicians, or they will become clinicians in the most limited sense. Medical education and experience make a legitimate base for service in new fields or social and political action, but they do not legitimatize the neglect of clinical competence in individual medical acts. This distinction needs careful scrutiny by those who would have physicians cure the accumulated social ills of our times and who upbraid them for their failures to do this and to maintain professional competence as well. "If you try to act beyond your powers, you not only disgrace yourself in it, but you neglect the part which you could have filled with success."[19]

Individual physicians can, and indeed should, limit their ethical pretensions. The profession as a body can but should not. Physicians as a group must assume ethical responsibility which may bind each physician. The profession, as we have shown, must attempt to do as a body what individuals cannot do by themselves—namely, span the full range of ethical imperatives. The profession is bound to assume responsibility for the ethical behavior of its members, for setting the context which best guarantees good behavior and taking sanctions against members who fall from their high estate while at the same time effecting their rehabilitation. Physicians as individuals may eschew certain responsibilities as inappropriate, but the profession cannot.

Herein, then, lies the final guarantee for the patient and the community: the interplay of ethical responsibilities for each individual physician and of the whole body of physicians. Each physician must consciously define on several levels his or her personal moral responsibilities. The profession simultaneously must call for deep involvement of its members at all levels of ethical responsibility—the individual clinical medical transaction, the social consequences of medical acts and medical progress, the quality and availability of medical services, and the duties of its educated group to engage in the larger social issues confronting contemporary humanity. This reinforcement of the ethical perspective of the individual physician by a heightened ethical perception of the community of physicians is an essential ingredient of any professional ethical framework which hopes to cope with the current flux in values and goals afflicting modern society.

What will happen to the conscience and the values of the individual physician if the claims of society and the profession are given new ethical force? The law can insist that confidences be revealed in the interest of justice; if abortion is legalized, the physician as agent of society will be expected to provide this service; the same is true if euthanasia, personality and behavioral modification, and chemical sterilization should become public mandates. How shall we balance social and public mandates against the conscience of the individual physician? How will we safeguard the integrity of the physician's own values?

We have a terrifying example of the inability of physicians to withstand social pressures in the acts of unmitigated evil perpetrated by the physicians in German prison camps. These physicians abdicated conscience and choice so thoroughly that they participated in the most reprehensible acts, convinced that they were innocent bystanders. The individual conscience simply ceased to exist, and the individual physician became a mindless cipher. They were willingly conscripted into that "auxiliary bureaucracy" which Gabriel Marcel so scathingly deplores in *Man against Mass Society*.[20]

The very horror of this possibility should underscore how essential is the defense of the mind, conscience, and values of the individual physician and his or her patient in any system of medicine, ethics, or political organization. This is all the more reason for an axiologic approach, which always calls for an orderly analysis of the values underlying moral choices. The highest ethical call is still that of the conscience of an individual human person, a conscience which must be prepared at all times to take issue with social directives, corporate agreements, and political pressures. The dignity and the worth of the human being he or she treats must still remain the beacon that guides the physician's conscience in the ethical night before us. Marcel pinpoints this duty so peculiar to our times: "It is within the scope of each of us, within his own proper field, in his profession, to pursue an unrelaxing struggle for man, for the dignity of man against everything that today threatens to annihilate man and his dignity."[21]

We have attempted a brief analysis of some of the limitations and omissions in traditional medical ethics as embodied in the Hippocratic corpus and its later exemplifications. These limitations are largely in the realm of social and corporate ethics, realms of increasing significance in an egalitarian, highly structured, and exquisitely interlocked social order.

The individual physician needs more explicit guidelines than traditional codes afford to meet today's new problems. The Hippocratic ethic is one of the most admirable codes in the history of man. But even its ethical sensibilities and high moral tone are insufficient for the complexities of today's problems.

An evolving, constantly refurbished system of medical ethics is requisite in the twentieth century. An axiologic, rather than a deontologic, bias is more in harmony with the questions raised in a world society whose values are in continual flux and reexamination. There is ample opportunity for a critical reappraisal of the Hippocratic ethic and for the elaboration of a fuller and more comprehensive medical ethic suited to our profession as it nears the twenty-first century. This fuller ethic will build upon the noble precepts set forth so long ago in the Hippocratic corpus. It will explicate, complement, and develop those precepts, but it must not be delimited in its evolution by an unwarranted reluctance to question even so ancient and honorable a code as that of the Hippocratic writings.

Notes

1. American Academy of Arts and Sciences, *Proceedings* 98(2) (1969); E. D. Pellegrino, "The Necessity, Promise, and Dangers of Human Experimentation." In *Experiments with Man, World Council Studies, no. 6* (New York: World Council of Churches, Geneva, and Friendship Press, 1969); "New Dimensions in Legal and Ethical Concepts for Human Research," *Annual of the New York Academy of Arts and Sciences* 169 (1970): 293–593.

2. Ibid.; E. F. Torrey, *Ethical Issues in Medicine* (Boston: Little, Brown and Co., 1968).

3. H. E. Siegerist, *The History of Medicine,* vol. 11 (New York: Oxford University Press, 1961), pp. 260, 298; W. A. Heidel, *Hippocratic Medicine: Its Spirit and Method* (New York: Columbia University Press, 1941), p. 149.

4. W. H. S. Jones, ed. and trans., *Hippocrates* (Cambridge, MA: Harvard University Press, 1923), vol. 1, 229–301.

5. Ibid., vol. 2, 263–265.

6. Ibid., vol. 1, 299–301.

7. C. Leake, ed., *Percival's Medical Ethics* (Baltimore: William Wilkins, 1927), p. 291.

8. Jones, *Hippocrates,* vol. 2, 263–265.

9. Ibid., vol. 1, 299–301.

10. Ford et al., *The Doctor's Perspective* (New York: Year Book, 1967).

11. T. S. Eliot, "The Rock." In *The Complete Poems and Plays, 1909–1950* (New York: Harcourt and Brace, 1952), p. 101.

12. Jones, *Hippocrates,* vol. 2, 263–265.

13. M. Michler, "Medical Ethics in Hippocratic Bone Surgery." *Bulletin of the History of Medicine* 42 (1968): 297–311.

14. Jones, *Hippocrates,* vol. 1, 299–301.

15. Ibid., vol. 2, 263–265.

16. Ibid.

17. Ibid., vol. 1, 299–301.

18. C. Truett, A. W. Douville, B. Fagel, et al., "The Medical Curriculum and Human Values." *Journal of the American Medical Association* 209 (1969): 1341–1345

19. W. Oates, ed., *The Stoic and Epicurean Philosophers* (New York: Modern Library, 1957), p. 480.

20. G. Marcel, *Man against Mass Society* (Chicago: Henry Regnery, 1962), p. 180.

21. Ibid.

NINETEEN

Medical Ethics

Entering the Post-Hippocratic Era

The pace and depth of the transformations now occurring in the ages-old structure of medical ethics are truly unprecedented. More change has taken place in the last 15 years than in the entire previous history of medicine and the health professions. The ancient edifice of Hippocratic ethics has been disassembled, and we are entering what can without exaggeration be called the "post-Hippocratic" era.

What do these changes portend for the future of medical ethics? What are their origins? What will medical ethics look like in the twenty-first century? What can be salvaged from the past? What must be discarded? Should the ancient edifice be restored? Will physicians ever again agree on the set of obligations, duties, or virtues that ought to define the ethical physician?[1]

Answers to these questions constitute the most important agenda for medical ethics in the years ahead. How we answer them will define what it is to be a physician, and that answer will have an enormous influence on what physicians do and what patients can expect when they seek help from our profession.

It would be foolhardy to suggest that this brief essay will answer questions of such moment. However, I believe there is value in examining the nature of the changes and challenges confronting the Hippocratic tradition and in suggesting what elements seem likely to be retained, what ones are likely to be abandoned, and what the tentative shape of medical ethics will be as we enter this new era.

424

Sources of the Metamorphosis of Medical Ethics

The metamorphosis in medical ethics today has two sources: the first is the extraordinary expansion of capabilities that scientific advance has conferred on medicine; the second is the convergence of powerful socio-economic and political forces peculiar to our times. The first has given rise to biomedical ethics. The second gives rise to medical ethics proper—the obligation of physicians to sick people, that is to say, the ethics of the physician as physician.

The ethical challenges arising out of medical progress are now widely discussed and debated among physicians, ethicists, lawyers, and the general public. The quandaries of in vitro fertilization, surrogate parenting, gene mapping, behavior modification, withdrawal of life-sustaining treatment, organ transplantation, artificial hearts, etc., are the subject of a vast and growing literature. These will not detain us here—not because they are not of crucial importance, but because the changes taking place in the structure of the profession itself are even more important. This is the realm of medical ethics proper, the range of obligations, duties, principles, and guidelines that defines ethical conduct in the relations between physician and patient and physician and society. It is this segment of our post-Hippocratic journey on which I wish to concentrate.

The changes being effected in medical, as distinguished from biomedical, ethics are less the result of scientific advance than of sociopolitical and economic forces that have altered the societal fabric within which medicine exists. Only some of the more powerful forces need to be mentioned: the rise of participatory democracy in every walk of life; the civil rights, women's, and consumer rights movements; the growing distrust of institutions, authority, and elitism; the entry of legal and economic considerations into medical decisions; and, perhaps most powerful of all, the moral heterogeneity of American society.

These forces that have stirred up controversy and change in American life—and in other countries as well—are reshaping society's and the medical profession's notion of what a physician should be, what is expected of him or her, and whether there is anything ethically unique about the medical profession.

These questions would have amazed our medical forebears perhaps as much as, or more than, the phenomenal progress of medical science. For them, professional ethics seemed to have been settled for all time by the immutable axioms of the Hippocratic *Oath* and the deontological treatises of the Hippocratic corpus. Our forebears could not have foreseen the ubiquity and power of the sociopolitical forces reshaping our society and their impact on the most sensitive phenomenon of medicine—the physician-patient relationship. This is the moral nucleus of medical ethics, the part most of us, until recently, felt was secured for all time by the Hippocratic ethos. Although we know that not every one of the Hippocratic precepts was respected by every physician in every era, the fundamental probity of the Hippocratic ethic was accepted as the standard of medical conduct for more than two millennia. Those who violated it were moral and professional pariahs. In spirit and often in specific content, the same standards of conduct were expected of the Indian and Chinese physician as well.[2,3]

In the last two decades, every one of the Hippocratic precepts has been challenged. Some have already been dropped, some changed, some reinterpreted, and some retained. The task of professional ethics today is the reconstruction of medical ethics from the ground up. A simple restoration of the ancient edifice, for which many physicians hope, will not be possible. Too much was not foreseen in the ancient code, too much that is pertinent today was left out, and too much lacked philosophical justification. Our challenge is to discern what of the old ethic should be retained, what should be modified, and what added without losing the morally viable elements of an ethos that has been among the most noble commitments that any group of humans has made to the welfare of others.

The Deconstruction of the Hippocratic Precepts

Let me begin by examining some of the drastic changes being effected in the ethical substance of the Hippocratic ethic. A few instances will suffice to illustrate the kind and extent of metamorphosis now taking place. I will concentrate on the *Oath*, its preamble, and eight ethical precepts, with only passing reference to the other deontologic treatises of the Hippocratic corpus.[4,5]

The Oath

The preamble of the *Oath* exhorts the student to treat his teacher as a parent, to share his substance with him, relieve his necessities, teach his sons the art, and to keep the secrets of that art within the brotherhood. These precepts are long out of use and properly so. This concept of medicine as a "brotherhood" has come under serious criticism as sexist, elitist, monopolistic, and wholly inappropriate in democratic societies. Medical knowledge is not the property of a fraternity. It belongs to the community for the service of the sick. The profession holds medical knowledge in trust. To isolate it from those for whom it is intended to benefit is to violate that trust. Medical ethics is a concern of the public as well as the profession. Whatever advantages the idea of a brotherhood might have had, it is outweighed by medicine's social orientation.

Precept 1

The most serious and most problematic challenge to the Hippocratic ethic has been directed at the first of the truly ethical precepts of the *Oath:* "I will use treatment to help the sick, according to my ability and judgement but never with a view to injury or wrong-doing."[6] This pledge points to what are identified today as the principles of beneficence and nonmaleficence.

No one disagrees with the latter part of this statement, which commits the physician to nonmaleficence. Indeed, many would reduce the whole of professional ethics to nonmaleficence as stated here and in the *Epidemics.*[7] It is the first part of this precept, the invocation of beneficence, according to the physician's judgment, that is the center of controversy. Most observers see in this precept the origins of the "paternalist" conception of the physician-patient relationship, which many physicians interpret as justification for a benign authoritarianism. Today, the paternalism model is being supplanted by an autonomy model in which the locus of decision making is shifted from the physician to the patient. On the autonomy model, respect for persons dictates that the physician follow the patient's values and wishes or those of a valid surrogate (for incompetent patients) in clinical decisions. The opposition of these two models points to an important distinction. Namely, the medical view of the patient's good is not necessarily synonymous with the patient's own view of his or her best interests.

Recently, David C. Thomasma and I have explored the concept of the patient's good in some detail.[8] The patient's good is a complex notion. It consists not only in the good that medicine can achieve, but also in the way a medical intervention fits the patient's notion of what is considered a good life—one consistent with the patient's values, both material and spiritual.

In our view, autonomy and beneficence need not be in conflict. Indeed, it is difficult to conceive of beneficence that violates the autonomy and respect for persons, which is so integrally tied to the very humanity of the patient. Thus, we speak of "beneficence-in-trust."

Paternalism, therefore, is not the equivalent of beneficence, because paternalism may violate the respect we must have for other persons as persons. Our patients have a moral claim on us to respect their freedom to live their lives as they see fit. That freedom should be limited only if it results in harm to third parties or involves violating some deeply held moral principle to which the physician is committed. The physician can justifiably withdraw from the care of the patient who asks him to violate his own conscience.

The opposition of the autonomy and the paternalism models has created a whole new domain of moral conflict. Although many physicians still feel that they know best, that patients cannot really comprehend the nature of a clinical decision, that illness impairs the patient's autonomy, and that, as a result, informed consent is an illusory concept, the weight of social and legal opinion is swinging increasingly in the direction of patient self-determination. So much is this the case that autonomy threatens to become an absolute principle. Its limits must be carefully delineated, while retaining the concept of respect for persons.

Precept 2

The second Hippocratic precept is the admonition against giving any deadly medicine: "Neither will I administer a poison to anybody when asked to do so, nor will I suggest such a course."[9] Many commentators take this to be a sanction against euthanasia. While the proscription against euthanasia is still generally respected, it has been abrogated in private and also publicly in some countries.[10,11] In the United States, one recent court decision carried the implication that physicians ought to assist competent patients who decide to end their lives.[12] There is a real likelihood that direct voluntary euthanasia will be legal in some states very soon. In California, a referendum that might make this possible missed being placed on the ballot this year (1988).[13]

Precept 3

The third Hippocratic precept is the admonition against abortion: "I will not give a woman a pessary to cause abortion." As is well known, this proscription has been widely abrogated by law in the United States and in many other countries. I will refer to this precept again below.

Precept 4

The fourth precept asks that the physician pursue his life and art with "purity and holiness." This precept reflects the ascetic elements of the Pythagorean philosophy, which inspired the author(s) of the *Oath*. It is doubtful if it was ever seriously honored by the majority of physicians. Today, we tend increasingly to separate personal morals from professional behavior, sometimes to an unfortunate degree. Yet, realistically, were we to apply such a precept, we would face the impracticality of regulating private morals—a dubious and impossible undertaking in a morally pluralistic society.

Precept 5

The fifth precept, "I will not use the knife, not even verily, on sufferers from stone," is usually interpreted as a warning against surgery or "cutting" for the stone, leaving it to ". . . practitioners of this sort of work." This precept is still well respected today, if we interpret it as a call for competence and specialization.[14,15] This is one part of the ancient tradition that is unaffected by the forces effecting changes in other parts of the Hippocratic ethic.

Precept 6

The sixth precept urges the physician to enter the patient's home for the benefit of the sick and to refrain from mischief and corruption. This is really a paraphrase of the first precept. Like it, the principles of both beneficence and nonmaleficence are enunciated together.

Precept 7

The seventh precept forbids seduction of the members of the household of the sick person. It is difficult to know the extent to which this admonition was, or is, honored; however, recently, a small number of psychiatrists have suggested that having sexual relations with their patients is morally permissible or even therapeutic.[16,17]

Precept 8

The eighth precept enjoins confidentiality with respect to ". . . whatsoever I shall see and hear in the course of my profession, as well as outside my profession. . . ."[18] Important as it is to physician-patient relations, there are good reasons why confidentiality has become less and less of an absolute. In an interdependent society, individual decisions may have injurious effects on others. In the interests of justice, a physician might be compelled to violate the confidentiality of a patient; for example, a commercial airline pilot or railroad engineer who uses drugs on the job; a husband seropositive for HIV infection who refuses to tell his pregnant wife; or a homicidal psychotic who threatens the life of another.

This cursory review is not intended to show that some physicians violate the Hippocratic precepts. That has always been true. Rather, what is significant is that the moral validity of most of the precepts themselves are questioned or judged to be ethically unsound by many ethicists and physicians. With the exception of the precepts of nonmaleficence and competence, little is left of the Hippocratic *Oath* that is held in common by all physicians today.

These transformations most clearly reveal the growing divergencies in fundamental philosophical and religious beliefs about political philosophies (e.g., autonomy, the elitist conception of Hippocratic ethics), sexual mores (e.g., sexual relations with patients), private morality (e.g., definition of a pure life), and about the meaning and purposes of human life (e.g., the precepts on abortion and euthanasia).

Similar difficulties can be pointed out in the ethical assertions in other works of the Hippocratic corpus—e.g., the *Physician, Law, Decorum, On the Art,* and *Ancient Medicine.*

For example, *Decorum* includes altruism or "disinterestedness"[19] as an essential virtue of the physician. Yet, today, there are not only surgeons who refuse to treat patients with HIV infection for fear of contagion,[20] but also obstetricians and orthopedists who withhold their services for fear of malpractice suits.[21,22] There are also many physicians who will not treat the poor.[23,24] Indeed, the current legitimation of physician self-interest may be the greatest challenge to professional ethics in our time.[25]

Elsewhere, other conflicts can be noted between the Hippocratic ethic and current ethical beliefs. In two places, for example, the physician is expressly advised not to tell the patient or his family about the severity of the illness and to act toward the patient as one who commands to one who obeys.[26,27] Both of these precepts are directly contrary to the emergent principle of autonomy.

Some Omissions in the Hippocratic Ethic

In addition to these examples of conflict between the ancient precepts and contemporary ethical thinking, there are some serious omissions in areas of great concern in contemporary society. Again, only some examples can be given.

One omission is the failure to mention questions of social ethics such as the possibility of a physician's competing obligations to society and to the individual patient. This problem is evident today in questions involving the physician's role in the rationing and allocation of health care resources.[28] In our time, the roles of bureaucrat, entrepreneur, proletarian, or scientist are being thrust upon physicians by necessity and by societal pressures. The ancient canons provide no guidelines on how to resolve some of the more acute conflicts that occur when these roles overlap with that of healer.

Another omission is in the realm of medical economics, which looms so large for physicians in capitalist as well as in collectivist countries. References in the Hippocratic works to care of the indigent are ambivalent and vary from book to book.[29,30] The problems of medical entrepreneurism, for-profit medicine, and investment in, and ownership of, medical facilities are peculiarly modern. Although Plato, in the *Republic*,[31] did make a distinction between the art of medicine and the art of making money, specific reference to the conflict between altruism and financial self-interest is missing in classical texts.

The Hippocratic corpus is also silent on the subject of the "health care team." The Hippocratic physician was assisted in the care of patients by a student or the patient's family. Because the professional nurse, dentist, and the many technicians necessary in modern medical care simply did not exist in ancient times, the ethics of team obligations, conflicts, and cooperation were not matters of ethical moment.

Finally, the Hippocratic ethic does not deal with the ways in which law and medical ethics may come into conflict. The extreme examples in our day are the Nazi physicians who actively participated in genocide or illicit human experiments,[32] the enlistment of psychiatrists in the removal of political enemies to asylums on the pretext of insanity,[33,34] or the participation of physicians in torture or executions.[35,36] Even more subtle instances of potential conflict between legal and moral justification are beginning to appear where abortion, surrogate motherhood, embryo freezing or "preembryo" experimentation, and the sale of organs and tissues are sanctioned by law. In these instances, the personal or professional ethics of the physician may be subject to overt or subtle pressures unimaginable to the Hippocratic physician. The modern physician must be constantly reminded that the law and ethics are two separate domains and that moral accountability at times transcends law and social custom.

There are serious problems in reliance on a set of texts that is 2500 years old. First is the problem of language. The discrepancies in ancient and modern meaning and usage are notorious. Second is the difference between the textual meaning as a whole as it was taken up in ancient times and as it is perceived today. Finally, there is the overlay of commentaries and interpretations that may obfuscate rather than illuminate the ancient tradition. These textual difficulties constitute another good reason for rethinking the ancient codal foundations of professional ethics.

I list these omissions in the Hippocratic ethic not to deprecate that noble edifice. It has served humankind long and well. Indeed, the ethics of medicine, when it is faithfully observed, is one of the higher achievements of humanity. We in medicine should be proud that medicine was the first profession to build its art on a truly ethical framework.

The question we are faced with today is how to reconstruct the moral foundations of a professional ethic that will more explicitly take into account the metamorphoses and omissions I have just outlined. If, as I have suggested, we are now already in the post-Hippocratic era, how do we find our way into the future? Is it still possible in a morally heterogeneous society to find some set of common moral norms that will bind all physicians? Or is the whole project of professional ethics effectively at an end?

I would like to suggest some steps on the way to a restructured medical ethics equal to the challenges of the twenty-first century. I shall touch only on professional ethics—not on the vast array of bioethical quandaries generated by medical progress.

Restructuring the Moral Foundations of Medicine

The steps toward a reconstruction of professional ethics are three: (1) establishing a moral philosophy of medicine, (2) salvaging what is still viable from the Hippocratic ethic, and (3) adding certain missing elements.

The Need for a Moral Philosophy of Medicine

Given the moral heterogeneity of modern societies and the cosmopolitan character of scientific medicine, any sound moral philosophy of medicine will need to be "internal" to medicine itself. It cannot be derived solely from any external philosophical system as in the past. Such a moral philosophy would be based in four things: the phenomena of human illness, the special nature of medical knowledge, the moral nature of clinical decisions, and the claim of medicine to be a profession. Until recently, professional ethics consisted largely of moral assertions and statements defining the moral behavior physicians should exhibit. These assertions have been made, however, without explicit or formal moral argumentation. This is the genre to which the Hippocratic ethic belongs, as do most subsequent treatises and codifications of medical ethics up to our day. In most cases, the philosophical presuppositions inherent in these moral pronouncements were derived from philosophical systems external to medicine itself.

Medical ethics as a formal discipline began seriously only two decades ago when the moral assertions that had sufficed for so many centuries became problematic. For the first time, these assertions were subjected to formal analysis and treated as a special case of general ethics. Professional philosophers who ignored medical ethics for most of medicine's history sought clarification of its content in terms of prima facie principles of beneficence, autonomy, and nonmaleficence from which they derived the secondary principles of confidentially, truthtelling, and fidelity to promises. This is the analytical approach of Anglo-American ethics based largely in the philosophies of Hume, Kant, and J. S. Mill.

Salubrious as it has been, the current approach to professional ethics has certain deficiencies. It leaves an inferential gap between principles and their application in concrete clinical cases. It is not convincing to physicians, because it is derived from philosophies external to medicine. Moreover, as it functions today, principle-based ethics does not deal directly with the role-specific obligations of physicians, nurses, hospital administrators, etc. Finally, Anglo-American ethics pays little attention to the ethics of virtue.

All of this points to the need for a moral philosophy specific to medicine. Such a philosophy would be prior to medical ethics. It should provide philosophical foundations for defining what constitutes good medicine, the good physician, and the moral obligations that derive from these definitions. A moral philosophy of medicine would itself be grounded in a philosophy of the nature of health, illness, suffering, and healing; the logic and epistemology of medical knowledge; and, especially, in the nature of the physician-patient relationship. The dominant mode of medical ethics today does well at clarifying some of the questions, but to answer them adequately requires a fully developed theory of medicine and medical morality.

Such a theory of medicine and medical morals exists only in fragmentary and suggestive forms in the history of medicine. In the past, the philosophic foundations of medicine were drawn from the dominant philosophical schools of the times. Hellenic and Roman medicine relied on remnants of all the major schools of Greek philosophy. Medieval medicine was shaped by the Christian, Jewish, and Moslem religions. Since the eighteenth century, Anglo-American medical ethics has been based in the philosophies of Locke, Bentham, Hume, and J. S. Mill. Remarkably, even the physicians who were philosophers, such as Locke, Jaspers, or William James, did not develop moral philosophies of medicine.

The first genuine suggestion of a moral philosophy specific to medicine is found in the first century A.D. in the work of the physician/pharmacist Scribonius Largus. Here, for the first time, we encounter the words "humanity," "compassion," and "profession."[37] Scribonius insists that these qualities are intrinsic to being a physician. Without them, the physician ceases to be a physician. Scribonius' conception was itself derived from Panaetius' Stoic teachings on role-specific duties as transmitted to the Roman world in Cicero's *De Officiis*.[38] On this view, each role in life comes with certain specific duties. It is the derivation of these duties that constitutes the "internal" morality of medicine—a set of obligations drawn from the nature of clinical medicine as a special kind of human activity.

What Is Still Viable in the Hippocratic Ethic?

Even though we lack the first essential step of a moral philosophy, we can take the next step in the reconstruction of professional ethics by salvaging the still-viable elements of the old edifice. Here are some examples of what I mean:

As we saw above, the most important principles of the *Oath* are contained in its first genuinely ethical precept—the correlative principles of beneficence and nonmaleficence. These must remain as the cornerstone of any new professional ethic. Without these ordering principles, no ethical restraint can be placed on the use of medical knowledge.

The other principle still viable in the *Oath* is competence. This is even more strongly enjoined in the Hippocratic treatises *Physician, Law,*

Decorum, On the Art, and *On Ancient Medicine.* Competence, like beneficence, is "internal" to medicine as an activity. Without competence, none
of the healing purposes of medicine can be achieved.

These principles must be enhanced by the virtue of altruism, especially noted in *Decorum.*[39] Together, they are essential if the physician is
to serve the telos of medicine, which is healing. Additional virtues like
honesty and tolerance, advised in the deontological books, complete that
portion of the Hippocratic ethic that is still viable. The lesser virtues of
calmness, a regular life, and decorous behavior referenced in the *Physician* and *Law* are important to the definition of the good physician, but
they are not as crucial as altruism, honesty, and tolerance.

Unfortunately, given the transformations in social mores, universal
agreement among physicians on such fundamental tenets as the prohibitions against abortion, euthanasia, breaking confidentiality, and leading
an "impure" life is not likely to be resuscitated. Many hold that these precepts are still valid, but henceforth we cannot expect sufficient agreement
by the majority of physicians to include them in a common professional
morality. To insist on such conformity is to divide the profession further
and to make the task of reconstruction virtually impossible.

In the post-Hippocratic era, we must expect a two-part medical ethic.
One part would consist of those precepts drawn from the nature of medicine to which all physicians might subscribe; the other part would vary
depending upon fundamental philosophical and theological beliefs.

In designing the portion that will be common, we can draw on those
parts of the Hippocratic corpus that are still viable. Some precepts will
need to be modified, and others added. For example, we must retain the
emphasis on beneficence but not the authoritarian strain of the *Oath.* Respect for the autonomy of the patient must be a clear commitment. We
must think of the conflation of beneficence and autonomy so that they are
not in conflict but mutually reinforcing. I would propose that we think of
beneficence as held "in trust," responsive to the patient's wishes, while still
motivated by a primary regard for his or her welfare.

The Addition of Missing Elements

Any new professional ethic would have to include some of the following: (1) obligations to members of the health care team, (2) rejection of

roles that conflict with the good of the patient, (3) a moral right of the physician to refuse to cooperate with a patient, institution, or policy that violates his or her own moral values, (4) a willingness under these conditions to withdraw from the care of the patient, (5) a moral right of the physician to the "discretionary space" necessary to act in the best interests of the patient lest this space be narrowed by legislation and law to the extent that the patient suffers, and (6) a commitment by the entire profession to act as the advocate for the best interests of the sick whenever and wherever those interests are threatened by law, economics, or social convention. David Thomasma and I have recently proposed a set of commitments that we believe could form the basis for a generally accepted code of ethics suitable for the post-Hippocratic era.[40]

Conclusion

The *Oath* and deontological writings of the Hippocratic corpus have formed the foundation of one of the most durable ethical codes in human history. The Hippocratic ethic has raised the moral sensitivities and constrained the behavior of physicians for centuries. Its prescriptions and proscriptions have united the world's physicians across religious, cultural, and national barriers. As a result, the care of the sick has entailed obligations of beneficence of the highest order.

In the last two decades, a series of social, economic, and political forces have converged to weaken this ancient edifice. Every element in the Hippocratic ethic is under scrutiny as a result. We can truly be said to be entering the post-Hippocratic era.

What this era portends for medical ethics and, more significantly, for the care of the sick is just becoming manifest. Public and profession alike have a stake in the outcome. Our task together is to examine what has been bequeathed to us by the past, to alter what cannot be morally justified, to retain what is morally viable, and to refashion a new edifice that neither discards all of the past nor accepts all of the new.

The post-Hippocratic era need not be viewed as the end of medical morality but as the beginning of an era of more responsible, more adult, more open, and more morally responsive relations between the sick and those who offer to help and heal them.

References

1. E. D. Pellegrino. "Toward a Reconstruction of Medical Morality: The Primacy of the Act of Profession and the Fact of Illness." *J Med Philos* 4 (1979): 32–56.
2. A. Menon and H. F. Haberman. "Oath of Initiation (from the Caraka Samhita)." *Med Hist* 14 (1970): 295–296. Reprinted in: W. T. Reich. *The Encyclopedia of Bioethics* (New York: Free Press, 1978), pp. 1732–1733.
3. I. Veith. *The Yellow Emperor's Classic of Internal Medicine (Huang-ti nei ching)* (Berkeley: University of California Press, 1966).
4. Hippocrates. (*Oath, Physician, Precepts, Decorum, Law, On the Art, Ancient Medicine, Epidemics.*) Vols. 1–2. Translated by W. H. S. Jones. Loeb Classical Library (Cambridge, MA: Harvard University Press, 1923–1931).
5. O. Temkin and C. L. Temkin, eds. *Ancient Medicine: Selected Papers of L. Edelstein* (Baltimore: Johns Hopkins University Press, 1967), pp. 328–329.
6. Hippocrates. (*Oath.*) Vol. 1:299.
7. *Idem. (Epidemics.)* Vol. 1:165.
8. E. D. Pellegrino and D. C. Thomasma. *For the Patient's Good: The Restoration of Beneficence in Health Care* (New York: Oxford University Press, 1988).
9. Hippocrates. (*Oath.*) Vol. 1:299.
10. "Final Report of the Netherlands State Committee on Euthanasia: An English Summary." *Bioethics* 1 (1987): 163–174.
11. J. Mathews. "Doctors Admit Euthanasia, Group Says." *New York Times,* February 26, 1988: A6.
12. *Bouvia v Superior Court (Glenchur),* 225 Cal. Rptr. 297 (1986).
13. K. Bishop. "California Euthanasia Plan Fails." *New York Times,* May 18, 1988: D30.
14. W. H. S. Jones. *The Doctor's Oath: An Essay on Medicine* (Cambridge, MA: Cambridge University Press, 1924).
15. O. Temkin and C. L. Temkin, eds. *Ancient Medicine,* pp. 26–32.
16. J. Black. "Pelvic Therapy." *New Times* 2 (1978): 52–56.
17. Six percent of U.S. psychiatrists admit to sexual relations with patients. *Washington Post,* August 31, 1986: A9a.
18. Hippocrates. (*Oath.*) Vol. 1:301.
19. *Idem. (Decorum.)* Vol. 2:287.
20. P. J. Guy. "AIDS: A Doctor's Duty." *Br Med J* 294 (1987): 445.
21. D. Clendinen. "Doctors in Georgia City Strike Back over Suits." *New York Times,* May 14, 1986: A1a.
22. "Orthopedic Surgeons and Obstetricians at Mass. Hospitals Reject New Patients." *Washington Post,* February 4, 1986: A5c.

23. J. E. Davis. "National Initiatives for Care of the Medically Needy." *JAMA* 259 (1988): 3171–3173.

24. G. D. Lundberg. "American Medicine's Problems, Opportunities, and Enemies." *JAMA* 259 (1988): 3174.

25. E. D. Pellegrino. "Altruism, Self-Interest and Medical Ethics." *JAMA* 259 (1987): 1939–1940.

26. Hippocrates. (*Decorum.*) Vol. 2:297–299.

27. *Idem.* (*The Art.*) Vol. 2:201–203.

28. E. D. Pellegrino. "Rationing Health Care: The Ethics of Medical Gate-Keeping." *J Contemp Health Law Policy* 2 (1986): 23–45.

29. Hippocrates. (*Precepts.*) Vol. 1:317–319.

30. *Idem.* (*Decorum.*) Vol. 2:287.

31. E. Hamilton and H. Cairns, eds. *Collected Dialogues of Plato.* Bollinger Series (Princeton, NJ: Princeton University Press, 1961), pp. 341c–346.

32. R. J. Lifton. *The Nazi Doctors* (New York: Basic Books, 1986).

33. S. Bloch and P. Reddaway. *Psychiatric Terror: How Soviet Psychiatry Is Used to Suppress Dissent* (New York: Basic Books, 1977).

34. A. Koryagin. "Unwilling Patients." *Lancet* 1 (1981): 821–824.

35. British Medical Association. *The Torture Report: A Report of a Working Party of the British Medical Association Investigating the Involvement of Doctors in Torture* (London: British Medical Association, 1986).

36. M. Rayner. "Turning a Blind Eye? Medical Accountability and the Prevention of Torture in South Africa." (Washington, DC: AAAS, 1987).

37. S. Sconocchia, ed. *Scribonii Largi compositiones* (Leipzig: B.G. Teubner, 1983).

38. J. Biggenbotham, trans. *On Moral Obligation: A New Translation of Cicero's De Officiis* (London: Faber and Faber, 1967).

39. Hippocrates. (*Decorum.*) Vol. 2:287.

40. E. D. Pellegrino and D. C. Thomasma. *For the Patient's Good,* pp. 205–206.

APPENDIX

Biography of Edmund D. Pellegrino

Formerly director of the Kennedy Institute of Ethics (1983–1989) and the Center for the Advanced Study of Ethics (1989–1994) at Georgetown University, Dr. Pellegrino has been Professor Emeritus of Medicine and Medical Ethics at the Center for Clinical Bioethics at Georgetown University Medical Center since 2001. He is currently the chairman of the President's Council on Bioethics.

From 1982 to 2001, Dr. Pellegrino was John Carroll Professor of Medicine and Medical Ethics at the Center for Clinical Bioethics at Georgetown University Medical Center. Prior to that position, he was President and Professor of Philosophy and Biology of the Catholic University of America in Washington, DC (1978–1982).

During his distinguished academic career, Edmund Pellegrino held positions in various other academic institutions. From 1975 to 1978 he was Professor of Medicine at Yale University and President and Chairman of the Board of Directors at the Yale–New Haven Medical Center in Connecticut. Between 1973 and 1975 he held the position of Chancellor and Vice President for Health Affairs at the University of Tennessee and Professor of Medicine and Medical Humanities at the University of Tennessee Center for the Health Sciences. From 1966 to 1973 he was Vice President for the Health Sciences, Dean of the School of Medicine, Director of the Health Sciences Center, and Professor of Medicine at the State University of New York, Stony Brook. He held the position of Professor and Chairman of the Department of Medicine at the University of Kentucky Medical Center in Lexington between 1959 and 1966.

Dr. Pellegrino graduated from St. John's University with a B.S. in 1937; he received his M.D. from New York University in 1944. He is the recipient of 46 honorary doctorates in addition to various other awards and honors, among them the Abraham Flexner Award of the Association of American Medical Colleges, the Benjamin Rush Award from the American Medical Association, and the Laetare Award of the University of Notre Dame.

He is a fellow or a member of twenty professional, scientific, and honorary societies, which include the Institute of Medicine of the National

Academy of Sciences, the American Clinical and Climatological Association, the Association of American Physicians, and the American Osler Society. He is also a Master of the American College of Physicians.

Although a physician by training, Dr. Pellegrino's interests go far beyond the field of medical practice. His research interests focus on various topics in the philosophy of medicine, the history of medicine, professional ethics, the Hippocratic tradition, and the patient-physician relationship. In addition to his crucial role in the development and the framing of the fields of bioethics and the philosophy of medicine, Dr. Pellegrino, through his work for ten years as Director of the Institute on Human Values in Medicine and as a founding member of the Society for Health and Human Values, fostered the development of programs in medical humanities in medical schools in the United States.

Throughout his career, Dr. Pellegrino has been a prolific author. He has published more than 550 articles and authored, co-authored, or edited twenty-four books. His most important works are *Humanism and the Physician* (1979) and, in collaboration with David C. Thomasma, *A Philosophical Basis of Medical Practice* (1981), *For the Patient's Good* (1988), *The Virtues in Medical Practice* (1993), *The Christian Virtues in Medical Practice* (1996), and *Helping and Healing* (1997).

He is the founding editor of the *Journal of Medicine and Philosophy*.

INDEX

EDMUND D. PELLEGRINO

has been Professor Emeritus of Medicine and Medical Ethics at
the Center for Clinical Bioethics at Georgetown University Medical
Center since 2001. The recipient of numerous honors and awards,
he has authored or co-authored twenty-four books and is the
founding editor of the *Journal of Medicine and Philosophy*.
In 2004, he was named to the International Bioethics Committee
of UNESCO, and in 2005 he became the chairman of the
President's Council on Bioethics.